D0906328

The Physical Therapist's Business Practice and Legal Guide

Sheila K. Nicholson, Esq, MBA, PT
Partner/Attorney
Quintairos, Prieto, Wood & Boyer, PA
Tampa, Florida

JONES AND BARTLETT PUBLISHERS
Sudbury, Massachusetts
BOSTON TORONTO LONDON SINGAPORE

World Headquarters
Jones and Bartlett Publishers
40 Tall Pine Drive
Sudbury, MA 01776
978-443-5000
info@jbpub.com
www.jbpub.com

Jones and Bartlett Publishers
Canada
6339 Ormindale Way
Mississauga, Ontario L5V 1J2
Canada

Jones and Bartlett Publishers
International
Barb House, Barb Mews
London W6 7PA
United Kingdom

Jones and Bartlett's books and products are available through most bookstores and online booksellers. To contact Jones and Bartlett Publishers directly, call 800-832-0034, fax 978-443-8000, or visit our website www.jbpub.com.

Substantial discounts on bulk quantities of Jones and Bartlett's publications are available to corporations, professional associations, and other qualified organizations. For details and specific discount information, contact the special sales department at Jones and Bartlett via the above contact information or send an email to specialsales@jbpub.com.

Library of Congress Cataloging-in-Publication Data

Nicholson, Sheila K.
The physical therapist's business practice and legal guide / Sheila K. Nicholson.
p. ; cm.
Includes index.
ISBN-13: 978-0-7637-4069-6
ISBN-10: 0-7637-4069-1
1. Physical therapists—Malpractice—United States. 2. Physical Therapy—Law and legislation—United States.
3. Insurance, Malpractice—United States. I. Title.
KF2915.T453N53 2008
344.7304'1—dc22

2007013278

6048

Production Credits
Executive Editor: David Cella
Editorial Assistant: Lisa Gordon
Production Director: Amy Rose
Production Editor: Renée Sekerak
Associate Marketing Manager: Jennifer Bengtson
Manufacturing and Inventory Coordinator: Amy Bacus
Cover Design: Kristin E. Ohlin
Composition: Paw Print Media
Printing and Binding: Malloy Incorporated
Cover Printing: Malloy Incorporated

Printed in the United States of America
11 10 09 08 07 10 9 8 7 6 5 4 3 2 1

Contents

Foreword

Generally speaking, lawsuits are usually defended through denial of liability and mitigation of damages. In order to deny liability, someone cannot have already confessed fault. While many people believe and practice admitting fault, you must understand litigation will not always treat you kindly for your acceptance of responsibility when something goes wrong.

Recognize that there is a new philosophy in health care to admit fault and take responsibility for one's mistake. Although this approach could help immediately diffuse someone's anger, it does not change the evidentiary rule that, in a court of law, admission can be used against you.

At trial, an opposing party, usually called a plaintiff, will be allowed to present to the jury your admission of fault with your apology. While I agree there would be fewer lawsuits if individuals took responsibility for their actions, I must caution against the verbalization or conduct of acceptance of fault for a bad outcome. As Joe Friday of the television show *Dragnet* would say, "anything you say can and will be used against you in a court of law."

While those words are a part of receiving your rights upon arrest, the phrase also holds true in a civil court of law. In criminal court your admission of fault (guilt) can be used against you for conviction and punishment of a crime, whereas, in civil court, the admission of fault can be used against you to substantiate liability and punishment will be given by a jury verdict of a monetary award. Thus, this is a warning that a request for forgiveness, an apology, or an acceptance of fault could be used against you in a court of law as an admission of fault. When that occurs, the case then becomes one of determining damages, not whether there is liability because the physical therapist, physical therapist assistant, or student has already confessed fault (liability) in that he or she breached some type of duty and caused some type of harm to the patient.

Preface

Seven years ago I took an incredible leap of faith and journeyed from being a clinically practicing physical therapist to a litigation attorney defending health care providers. Many have asked why and the answer is quite simple; I decided to battle for "the good guys" in a different role. At the outset I concede there are very legitimate claims against health care providers, but there are also, in my opinion, too many frivolous claims against health care providers. I would even venture to say there are some catastrophic health care injuries because of health care providers' negligence; however, in comparison to the number of lawsuits filed, the catastrophic claims are few and far between. Nonetheless, if you or a loved one is the victim, it does not matter that the number of catastrophic claims is low.

Furthermore, if you or a loved one was the victim of a health care provider's catastrophic mistake, you would likely want no limits to what a jury could award in compensation. In my opinion, the majority of the lawsuits seek compensation for risks (injuries) that naturally flow from the necessity of the health care providers' services, and as such, are not caused by the health care practitioner's negligence. These are nuisance lawsuits. So, you ask why would someone take the time to file such a lawsuit? The answer is simple, but insulting: money. Unfortunately, from a business perspective, many times it is less costly for a health care provider to settle these types of claims than it is to defend them. Like it or not, many times the physical therapist, physical therapist assistant, or student should practice so that any subsequent lawsuit has evidence for defense and mitigation of damages.

In that light, as the physical therapy profession continues to grow toward autonomous practice, I believe the profession and the physical therapist are going to face liability risks and liability exposure like never before. Further, despite having graduated from one of the finest physical therapy schools, I know firsthand that physical therapists, physical therapist assistants, and some students are ill-prepared for what likely lies ahead. Additionally, as I review the contents of doctoral physical therapy programs and transitional doctor of physical therapy programs, I still believe physical therapists will be ill-prepared for the liability risk exposure of the future. Thus, I now embark on a quest to educate physical therapists, physical therapist assistants, and students about the law, liability, and ways to mitigate risk exposure in the practice of physical therapy.

This book covers not only the current law, which is open to daily changes, but also reviews lawsuits that health care providers have experienced so that those lessons can be incorporated into physical therapy practice. Thus, this book's purpose is to provide the educational tools for you, the physical therapist, physical therapist assistant, or student, to integrate risk management practices into your daily patient care routine as your liability exposure increases with every patient and every treatment.

Sheila Nicholson

Acknowledgments

There are so many people who helped with the idea and ultimate writing of this book that it would take too much space to thank them all. However, I must thank Jack Bruggeman because he listened to one of my lectures on malpractice involving physical therapists and suggested I write it all down. Thus, this book now exists.

I must also thank my family, especially my mother and younger brother, Glenn, who have encouraged me to follow all of my dreams and believed I could do anything I tried. However, no one has influenced this book more than my niece, Taylor; you have the most incredible heart for inspiring me to be a better person every day.

For the individuals who read, edited, and made suggestions to make this book better, a most heartfelt thank you. Lastly, I could not have finished this book without some individuals who tirelessly gave of their time, energy, and knowledge: Adam Fleischmann, Esquire; Diana Ickes, PTA; Margaret Nonnemacher, DPT; and Professor Becky Morgan, BSBA, JD—thank you.

Introduction

HOW TO USE THIS BOOK

Hopefully, this book contains information that will assist in keeping you out of liability's way. Or, if you must cross paths with a lawsuit, the knowledge and tools provided here, if followed and applied, may help mitigate your liability exposure and subsequent damages. Everyone makes mistakes, many of which are purely honest mistakes. However, we live in a world that has become very litigious and individuals seek reparation for your "honest mistakes" through our judicial system.

The judicial system is large, daunting, and complicated. However, the basic right giving an individual the right to sue was created in 1791 in Amendment VII of the Constitution of the United States, which provided, "[i]n [s]uits at common law, where the value in controversy shall exceed twenty dollars, the right of trial by jury shall be preserved, and no fact tried by jury, shall be otherwise re-examined in any [c]ourt of the United States, than according to the rules of the common law."[1] Thus, citizens of the United States have the right to seek compensation in a court of law for conduct and/or circumstances deemed wrong.

Physical therapists and physical therapist assistants have been fairly insulated from lawsuits arising out of the practice of physical therapy; however, the profession is currently evolving into autonomous practice, which, for this book, will be called entry-level practice into the health care system. Autonomous practice, part of Vision 2020, will also likely unintentionally bring with it greater exposure to liability lawsuits. Vision 2020 has begun and with it comes greater expectations, responsibilities, and rewards for physical therapists and physical therapist assistants. However, with it also comes a greater risk of liability in that physical therapists have become practitioners whom patients visit first before a physician has conducted a differential diagnosis. In that regard, the physical therapist must learn and conduct a thorough examination that rules in and rules out diagnoses before developing appropriate plans of treatment. Thus, the physical therapist, as an entryway into the health care system, becomes a primary care provider and concomitantly exposes him- or herself to greater risk of liability.

This book is intended to give the physical therapist, physical therapist assistant, and student an overall understanding of the changes occurring in the physical therapy profession and how these changes will undoubtedly impact their legal exposure. This book will also provide the physical therapist, physical therapist assistant, and student with a thorough review of the legal profession as well as ways to manage the risk exposure.

NOTES

[1] Constitution of the United States, Amendment VII.

CHAPTER 1

The Evolution of Physical Therapy

Physical therapists and physical therapist assistants are a part of the health care team that includes physicians, nurses, occupational therapists, speech language pathologists, and other ancillary services. Physical therapy services are provided to patients every day within the United States and internationally. Included and critical to the health care team is the patient; although the patient is often overlooked or forgotten as an integral member of any health care team.

Physical therapists specifically evaluate patients and, along with physical therapist assistants, provide treatment to individuals that primarily focuses on movement, reduction of pain, restoration of function, and prevention of disability.[1] The population of patients evaluated and treated in physical therapy can vary in range of age from a newborn to the elderly. The most predominant clinical settings where physical therapists, physical therapist assistants, and students provide care include hospitals, outpatient clinics, private practices, nursing homes, assisted living facilities, home health, school systems and sport centers.

Traditionally, to receive an evaluation and/or treatment from a physical therapist or physical therapist assistant, the patient had to have a physician's order, which is also known as a referral. A *referral* is defined as "[a] recommendation that a patient or client seek service from another health care provider or resource."[2] However, today the practice of physical therapy has evolved such that in some states, the physician referral for physical therapy is no longer necessary or only is required at certain stages in the physical therapy treatment process. Consequently, as the physical therapist becomes an entry-level health care practitioner, his or her potential to be sued, for the very services the profession has sought to provide without the requirements of a physician's referral, grows.

The American Physical Therapy Association (APTA) is the one national organization recognized to speak for the profession of physical therapy. The association's members are physical therapists, physical therapist assistants, and students who voluntarily join. To join the association, an individual must be accepted, currently enrolled, or a graduate of an accredited physical therapy or physical therapist assistant program.

As the organization for physical therapists and physical therapist assistants, the APTA's leadership has developed a vision statement that by the year 2020, among other things, physical therapists will practice in every state without the necessity of a physician's referral, called *direct access*, and will practice without the necessity of physician consultation, called *autonomous practice*. Thus, as the profession of physical therapy approaches its centennial, it is once again undergoing major changes. This chapter will examine the evolution of physical therapy as a profession and how the current changes and vision of the association likely will lead to greater liability risk exposure for physical therapists and physical therapist assistants.

KEY CONCEPTS

Historical perspective of physical therapy
American Physical Therapy Association (APTA)
APTA specializations
Vision 2020
Six key elements of Vision 2020
Core values of professionalism
Entry-level health care practitioner
Education requirements for physical therapists and physical therapist assistants
Commission on the Accreditation of Physical Therapy Education (CAPTE)
Exposure to lawsuits
Misdiagnosed patient

WHAT IS PHYSICAL THERAPY?

Physical therapy is defined as "the treatment or management of physical disabilities, malfunction, or pain by exercises, massage, hydrotherapy, etc., without the use of medicines, surgery or radiation."[3] The APTA further defines physical therapy as follows:

- Physical therapists are experts in how the musculoskeletal and neuromuscular systems function.
- Physical therapist services are cost-effective. Early physical therapy intervention prevents more costly treatment later, can result in a faster recovery, and reduces costs associated with lost time from work.

- Patients pay less when they have direct access to physical therapy services. However, there can be a temptation under managed care to terminate services prematurely. A study conducted to determine whether direct access to physical therapy services was cost-effective found that patients who went directly to a physical therapist had fewer episodes of care, and services were ultimately less costly.[4]

Physical therapy is provided by physical therapists, physical therapist assistants, and sometimes physical therapy students. The qualifications of a physical therapist and physical therapist assistant will be discussed later in Chapter 4.

SERVICES PROVIDED IN PHYSICAL THERAPY

Depending on the clinical setting, the physical therapist or physical therapist assistant may provide treatment for:

- Back conditions
- Knee problems
- Shoulder/arm conditions
- Neck conditions
- Sprains and muscle strains
- Ankle/foot problems
- Carpal tunnel syndrome, hand/wrist problems
- Hip fracture
- Postsurgical rehabilitation
- Rehabilitation after a serious injury (e.g., broken bones, head injury)
- Stroke rehabilitation
- Problems with balance
- Disabilities in newborns
- Burn rehabilitation
- Pre-/postnatal programs
- Incontinence
- Women's health[5]

PHYSICAL THERAPY EVOLUTION

The profession of physical therapy in the United States developed during World War I between 1914 to 1917. This development was in response to the need to treat soldiers' injuries as a result of the war. The first (physical) therapists graduated from

Reed College and Walter Reed Hospital and were known as *reconstruction aides*. The original "reconstruction aides" were individuals degreed in other academic areas; subsequent to the degree, these individuals underwent additional training in order to perform physical therapy services.

As the profession developed, physical therapists primarily treated patients with poliomyelitis, which ravaged the United States between 1920 and 1930. Poliomyelitis was "an acute viral disease, usually affecting children and young adults, caused by any of three polioviruses, characterized by inflammation of the motor neurons of the brain stem and spinal cord, and resulting in a motor paralysis, followed by muscular atrophy and often permanent deformities."[6] In 1921, this new group of health care providers, physical therapists, decided to form a professional organization for physical therapists and called it the American Women's Physical Therapeutic Association.[7] The first president of the American Women's Physical Therapeutic Association was Mary McMillan.[8] Then in 1939 came World War II and because of advances in medicine, there were more survivors with injuries as a result of the war. These survivors with war disabilities required treatment, which was provided by the physical therapists. By the end of the 1930s, the American Women's Physical Therapeutic Association changed its name to the American Physiotherapy Association.[9]

In 1946 the Hospital Survey and Construction Act, also known as the Hill Burton Act, led to more physical therapists practicing in hospitals. By the end of the 1940s, the professional organization representing physical therapists again changed its name, this time to the American Physical Therapy Association (APTA).[10] The Korean War came with more soldier disabilities that required physical therapy treatment. The treatment of soldiers' injuries likely prevented the extinction of physical therapy at this point in time because the Salk vaccine had been developed and essentially eliminated poliomyelitis from the United States.

Physical therapy continued to evolve and develop. This development was primarily due to injuries sustained by soldiers during wars and advances in medicine that kept the soldiers from dying from these injuries. This dynamic evolution made the physical therapists develop educational and training programs that lead to physical therapy becoming a profession. One of the greatest hallmarks in the physical therapy profession came in 1967 when amendments to the Social Security Act added definitions for outpatient physical therapy services. This meant the Social Security organization recognized physical therapy services as a health care provider for reimbursement. From that time forward, the physical therapy profession has continued to expand treatment areas, many of which are based on medical advances. This growth has led to the need for specializations.

The APTA currently recognizes the following specialty sections as part of the professional organization of physical therapy:

- Acute care
- Aquatic physical therapy
- Cardiopulmonary and pulmonary
- Clinical electro and wound management
- Education
- Federal
- Geriatrics
- Hand
- Health policy and administration
- Neurology
- Oncology
- Orthopedic
- Pediatric
- Private practice
- Research
- Sports physical therapy
- Women's health[11]

Today, the profession of physical therapy has evolved to treat not only multiple types of diverse injuries, but also to prevent the dehabilitation associated with a multitude of disease processes. It also should be noted that the profession of physical therapy is international. Outside of the United States, the profession is referred to as *physiotherapy* and physical therapists are called *physiotherapists*. As history has demonstrated, physical therapists and physical therapist assistants have developed from the early days of essentially being technicians or extenders of prescribed health care, to today becoming entry-level health care practitioners.

TODAY'S PHYSICAL THERAPY

Today, it is common practice for physical therapists to receive physician referrals that simply prescribe: "Evaluate and treat as indicated." Thus, physicians no longer are dictating specifically what the physical therapists should do with a patient, but rather are leaving the evaluation and treatment decisions to the knowledge, judgment, and discretion of the physical therapists.

This growth and elevating responsibility in patient care has led the APTA to codify and develop a direction for this continual growth using a vision statement known as Vision 2020. Generally speaking, a *vision statement* is an organization's destination reduced to words; it usually is the organization's global goal. This global goal ultimately answers the question, "What will success look like for this organization?"[12] Other documents used in conjunction with a vision statement are mission statements and strategic plans. A *strategic plan* is the "blueprint" for an organization while the *mission statement* tells why the organization exists, the business it conducts, and the values of the organization that guide it.[13]

The year 2020, the year for accomplishing the APTA's current vision, is fast approaching, necessitating further changes in the preparation of students to become physical therapists and physical therapist assistants. In addition, it requires all physical therapists and physical therapist assistants to renew their commitment to the profession. Finally, the obtainment of Vision 2020 will require all physical therapists and physical therapist assistants to develop a greater understanding of risk management.

With this growth and development, understanding risk management is essential information every physical therapist, physical therapist assistant, and student must comprehend, because today's society has become extremely litigious. This growth and development, in combination with Vision 2020, and/or society's litigious nature, makes it even more important for physical therapists, physical therapist assistants, and students to understand risk management. Thus, with the combination of all these changes, it is imperative physical therapists, physical therapist assistants, and students understand, comprehend, and implement risk management techniques.

While some physical therapists and physical therapist assistants have heard of Vision 2020, it is disheartening and uncomfortable to realize that, as this book is written, many practicing physical therapists and physical therapist assistants are unaware and uninformed as to what Vision 2020 means and how progress toward its goals will impact each therapist's practice. Therefore, the following pages will review some of the highlights of Vision 2020, including its goals, which, although unintentional, will likely impact and lead to physical therapists, physical therapist assistants, and students having greater liability risk exposure.

VISION 2020

The APTA's current vision statement is that "[b]y 2020, physical therapy will be provided by physical therapists who are doctors of physical therapy, recognized by consumers and other health care professionals as practitioners of choice to whom consumers have direct access for the diagnosis of, interventions for, and prevention of impairments, functional limitations, and disabilities related to movement, function, and health."[14] For the vision, there are six key elements articulated. The "six key elements" of Vision 2020 are:

1. Autonomous practice
2. Direct access
3. Doctor of physical therapy
4. Evidence-based practice
5. Practitioner of choice
6. Professionalism[15]

An examination of each key element is critical to understanding how this development and growth of the physical therapy profession will likely concomitantly lead to an increased risk of lawsuits from patients. Accordingly, an understanding of what is expected of a physical therapist under an entry-level health care practitioner standard of care as defined in Vision 2020, and how physical therapists may violate that expectation, resulting in a lawsuit, is essential.

Autonomous Practice

Autonomous practice essentially means practice without constraints from others. The "others" could be other health care practitioners or third-party payors of service. *Autonomous* is defined as "not controlled by others or by outside forces; independent in mind or judgment; [and] self-directed."[16] As such, a physical therapist who evaluates a patient without input from any other health care practitioner, designs a treatment plan without any other health care practitioner's input, and reevaluates the effectiveness of the treatment plan without input from any other health care practitioner is surely considered to be practicing autonomously. What is imperative to understand from a legal perspective is that autonomous practice means the physical therapist is solely responsible for the patient's physical therapy diagnosis, evaluation, treatment(s), and outcome(s) from the treatment. No longer will a lawyer (plaintiff or defense) be able to include the physician in the chain of responsibility for the patient with regard to liability for a patient's outcome. Thus, the physical therapist will be 100 percent accountable for his or her decisions and actions if a patient decides to sue for what happened as a result of the physical therapy services. Consequently, with increasing autonomy comes increased liability exposure.

Direct Access

Direct access means a state's licensure laws allow the physical therapist to evaluate and treat a patient without the requirement of a physician's referral (also known as a physician's order). Based on the most recent data from the APTA, Nebraska was the first state to have some type of direct access, which occurred in 1957.[17] Since that time, 43 states now have some type of direct access.[18] Two of the greatest factors discussed when considering direct access for physical therapy services have been:

1. Whether physical therapists are qualified to deliver physical therapy services without the direction and oversight of a physician
2. Whether there would be an increase in costs for the delivery of physical therapy services

According to data from the APTA, physical therapists are qualified to deliver services without the necessity of a physician's referral because physical therapists recognize the parameters associated within their scope of practice.[19] Further, in the same publication, the APTA promotes a study done by Jean Mitchell of Georgetown University and Gregory de Lissovoy of Johns Hopkins University wherein the authors found there were more physical therapy claims billed when the services were referred by a physician as compared to fewer claims billed when the physical therapist was working under a direct access scenario.[20]

Thus, it appears physical therapy services may be overutilized by other health care practitioners who have the ability to bill for services under physical therapy codes. This realization is further supported by the Department of Health and Human Services' Office of Inspector General's (OIG) report in May 2006 that found approximately 91 percent of physical therapy services billed by physicians to Medicare beneficiaries in the first 6 months of 2002 did not meet program requirements, which resulted in improper payments of approximately $136 million.[21]

This data supports the concept that physical therapists under direct access would not abuse the reimbursement system. However, at this time it is difficult to know the impact of direct access on liability claims because states with direct access still have some form of physician control over the services and not all practicing physical therapists and physical therapist assistants carry malpractice insurance. Hence, if a physical therapist or physical therapist assistant is sued and has no professional liability insurance, the likelihood that the claim would be reported for tracking statistics is slim to none.

Consequently, physical therapists, physical therapist assistants, and students should read the opinions that professional malpractice claims have not risen as a result of direct access to physical therapy with some skepticism. This is especially true in light of the 2006 CNA insurance claim study that was released. According to the CNA report, in 1995, 59 claims led to insurance payment for coverage of an alleged physical therapist's, physical therapist assistant's, or student's professional malpractice; and in 2004, there were 119 claims.[22] In a span of nine years, physical therapy malpractice claims have at least doubled. Recall though, not all physical therapists, physical therapist assistants, or students carried professional malpractice insurance; therefore, it is likely employers of physical therapists, physical therapist assistants, and students may have paid more for claims not reported or accounted for in this study because this study only represents claims that were paid through CNA insurance.

Doctor of Physical Therapy

Doctor of physical therapy simply means that by the year 2020, practicing physical therapists will have obtained a doctoral degree in physical therapy. As many therapists know, there are currently two types of doctoral degrees available in physical therapy: (1) an academic doctoral degree from a university or institution accredited by the Commission on the Accreditation of Physical Therapy Education (CAPTE); or (2) a transitional doctoral degree in physical therapy from a transitional doctor of physical therapy program that may be CAPTE-accredited. The doctoral programs are referred to as a DPT (doctor of physical therapy) or tDPT (transitional doctor of physical therapy) program. This particular key element of Vision 2020 did not address the role or growth of the physical therapist assistant.

Evidence-Based Practice

Evidence-based practice means that the patient's treatment plan is based on research that has substantiated a likelihood that the treatment, based on the physical therapy evaluation findings, will be the most cost-effective and beneficial treatment. Thus, this type of practice means that physical therapists, physical therapist assistants, and students must constantly and continuously educate themselves and review research for evidence that the treatments being rendered to patients are actually beneficial and effective. To assist with obtainment of this goal, the APTA developed what is called "hooked on evidence." Hooked on evidence already has evolved into a program called "Open Door: APTA's portal to evidence-based practice" available to APTA members.[23]

Practitioner of Choice

Practitioner of choice is probably the most intangible and theoretical element contained within Vision 2020. Essentially it means that physical therapists and physical therapist assistants will be the consumers' first choice for treatment of movement dysfunction, dysfunction related to pain, and restoration of function due to diseases and disabilities. There are other professionals who claim an ability to also treat many of the same problems physical therapy services treat, such as athletic trainers, massage therapists, exercise physiologists, chiropractors, and personal trainers, to name a few. These other professionals often market their provision of services as similar or akin to physical therapy. Thus, being the practitioner of choice means the consumer would choose physical therapists and physical therapist assistants for physical therapy services over these other professionals because of the recognition that physical therapists and physical therapist assistants are more educated, have greater skills and training, and utilize research to support treatment decisions.

Professionalism

Professionalism is defined as "professional character, spirit, or methods. [T]he standing practice or methods of a professional as distinguished from an amateur."[24] The APTA has identified seven "core values" of professionalism in physical therapy as:

1. Accountability
2. Altruism
3. Compassion/Caring
4. Excellence
5. Integrity
6. Professional duty
7. Social responsibility[25]

Further, the APTA defined each core value and provided sample indicators of the value. These will be discussed in greater detail in Chapter 16. Although most individuals easily can recognize professional and unprofessional conduct, few can articulate a clear and concise definition.

As a result of this evolution in physical therapy toward the APTA's Vision 2020, physical therapists and physical therapist assistants undoubtedly will be exposed to more liability risk. This increased liability risk will be carried solo because no other health care practitioners will be overseeing or coordinating the care and treatment received by the patient. Hence, physical therapists and physical therapist assistants now must develop methods and implement systems to enhance risk management as an entry-level health care practitioner.

ENTRY-LEVEL HEALTH CARE PRACTITIONER

What does being an entry-level health care practitioner mean? It means the patient is coming to the physical therapist first for an evaluation and diagnosis of whatever ails him or her. Based on the physical therapy evaluation, the physical therapist may need to refer the patient for further testing or refer the patient to another health care provider for evaluation. Remember, not every patient is appropriate for physical therapy services. If, at the conclusion of the physical therapy evaluation, the physical therapist believes the patient has a problem that is within the physical therapist's scope of practice or expertise, then the physical therapist likely will develop and implement a plan of treatment without any other health care provider's input. However, if the physical therapist is wrong, and the patient sues, the physical therapist could be held liable for his or her action(s) and/or omission(s).

In contrast, when a patient goes to physical therapy with a physician's referral, the physician's referral (prescription) implicitly "clears" the patient for physical therapy services. The same might be implied when the physician signs the plan of care for a patient's physical therapy treatment. In these situations, the physician also is responsible for the overall services delivered to the patient pursuant to the prescription. This schematic of liability responsibility has been attractive to plaintiffs' attorneys because usually a physician carries greater amounts of insurance than a physical therapist or physical therapist assistant.

In fact, there are cases that discuss factual situations involving a physical therapist or physical therapist assistant wherein the physical therapist or physical therapist assistant was not named as a defendant. This lack of individually naming the physical therapist or physical therapist assistant in the lawsuit despite the individual being intimately involved with the factual scenario is because the physical therapist or physical therapist assistant did not have professional malpractice insurance. However, when only the physical therapist is responsible for the services being delivered to the patient, then the physical therapist will be the only available individual to name as a defendant and will bear the complete and sole responsibility for liability for a patient's alleged harm.

Additionally, if the physical therapist delegates any provision of services to a subordinate, aide, or physical therapist assistant, which later becomes the issue of the lawsuit, then the physical therapist is going to not only be responsible for the overall delivery of services, but the physical therapist also will be liable for the services delivered by the subordinate. To complicate the discussion even further, if a physical therapist was the owner of a clinic that employed other physical therapists and physical therapist assistants, then the owner of the clinic also is likely to be named as a defendant in the lawsuit because the owner ultimately is responsible for everything that occurs within the clinic regardless of whether he or she was the primary evaluating or treating therapist.

The entry-level health care practitioner likely will be the ultimate party responsible for the services delivered to a patient, and a clinic owner also will bear liability if the alleged conduct or omission for the care was rendered in his or her privately owned clinic. One of the most worrisome areas of potential professional physical therapy malpractice will be if the entry-level health care practicing physical therapist misdiagnoses a patient.

Example of a Misdiagnosed Patient

As an entry-level health care practitioner, there is no one overseeing the evaluation or services the physical therapist provides. As an example, recall the comfort associated with knowing, as a student of physical therapy, that there was always a clinical instructor overseeing and reviewing the physical therapy evaluations and the plans of care established.

Likewise the physical therapist assistant student always had the watchful eye of the clinical instructor. The clinical instructor was ultimately the actual responsible party for the provision of care that either the physical therapist or physical therapist assistant student provided. Further, whoever employed the clinical instructor also bore liability for the services the student provided. Thus, as an entry-level health care practitioner who is no longer a student, the layers of responsible persons will be gone and the physical therapist now will be standing alone on how he or she actually performed the evaluation, including what he or she decided to evaluate and what he or she omitted from the evaluation. A case that demonstrates how daunting this skill can be is *Wyckoff v. Jujamcyn Theaters, Inc.*, 784 N.Y.S.2d 26 (NY Sup. Ct. App. Div. 2004).

In the *Wyckoff* case, a consumer went to a New York theater and fell on the premises, sustaining personal injuries.[26] As with most cases, the issue being resolved by the appellate court was not directly on point for the discussion at hand. However, many cases that do not provide points directly on issues still contain useful information and language that can be beneficial in other cases. This useful information can then also provide a portal to areas of potential liability risk exposure. The *Wyckoff* case was ultimately decided on whether the theater was negligent in its premises maintenance; however, in the body of the case were allegations that the consumer's injuries were exacerbated as a result of the failure to properly diagnose a cervical fracture.[27]

The *Wyckoff* plaintiff not only sued the theater, but also sued the hospital and the physician for an alleged failure to diagnosis a neck fracture. As a result of the failure to diagnose, the consumer (patient) underwent physical therapy services for 1 week with an unstablized neck fracture.[28] Thus, the physical therapist who evaluated and treated this patient failed to identify there was an unstablized neck fracture and implemented a plan of care for the treatment of the patient's complaints. Thereafter, the patient suffered residual weakness, allegedly as a result of the failure to diagnose and stabilize the neck fracture and concurrent treatments with physical therapy.[29]

In the *Wyckoff* case, the hospital and the physician were sued along with the theater.[30] There is nothing in this case to indicate the physical therapist was also sued. However, if this patient had presented to the physical therapist and the physical therapist was an entry-level health care practitioner, it is likely the physical therapist may have missed the same diagnosis as did the physician. If this latter scenario were true, the physical therapist as an entry-level health care practitioner would have missed the diagnosis and there would be no one to blame but the entry-level health care practicing physical therapist. As a result, the plaintiff would then directly sue the physical therapist only because the physician would not have even entered the picture as an evaluator or prescriber of treatment.

Looking at this last case further in a hypothetical situation, if the patient presented to a physical therapy clinic and the physical therapist conducted an evaluation of the patient, the likelihood is that during the evaluation, the physical therapist would ask the patient to move the cervical spine and obtain range-of-motion measurements. Perhaps the most astute clinician would gain enough information through the taking of a history and physical to avoid any evaluation and immediately refer the patient to a primary care physician or local emergency room for emergent evaluation. However, if, as appeared in this case, the instability of the cervical spine was difficult to ascertain, it is likely a physical therapist would complete the evaluation, as was done in this case, and implement a plan of treatment for any identified problems. Thus, had this case been as this hypothetical outlines, the entry-level health care physical therapist arguably would have just assumed liability for the exacerbation of whatever injury was sustained in the fall at the theater.

Now, does this mean as an entry-level health care practitioner that every patient who presents to a physical therapy clinic for evaluation and treatment should be referred for radiograph studies or to the primary care physician for clearance before treatment? No, but it does mean as the entry-level health care practitioner, the physical therapist needs to be prepared to do a thorough health assessment and questionnaire and, if in doubt, refer. As this case illustrated, it is unfortunately common for even a physician to misdiagnose patients. The difference is when a physician misdiagnoses and the physical therapist treats the patient, the physician potentially has liability for the referral to physical therapy. Whereas the entry-level health care practitioner—the physical therapist—who misdiagnoses a patient and treats the patient in a contradictory fashion will bear full liability for a malpractice claim.

Another example of a case, this time where the physical therapist appropriately diagnosed and referred a patient, is *Bailey v. Haynes*, 856 So.2d 1207 (LA. 2003). As already explained, with most cases, the point, or in law called the issue of the case on appeal for this particular case was whether the cause of action had been brought within the applicable statute of limitations.[31] The concept of statute of limitations will be discussed in Chapter 5. However, this case provides illustration of a physical therapist who accurately and appropriately diagnosed cerebral palsy in a child.[32]

Based on the timing of the physical therapist's diagnosis of cerebral palsy, the court ruled it was the physical therapist's diagnosis that gave sufficient knowledge to the mother that there might have been negligence involved during the delivery of her baby.[33] To provide this kind of information to the mother, the physical therapist evaluated the child, diagnosed the child, and gave the mother sufficient information so that the mother could then bring a lawsuit for the alleged negligence of the physician involved in the delivery of the baby. This would also be an example of how a physical therapist could be utilized as an expert witness, which will be discussed later in Chapter 17.

EDUCATIONAL TRAINING FOR THE PHYSICAL THERAPIST AND PHYSICAL THERAPIST ASSISTANT

In order to practice as a physical therapist or physical therapist assistant, an individual must be licensed. (Note: There are still a few states where physical therapist assistants are not licensed.) Each state promulgates its licensure requirements for the physical therapists and physical therapist assistants who practice within its state. Hence, there is no national licensure, only licensure by a particular state. A physical therapist or physical therapist assistant may be licensed by as many states as he or she chooses.

Before someone even can apply for a physical therapist or physical therapist assistant license, he or she first must graduate from a school that has been accredited for the provision of physical therapy education. The body responsible for accrediting physical therapy and physical therapist assistant programs is the Commission on Accreditation in Physical Therapy Education (CAPTE).

Currently CAPTE accredits programs graduating physical therapists at the master's and doctoral level and programs graduating physical therapist assistants at the associate's degree level.[34] CAPTE's mission is "to serve the public by establishing and applying standards that assure quality and continuous improvement in the entry-level preparation of physical therapists and physical therapist assistants and that reflect the evolving nature of education, research and practice."[35]

EVOLUTION IN EDUCATIONAL TRAINING

As discussed previously, the first physical therapists in the United States were reconstruction aides. The reconstruction aides had other degrees before receiving training in physical therapy. As the level of physical therapy practice evolved, the education evolved such that physical therapy was taught only at certain institutions. These institutions' programs were very specific and had limited admissions initially for an individual's junior and senior year of a baccalaureate degree. Over time, the APTA and the CAPTE promoted that the education of physical therapists needed to be elevated to a master's degree level; thus, the body of knowledge and skills to master required more academic time.

With the progression toward a master's-level educational standard, students would obtain a baccalaureate degree that included certain physical therapy prerequisites before entering physical therapy school for specialized education and skills training to graduate with a master's degree. Initially there was a delay in the implementation of physical therapists being master's-level prepared. Nonetheless, this progression was again undertaken and as of January 1, 2002, CAPTE was no longer accrediting baccalaureate physical therapy programs.[36] The rationale for this progression was that the amount of information a physical therapy program needed to impart on students was simply too voluminous to provide in a baccalaureate program. Today, most of the master's-level programs have or are now progressing to the doctoral level.

Lastly, physical therapist assistants are now educated at the associate's degree level. Just like physical therapy programs, physical therapist assistants programs are accredited through CAPTE. As physical therapists evolve toward APTA's Vision 2020, there is controversy over the future role of the physical therapist assistant and as this book is written, no real answers yet exist.

As of November 28, 2006, there were 43 institutions that offered master's-level physical therapy programs and 166 institutions that offered doctoral-level physical therapy programs.[37] There was also one institution under development of a doctoral physical therapy program.[38] For physical therapist assistants there were 221 institutions supporting 233 programs.[39] There were also 13 institutions developing physical therapist assistants programs.[40] For a current listing of institutions offering the different programs, go to the APTA's Web site, www.apta.org.

AMERICAN PHYSICAL THERAPY ASSOCIATION

As the profession of physical therapy has evolved, so has the organization that represents physical therapists and physical therapist assistants. As previously discussed, the organization is the American Physical Therapy Association (APTA). This organization now has evolved to having a national office in Alexandria, Virginia, as well as a chapter office (now called a component of the organization) in almost every state.

To become a member of the APTA, an individual must have been accepted to, enrolled in, or graduated from an accredited physical therapy or physical therapy assistant program. If the physical therapy or physical therapy assistant program has been granted cadency status by the CAPTE and has been accredited by graduation, the physical therapist or physical therapist assistant is eligible for membership. Membership is voluntary and not mandatory for licensure. The cost of membership dues includes mandatory concurrent joining of the national association as well as the state association where the physical therapist or physical therapist assistant identifies as his or her residency. As of 2007, the national annual dues were as follows:

Physical therapists	$280.00
Physical therapist assistants	$185.00
Student (physical therapist or physical therapist assistant)	$ 80.00
Physical therapy postprofessional student	$150.00

To the national dues, the physical therapist, physical therapist assistant, or student must then add the dues for membership in his or her state association of the APTA. Then to that total the physical therapist, physical therapist assistant, or student must add the dues for any section he or she chooses to belong to for any given year. The state dues structure will be provided later with the addresses of each state's (component's) address. At the conclusion of this chapter, the dues for each section's membership will be provided. A physical therapist or physical therapist assistant also can belong to more than one chapter (component) by paying what is called *corresponding dues* to the second or additional chapters that the physical therapist or physical therapist assistant wants to join.

The operation of the APTA is beyond the scope of this book; however, the contact information for the APTA and each component, if it exists, is provided here as a reference:

American Physical Therapy Association
1111 North Fairfax Street
Alexandria, Virginia 22314-1488
(703) 684-2782
(800) 999-2782
Fax: (703) 684-7343
www.apta.org

Alabama
Alabama Physical Therapy Association
P.O. Box 660551
Birmingham, Alabama 35266-0551
www.ptalabama.org

Physical therapists	$140.00 per year
Physical therapist assistants	$ 65.00 per year
Student (physical therapist or physical therapist assistant)	$ 5.00 per year
Physical therapy postprofessional student	$ 5.00 per year
Corresponding dues	$ 65.00 per year

Alaska
Alaska Physical Therapy Association
P.O. Box 140351
Anchorage, Alaska 99514-0351
(907) 244-7463 (as of the writing of the book there is no website)

Physical therapists	$ 75.00 per year
Physical therapist assistants	$ 30.00 per year
Student (physical therapist or physical therapist assistant)	$ 8.00 per year
Physical therapy postprofessional student	$ 30.00 per year
Corresponding dues	$ 75.00 per year

Arizona
Arizona Physical Therapy Association
4035 East Fanfol Drive
Phoenix, Arizona 85028-5103
www.aptaaz.org

Physical therapists	$140.00 per year
Physical therapist assistants	$ 84.00 per year
Student (physical therapist or physical therapist assistant)	$ 0.00 per year
Physical therapy postprofessional student	$ 50.00 per year
Corresponding dues	$140.00 per year

Arkansas

Arkansas Physical Therapy Association
1401 West 6th Street
Little Rock, Arkansas 72201-2901
www.arpta.org

Physical therapists	$115.00 per year
Physical therapist assistants	$ 55.00 per year
Student (physical therapist or physical therapist assistant)	$ 0.00 per year
Physical therapy postprofessional student	$ 50.00 per year
Corresponding dues	$ 50.00 per year

California

California Physical Therapy Association
2880 Gateway Oaks Drive, Suite 140
Sacramento, California 95833
www.ccapta.org

Physical therapists	$245.00 per year
Physical therapist assistants	$156.00 per year
Student (physical therapist or physical therapist assistant)	$ 23.00 per year
Physical therapy postprofessional student	$100.00 per year
Corresponding dues	$120.00 per year

Colorado

Colorado Physical Therapy Association
7400 East Arapahoe Road, Suite 211
Centennial, Colorado 80112-1281
www.aptaco.org

Physical therapists	$140.00 per year
Physical therapist assistants	$ 85.00 per year
Student (physical therapist or physical therapist assistant)	$ 20.00 per year
Physical therapy postprofessional student	$ 65.00 per year
Corresponding dues	$ 65.00 per year

Connecticut

Connecticut Physical Therapy Association
Administrative Offices
15 North River Road
Tolland, Connecticut 06084-2705
www.ctpt.org

Physical therapists	$120.00 per year
Physical therapist assistants	$ 60.00 per year
Student (physical therapist or physical therapist assistant)	$ 10.00 per year
Physical therapy postprofessional student	$ 10.00 per year
Corresponding dues	$ 60.00 per year

Delaware

Delaware Physical Therapy Association
120 Churchill Lane
Wilmington, Delaware 19808-4319
www.dptaonline.com

Physical therapists	$ 90.00 per year
Physical therapist assistants	$ 40.00 per year
Student (physical therapist or physical therapist assistant)	$ 15.00 per year
Physical therapy postprofessional student	$ 15.00 per year
Corresponding dues	$ 50.00 per year

District of Columbia

District of Columbia Physical Therapy Association
120 Irving Street, NW
Washington, DC 20010-2921
www.dcpta.com

Physical therapists	$ 75.00 per year
Physical therapist assistants	$ 25.00 per year
Student (physical therapist or physical therapist assistant)	$ 25.00 per year
Physical therapy postprofessional student	$ 25.00 per year
Corresponding dues	$ 25.00 per year

Florida

Florida Physical Therapy Association
2104 Delta Way, Suite 7
Tallahassee, Florida 32303-4236
www.fpta.org

Physical therapists	$160.00 per year
Physical therapist assistants	$110.00 per year
Student (physical therapist or physical therapist assistant)	$ 10.00 per year
Physical therapy postprofessional student	$100.00 per year
Corresponding dues	$125.00 per year

Georgia

Georgia Physical Therapy Association
1260 Winchester Parkway, Suite 205
Smyrna, Georgia 30080-6546
www.ptagonline.org

Physical therapists	$105.00 per year
Physical therapist assistants	$ 52.50 per year
Student (physical therapist or physical therapist assistant)	$ 7.00 per year
Physical therapy postprofessional student	$105.00 per year
Corresponding dues	$ 70.00 per year

Hawaii

Hawaii Physical Therapy Association
1360 Beretania Street, 301
Honolulu, Hawaii 96814
www.hapta.org

Physical therapists	$120.00 per year
Physical therapist assistants	$ 50.00 per year
Student (physical therapist or physical therapist assistant)	$ 15.00 per year
Physical therapy postprofessional student	$ 75.00 per year
Corresponding dues	$ 25.00 per year

Idaho

Idaho Physical Therapy Association
4220 Bodenheimer Street
Boise, Idaho 83703-4202
www.idaho.org

Physical therapists	$ 95.00 per year
Physical therapist assistants	$ 70.00 per year
Student (physical therapist or physical therapist assistant)	$ 20.00 per year
Physical therapy postprofessional student	$ 20.00 per year
Corresponding dues	$ 10.00 per year

Illinois

Illinois Physical Therapy Association
1010 Jorie Boulevard, Suite 134
Oak Brook, Illinois 60523-4441
www.ipta.org

Physical therapists	$150.00 per year
Physical therapist assistants	$ 75.00 per year
Student (physical therapist or physical therapist assistant)	$ 10.00 per year
Physical therapy postprofessional student	$ 90.00 per year
Corresponding dues	$150.00 per year

Indiana

Indiana Physical Therapy Association
P.O. Box 26692
Indianapolis, Indiana 46226-0692
www.inapta.org

Physical therapists	$120.00 per year
Physical therapist assistants	$ 65.00 per year
Student (physical therapist or physical therapist assistant)	$ 0.00 per year
Physical therapy postprofessional student	$ 0.00 per year
Corresponding dues	$120.00 per year

Iowa

Iowa Physical Therapy Association
1228 8th South, Suite 106
West Des Moines, Iowa 50265-2624
www.iowaapta.org

Physical therapists	$143.00 per year
Physical therapist assistants	$ 69.00 per year
Student (physical therapist or physical therapist assistant)	$ 20.00 per year
Physical therapy postprofessional student	$ 65.00 per year
Corresponding dues	$ 70.00 per year

Kansas

Kansas Physical Therapy Association
214 SW 6th Avenue, Suite 205
Topeka, Kansas 66603-3780
www.kpta.com

Physical therapists	$ 80.00 per year
Physical therapist assistants	$ 45.00 per year
Student (physical therapist or physical therapist assistant)	$ 10.00 per year
Physical therapy postprofessional student	$ 30.00 per year
Corresponding dues	$ 40.00 per year

Kentucky
Kentucky Physical Therapy Association
15847 Teal Road
Verona, Kentucky 41092-8229
www.KPTA.org

Physical therapists	$105.00 per year
Physical therapist assistants	$ 75.00 per year
Student (physical therapist or physical therapist assistant)	$ 0.00 per year
Physical therapy postprofessional student	$ 50.00 per year
Corresponding dues	$105.00 per year

Louisiana
Louisiana Physical Therapy Association
8550 United Plaza Boulevard, Suite 1001A
Baton Rogue, Louisiana 70809-2256
www.lpta.org

Physical therapists	$125.00 per year
Physical therapist assistants	$ 94.00 per year
Student (physical therapist or physical therapist assistant)	$ 0.00 per year
Physical therapy postprofessional student	$ 25.00 per year
Corresponding dues	$ 50.00 per year

Maine
Maine Physical Therapy Association
P.O. Box 1783
Portland, Maine 04104-1783
www.maineapta.org

Physical therapists	$ 70.00 per year
Physical therapist assistants	$ 35.00 per year
Student (physical therapist or physical therapist assistant)	$ 0.00 per year
Physical therapy postprofessional student	$ 25.00 per year
Corresponding dues	$ 15.00 per year

Maryland

Maryland Physical Therapy Association
1111 North Fairfax Street
Alexandria, Virginia 22314-1484
www.aptamd.org

Physical therapists	$120.00 per year
Physical therapist assistants	$ 60.00 per year
Student (physical therapist or physical therapist assistant)	$ 0.00 per year
Physical therapy postprofessional student	$ 75.00 per year
Corresponding dues	$ 60.00 per year

Massachusetts

Massachusetts Physical Therapy Association
34 Atlantic Street
Gloucester, Massachusetts 01930-1625
www.aptaofma.org

Physical therapists	$120.00 per year
Physical therapist assistants	$ 60.00 per year
Student (physical therapist or physical therapist assistant)	$ 24.00 per year
Physical therapy postprofessional student	$ 60.00 per year
Corresponding dues	$120.00 per year

Michigan

Michigan Physical Therapy Association
3300 Washtenaw Avenue, Suite 220
Ann Arbor, Michigan 48104-4292
www.mpta.org

Physical therapists	$125.00 per year
Physical therapist assistants	$ 65.00 per year
Student (physical therapist or physical therapist assistant)	$ 10.00 per year
Physical therapy postprofessional student	$100.00 per year
Corresponding dues	$100.00 per year

Minnesota

Minnesota Physical Therapy Association
1711 West County Road B, Suite 102S
Roseville, Minnesota 55113-4036
www.mnapta.org

Physical therapists	$140.00 per year
Physical therapist assistants	$ 60.00 per year
Student (physical therapist or physical therapist assistant)	$ 10.00 per year
Physical therapy postprofessional student	$ 10.00 per year
Corresponding dues	$ 50.00 per year

Mississippi

Mississippi Physical Therapy Association
P.O. Box 4195
Jackson, Mississippi 39296-4195
www.mpta.org

Physical therapists	$100.00 per year
Physical therapist assistants	$ 50.00 per year
Student (physical therapist or physical therapist assistant)	$ 10.00 per year
Physical therapy postprofessional student	$ 10.00 per year
Corresponding dues	$ 50.00 per year

Missouri

Missouri Physical Therapy Association
205 East Capitol, Suite 100
Jefferson City, Missouri 65101-3166
www.mopt.org

Physical therapists	$110.00 per year
Physical therapist assistants	$ 85.00 per year
Student (physical therapist or physical therapist assistant)	$ 10.00 per year
Physical therapy postprofessional student	$ 50.00 per year
Corresponding dues	$ 40.00 per year

Montana

Montana Physical Therapy Association
P.O. Box 8575
Missoula, Montana 59807-8575
www.MAPTA.org

Physical therapists	$100.00 per year
Physical therapist assistants	$ 50.00 per year
Student (physical therapist or physical therapist assistant)	$ 0.00 per year
Physical therapy postprofessional student	$ 50.00 per year
Corresponding dues	$ 50.00 per year

Nebraska

Nebraska Physical Therapy Association
P.O. Box 540427
Omaha, Nebraska 68154-0427
www.npta.org

Physical therapists	$ 75.00 per year
Physical therapist assistants	$ 40.00 per year
Student (physical therapist or physical therapist assistant)	$ 0.00 per year
Physical therapy postprofessional student	$ 0.00 per year
Corresponding dues	$ 75.00 per year

Nevada

Nevada Physical Therapy Association
8665 West Flamingo Road, Suite 131
Las Vegas, Nevada 89147-8663
www.NVapta.org

Physical therapists	$100.00 per year
Physical therapist assistants	$ 80.00 per year
Student (physical therapist or physical therapist assistant)	$ 0.00 per year
Physical therapy postprofessional student	$ 50.00 per year
Corresponding dues	$ 50.00 per year

New Hampshire

New Hampshire Physical Therapy Association
P.O. Box 978
Manchester, New Hampshire 03105-0978
www.nhapta.org

Physical therapists	$ 75.00 per year
Physical therapist assistants	$ 40.00 per year
Student (physical therapist or physical therapist assistant)	$ 10.00 per year
Physical therapy postprofessional student	$ 10.00 per year
Corresponding dues	$ 15.00 per year

New Jersey

New Jersey Physical Therapy Association
1100 US Highway 130, Suite 3
Robbinsville, New Jersey 08691-1108
www.aptanj.org

Physical therapists	$145.00 per year
Physical therapist assistants	$ 80.00 per year
Student (physical therapist or physical therapist assistant)	$ 15.00 per year
Physical therapy postprofessional student	$ 75.00 per year
Corresponding dues	$ 50.00 per year

New Mexico
New Mexico Physical Therapy Association
c/o New Mexico Chapter Executive Office
1111 North Fairfax Street
Alexandria, Virginia 22314
www.nmapta.org

Physical therapists	$ 60.00 per year
Physical therapist assistants	$ 30.00 per year
Student (physical therapist or physical therapist assistant)	$ 5.00 per year
Physical therapy postprofessional student	$ 5.00 per year
Corresponding dues	$ 30.00 per year

New York
New York Physical Therapy Association
5 Palisades Drive, Suite 330
Albany, New York 12205-6433
www.nypta.org

Physical therapists	$180.00 per year
Physical therapist assistants	$115.00 per year
Student (physical therapist or physical therapist assistant)	$ 5.00 per year
Physical therapy postprofessional student	$110.00 per year
Corresponding dues	$180.00 per year

North Carolina
North Carolina Physical Therapy Association
316 West Milbrook Road 105
Raleigh, North Carolina 27609-4482
www.ncpt.org

Physical therapists	$105.00 per year
Physical therapist assistants	$ 70.00 per year
Student (physical therapist or physical therapist assistant)	$ 0.00 per year
Physical therapy postprofessional student	$ 0.00 per year
Corresponding dues	$ 50.00 per year

North Dakota

North Dakota Physical Therapy Association
University of North Dakota
Department of Physical Therapy
Grand Falls, North Dakota 58202
www.med.und.nodak.edu/depts/pt/ndpta/welcome.htm

Physical therapists	$ 45.00 per year
Physical therapist assistants	$ 25.00 per year
Student (physical therapist or physical therapist assistant)	$ 0.00 per year
Physical therapy postprofessional student	$ 45.00 per year
Corresponding dues	$ 23.00 per year

Ohio

Ohio Physical Therapy Association
1085 Beecher Crossing North, Suite B
Gahanna, Ohio 43230-4563
www.ohiopt.org

Physical therapists	$170.00 per year
Physical therapist assistants	$ 99.00 per year
Student (physical therapist or physical therapist assistant)	$ 10.00 per year
Physical therapy postprofessional student	$ 50.00 per year
Corresponding dues	$ 48.00 per year

Oklahoma

Oklahoma Physical Therapy Association
P.O. Box 5354
Edmond, Oklahoma 73083-5354
www.okpt.org

Physical therapists	$100.00 per year
Physical therapist assistants	$ 65.00 per year
Student (physical therapist or physical therapist assistant)	$ 10.00 per year
Physical therapy postprofessional student	$ 10.00 per year
Corresponding dues	$ 20.00 per year

Oregon

Oregon Physical Therapy Association
147 SE 102nd
Portland, Oregon 97216-2703
www.opta.org

Physical therapists	$100.00 per year
Physical therapist assistants	$ 55.00 per year
Student (physical therapist or physical therapist assistant)	$ 15.00 per year
Physical therapy postprofessional student	$ 50.00 per year
Corresponding dues	$ 50.00 per year

Pennsylvania

Pennsylvania Physical Therapy Association
4646 Smith Street
Harrisburg, Pennsylvania 17109-1525
www.ppta.org

Physical therapists	$145.00 per year
Physical therapist assistants	$105.00 per year
Student (physical therapist or physical therapist assistant)	$ 5.00 per year
Physical therapy postprofessional student	$ 50.00 per year
Corresponding dues	$ 75.00 per year

Rhode Island

Rhode Island Physical Therapy Association
Rhode Island Administrative Office
15 North River Road
Tolland, Rhode Island 06084-2705
www.riapta.com

Physical therapists	$ 80.00 per year
Physical therapist assistants	$ 40.00 per year
Student (physical therapist or physical therapist assistant)	$ 10.00 per year
Physical therapy postprofessional student	$ 50.00 per year
Corresponding dues	$ 25.00 per year

South Carolina

South Carolina Physical Therapy Association
3581 Centre Circle, Suite 104
Fort Mill, South Carolina 29715-9742
www.scapta.org

Physical therapists	$100.00 per year
Physical therapist assistants	$ 60.00 per year
Student (physical therapist or physical therapist assistant)	$ 5.00 per year
Physical therapy postprofessional student	$100.00 per year
Corresponding dues	$ 50.00 per year

South Dakota
South Dakota Physical Therapy Association
P.O. Box 91146
Sioux Falls, South Dakota 57109-1146
www.sdpta.org

Physical therapists	$ 50.00 per year
Physical therapist assistants	$ 406.00 per year
Student (physical therapist or physical therapist assistant)	$ 25.00 per year
Physical therapy postprofessional student	$ 25.00 per year
Corresponding dues	$ 0.00 per year

Tennessee
Tennessee Physical Therapy Association
4205 Hillsboro Road, Suite 317
Nashville, Tennessee 37215-3336
www.tptaonline.org

Physical therapists	$100.00 per year
Physical therapist assistants	$ 67.00 per year
Student (physical therapist or physical therapist assistant)	$ 0.00 per year
Physical therapy postprofessional student	$ 25.00 per year
Corresponding dues	$ 25.00 per year

Texas
Texas Physical Therapy Association
701 Brazos Street, Suite 440
Austin, Texas 78701-3286
www.tpta.org

Physical therapists	$135.00 per year
Physical therapist assistants	$ 83.00 per year
Student (physical therapist or physical therapist assistant)	$ 10.00 per year
Physical therapy postprofessional student	$100.00 per year
Corresponding dues	$100.00 per year

Utah
Utah Physical Therapy Association
1551 Renaissance Towne Drive, Suite 350
Bountiful, Utah 84010-7674
www.uapta.org

Physical therapists	$100.00 per year
Physical therapist assistants	$ 25.00 per year
Student (physical therapist or physical therapist assistant)	$ 5.00 per year
Physical therapy postprofessional student	$100.00 per year
Corresponding dues	$ 0.00 per year

Vermont

Vermont Physical Therapy Association
995 Dorset Street
South Burlington, Vermont 05403-7503
www.vtapta.org

Physical therapists	$ 60.00 per year
Physical therapist assistants	$ 40.00 per year
Student (physical therapist or physical therapist assistant)	$ 0.00 per year
Physical therapy postprofessional student	$ 0.00 per year
Corresponding dues	$ 20.00 per year

Virginia

Virginia Physical Therapy Association
c/o APTA
1111 North Fairfax Street
Alexandria, Virginia 22314-1488
www.vpta.org

Physical therapists	$ 85.00 per year
Physical therapist assistants	$ 60.00 per year
Student (physical therapist or physical therapist assistant)	$ 0.00 per year
Physical therapy postprofessional student	$ 50.00 per year
Corresponding dues	$ 75.00 per year

Washington

Washington Physical Therapy Association
208 Rogers Street, NW
Olympia, Washington 98502-4940
www.ptwa.org

Physical therapists	$125.00 per year
Physical therapist assistants	$ 82.00 per year
Student (physical therapist or physical therapist assistant)	$ 0.00 per year
Physical therapy postprofessional student	$ 40.00 per year
Corresponding dues	$ 50.00 per year

West Virginia
West Virginia Physical Therapy Association
2110 Kanawha Boulevard East, Suite 5220
Charleston, West Virginia 25311-2217
www.wvpta.org

Physical therapists	$ 90.00 per year
Physical therapist assistants	$ 60.00 per year
Student (physical therapist or physical therapist assistant)	$ 10.00 per year
Physical therapy postprofessional student	$ 25.00 per year
Corresponding dues	$ 25.00 per year

Wisconsin
Wisconsin Physical Therapy Association
4781 Hayes Road, Suite 201
Madison, Wisconsin 53704
www.wpta.org

Physical therapists	$156.00 per year
Physical therapist assistants	$ 79.00 per year
Student (physical therapist or physical therapist assistant)	$ 15.00 per year
Physical therapy postprofessional student	$ 90.00 per year
Corresponding dues	$ 45.00 per year

Wyoming
Wyoming Physical Therapy Association
1536 East 4th Street
Casper, Wyoming 82601-3048
www.wypta.org

Physical therapists	$ 60.00 per year
Physical therapist assistants	$ 38.00 per year
Student (physical therapist or physical therapist assistant)	$ 30.00 per year
Physical therapy postprofessional student	$ 0.00 per year
Corresponding dues	$ 20.00 per year

Section dues are as follows:

Acute Care

Physical therapists	$ 35.00 per year
Physical therapist assistants	$ 17.00 per year
Student (physical therapist or physical therapist assistant)	$ 6.00 per year
Physical therapy postprofessional student	$ 6.00 per year

Aquatic Physical Therapy

Physical therapists	$ 45.00 per year
Physical therapist assistants	$ 35.00 per year
Student (physical therapist or physical therapist assistant)	$ 20.00 per year
Physical therapy postprofessional student	$ 20.00 per year

Cardiopulmonary and Pulmonary

Physical therapists	$ 40.00 per year
Physical therapist assistants	$ 20.00 per year
Student (physical therapist or physical therapist assistant)	$ 10.00 per year
Physical therapy postprofessional student	$ 10.00 per year

Clinical Electro and Wound Management

Physical therapists	$ 35.00 per year
Physical therapist assistants	$ 25.00 per year
Student (physical therapist or physical therapist assistant)	$ 5.00 per year
Physical therapy postprofessional student	$ 5.00 per year

Education

Physical therapists	$ 50.00 per year
Physical therapist assistants	$ 35.00 per year
Student (physical therapist or physical therapist assistant)	$ 15.00 per year
Physical therapy postprofessional student	$ 25.00 per year

Federal

Physical therapists	$ 25.00 per year
Physical therapist assistants	$ 18.00 per year
Student (physical therapist or physical therapist assistant)	$ 8.00 per year
Physical therapy postprofessional student	$ 15.00 per year

Geriatrics

Physical therapists	$ 45.00 per year
Physical therapist assistants	$ 35.00 per year
Student (physical therapist or physical therapist assistant)	$ 15.00 per year
Physical therapy postprofessional student	$ 15.00 per year

Hand

Physical therapists	$ 35.00 per year
Physical therapist assistants	$ 25.00 per year
Student (physical therapist or physical therapist assistant)	$ 10.00 per year
Physical therapy postprofessional student	$ 21.00 per year

Health Policy and Administration

Physical therapists	$ 50.00 per year
Physical therapist assistants	$ 30.00 per year
Student (physical therapist or physical therapist assistant)	$ 10.00 per year
Physical therapy postprofessional student	$ 30.00 per year

Neurology

Physical therapists	$ 40.00 per year
Physical therapist assistants	$ 20.00 per year
Student (physical therapist or physical therapist assistant)	$ 15.00 per year
Physical therapy postprofessional student	$ 15.00 per year

Oncology

Physical therapists	$ 35.00 per year
Physical therapist assistants	$ 20.00 per year
Student (physical therapist or physical therapist assistant)	$ 10.00 per year
Physical therapy postprofessional student	$ 10.00 per year

Orthopedic

Physical therapists	$ 50.00 per year
Physical therapist assistants	$ 30.00 per year
Student (physical therapist or physical therapist assistant)	$ 15.00 per year
Physical therapy postprofessional student	$ 15.00 per year

Pediatric

Physical therapists	$ 55.00 per year
Physical therapist assistants	$ 35.00 per year
Student (physical therapist or physical therapist assistant)	$ 20.00 per year
Physical therapy postprofessional student	$ 35.00 per year

Private Practice

Physical therapists	$175.00 per year
Physical therapist assistants	$105.00 per year
Student (physical therapist or physical therapist assistant)	$ 50.00 per year
Physical therapy postprofessional student	$150.00 per year

Research

Physical therapists	$ 35.00 per year
Physical therapist assistants	$ 25.00 per year
Student (physical therapist or physical therapist assistant)	$ 5.00 per year
Physical therapy postprofessional student	$ 5.00 per year

Sports Physical Therapy

Physical therapists	$ 50.00 per year
Physical therapist assistants	$ 40.00 per year
Student (physical therapist or physical therapist assistant)	$ 15.00 per year
Physical therapy postprofessional student	$ 15.00 per year

Women's Health

Physical therapists	$ 50.00 per year
Physical therapist assistants	$ 25.00 per year
Student (physical therapist or physical therapist assistant)	$ 25.00 per year
Physical therapy postprofessional student	$ 25.00 per year

PROFESSIONAL DESIGNATOR

The professional designator for physical therapists is currently under debate. In the 1970s and 1980s, the professional designator was RPT (Registered Physical Therapist) or LPT (Licensed Physical Therapist) and for the physical therapist assistants it was RPTA (Registered Physical Therapist Assistant) or LPTA (Licensed Physical Therapist Assistant). However, in the late 1980s and early 1990s, a movement of change occurred for the professional designator for physical therapist or physical therapist assistant to be PT or PTA. One of the primary rationales for this change was that an individual could not practice as a physical therapist or physical therapist assistant without being licensed or registered; hence, the additional letters made no difference and actually created some confusion because some therapists were using an "R" and some were using the "L."

Today the debate concerns whether to change the physical therapist designator to DPT in recognition of the doctoral degree. Much time, energy, and some cost are being spent to perhaps change the designator once again. However, from a historical perspective, the current debate seems to make a fallacy of the arguments that successfully changed the designator in the 1980s. Just like an "R" or "L" was unnecessary to communicate someone was a licensed physical therapist, it seems a "D" adds nothing to the communication that someone is a physical therapist and may actually create more confusion with consumers as personal trainers want to use the designator PT. When and how the debate will end is unknown as this book is written.

SUMMARY

In summation, the profession of physical therapy started as health care extenders or reconstruction aides to physicians in the delivery of treatment to soldiers injured as a result of wars. The education preparation of physical therapists has progressed from being a baccalaureate to master's to now most physical therapy programs are at the doctoral level. Only 20 percent of programs remain at the master's level and no programs remain at the baccalaureate level.[41]

The physical therapist assistant evolved to assist the physical therapist and play a vital role in the delivery of physical therapy services. With the evolution of the profession also has come the evolution of the organization representing physical therapists, physical therapist assistants, and students, the American Physical Therapy Association. Today the physical therapy profession is guided under the direction of the APTA and is working toward obtaining goals established under Vision 2020. One of the major goals is for the physical therapist to become an entry-level health care practitioner, which also will likely cause an increase in the frequency of professional malpractice claims. The malpractice claims will not only be brought against the physical therapist, but also physical therapist assistants and students.

DISCUSSION QUESTIONS

1. What is physical therapy?
2. Explain how physical therapy developed.
3. What were the key reasons physical therapy developed as a profession?
4. What is a vision statement?
5. What is Vision 2020?
6. What are the key elements of Vision 2020?
7. Explain each key element of Vision 2020.
8. Why is there a greater chance a physical therapist, physical therapist assistant, or student might be sued by his or her patient?
9. Discuss the two factors considered in granting direct access to physical therapy services.
10. Identify and discuss the core values of professionalism in physical therapy.
11. Explain the difference in liability exposure between treating a patient with a physician's referral or as an entry-level health care practitioner.

12. How has the educational preparation of physical therapists changed from the initial physical therapist to today?
13. What is the significance of the educational change to the physical therapy profession?
14. What, in your opinion, should the physical therapist professional designator be and why?

NOTES

[1] The American Physical Therapy Association web page at www.apta.org.
[2] *Guide to Physical Therapy Practice*, 682 (American Physical Therapy Association, 2nd ed., 2003).
[3] www.dictionary.com.
[4] The American Physical Therapy Association web page at www.apta.org, Areas of Interest, Professional Resources, Reimbursement, Info for Consumers, Physical Therapy & Your Insurance: A Patient's Guide to Getting the Best Coverage.
[5] *Id.*
[6] www.dictionary.com.
[7] The American Physical Therapy Association web page www.apta.org, Home, About APTA, History.
[8] *Id.*
[9] *Id.*
[10] *Id.*
[11] *Id.*
[12] Alliance for Nonprofit Management web page at www.allianceonline.org, Frequently Asked Questions, What Is a Vision Statement?
[13] *Id.*
[14] *Id.*
[15] *Id.*
[16] *The American Heritage Dictionary of the English Language*, (Houghton Mifflin Co., 4th Ed., 2000).
[17] American Physical Therapy Association, *Direct Access to Physical Therapist Services*, www.apta.org.
[18] *Id.*
[19] *Id.*
[20] Jean Mitchell and Gregory de Lissovoy, Cost Effectiveness of Direct Access to Physical Therapy, *Phys. Ther.* 77: 10–18 (1997).
[21] Department of Health & Human Services, Office of Inspector General, *Physical Therapy Billed by Physicians* OEI-09-02-00200 (May 1, 2006).
[22] Physical Therapy Claims Study, CNA HealthPro, 13 (December 4, 2006).
[23] The American Physical Therapy Association web page at www.apta.org, Research.
[24] www.dictionary.com.
[25] The American Physical Therapy Association web page at www.apta.org, Professionalism in Physical Therapy: Core Values.
[26] *Wyckoff v. Jujamcyn Theaters, Inc.*, 784 N.Y.S.2d 26, 27 (NY Sup. Ct. App. Div. 2004).

[27] *Id.*
[28] *Id.*
[29] *Id.*
[30] *Id.*
[31] *Baily v. Haynes*, 856 S.2d 1207 (La. 2003).
[32] *Id.*
[33] *Id.* at 1210.
[34] The American Physical Therapy Association web page at www.apta.org, Education, Accreditation (CAPTE), § 2.3.
[35] *Id.* at § 2.2.
[36] *Id.* at Education programs, Professional Physical Therapy.
[37] *Id.* at Accreditation (CAPTE), PTA Programs, PT & PTA Programs.
[38] *Id.*
[39] *Id.*
[40] *Id.*
[41] The American Physical Therapy Association web page at www.apta.org, Education, Accreditation (CAPTE), § 2.3.

CHAPTER 2

The Legal System

A basic understanding of the legal system is critical to mastering concepts in this book. Unlike physical therapy, in the profession of law, few things are concrete or "black and white." Law is a profession intertwined with actual laws, concepts, theories, and principles to which facts of cases are applied to determine outcomes for individual situations. Therefore, definitions of legal terms and concepts will be discussed throughout this book. Nevertheless, a foundation of the legal system is necessary to maximize the benefit of this book; the purpose of this chapter is to establish the groundwork necessary for subsequent chapters.

KEY CONCEPTS

Different types of law
Burdens of persuasion
Different court systems
Teston case
Federal court system
State court systems
Venue
Personal jurisdiction
Subject matter jurisdiction
Appeals

DIFFERENT TYPES OF LAW

Generally speaking, law can be divided into three types: criminal, civil, and administrative. The most-recognized type of law is probably criminal because there have been, and there will probably continue to be, television shows that tell these stories.

CRIMINAL LAW

Criminal law involves an attempt to punish a particular act that laws have been created to prohibit. Thus, in criminal law an attorney, called a *prosecutor*, represents either the victim or the state's interest in seeking punishment for a crime. The law(s) governing the prosecution of the criminal act have been enacted by that state's legislature. The laws, which are also called *statutes*, create the elements of the causes of action the state's prosecutor must prove.

An element of a cause of action is defined as, "[a] constituent part of a claim that must be proved for the claim to succeed."[1] As an example, the crime of murder is generally defined as "[t]he killing of a human being with malice aforethought."[2] (It should be noted this is an example and each state's definition or statute defining the crime of murder could be slightly different and have varying levels.) Hence, the elements of this cause of action would be:

1. A killing
2. Of a human being
3. With malice aforethought

Consequently, for a prosecutor to be successful in proving a defendant murdered someone, the prosecutor would have to prove each element of the crime; thus, all three elements would have to be proven.

The person or entity being prosecuted is called a *defendant* and has the right to be represented by counsel to defend charges brought forth through the prosecutor working for the state attorney's office (SAO). Sometimes a defendant can afford to have private counsel represent his or her interest. If a defendant cannot afford counsel, then the defendant's rights are represented and protected by the *public defender*. A public defender is "a lawyer or staff of lawyers, usually publicly appointed, whose duty is to represent indigent criminal defendants."[3]

Criminal law differs from civil law in many ways. Civil law attempts to compensate a victim for a particular act or omission to act in an attempt to make the victim wronged "whole again." It is possible for a scenario of facts to result in criminal prosecution as well as a civil lawsuit. The criminal prosecution would be to punish the act or omission to act because laws of the state prohibit the conduct, while the civil lawsuit would be an attempt to compensate the victim for his or her loss. The attorney representing the victim in a civil lawsuit is called the *plaintiff's attorney*, whereas the party being sued is represented again by defense counsel. Civil law also differs from criminal law relative to the causes of action sued upon.

Criminal law's causes of action are statutorily based (laws) whereas civil law involves various causes of action established through case law for intentional torts, contracts, property, or various types of negligence. There are even statutorily created rights under which plaintiffs can sue for the enforcement of damages related to failure to comply with certain statutes. One of the best examples of a statutorily created civil right is the Civil Rights Acts of 1964, 42 U.S.C. § 2000d, et. seq. According to this compilation of statutes, amongst other things, employers may not discriminate in their hiring practices based upon a person's race, color, or national origin.

Administrative law is the area of law that deals with the enforcement or punishment of violations of rules and regulations that govern various professions or services. The best example relative to this book is that each state has developed for its state a practice act that governs physical therapists and physical therapist assistants. Physical therapists and physical therapist assistants, as well as students, must abide by a state's practice act in order to practice physical therapy within that state. A violation of the rules and regulations as set forth in the practice act could lead to the individual having a complaint filed against his or her license.

Once an *administrative complaint* is filed, the department responsible for the administration of that state's practice act is charged with the responsibility to investigate and determine if probable cause exists for the matter to be referred to that state's board of physical therapy practice. If probable cause exists, then the board of physical therapy practice would determine whether to bring forth charges against the licensee. If charges are brought, the licensee would have an opportunity to present evidence and defend his or her license against the charges. It is possible, depending on the allegations in the administrative complaint, for a licensee to be reprimanded, a fine to be levied, or someone's license to be suspended or revoked for extreme or multiple offenses. There also can be a combination of sanctions against a licensee.

To further understand the different types of law, an in-depth discussion will follow. One of the greatest differences between civil and criminal law is the different "burdens of persuasion" that accompany the different types of law.

Burdens of Persuasion

Depending on the type of law—criminal, civil, or administrative—there are different burdens of proof or persuasion necessary in order to adjudicate guilt or liability. As previously discussed, in criminal law, the prosecutor must prove each element of the crime (cause of action) "beyond a reasonable doubt." *Reasonable doubt* is defined as "[t]he doubt that prevents one from being firmly convinced of a defendant's guilt, or the belief that there is a real possibility that a defendant is not guilty."[4]

Another way to quantitatively understand this standard of proof is that the prosecution must prove each element of the crime at approximately 90 percent. In other words, the standard of reasonable doubt does not require 100 percent proof positive; however, it does require that the evidence presented prove beyond reasonable doubt that the way the prosecutor presented evidence is the most likely, beyond reasonable doubt, way the events unfolded or occurred. From that, a jury can draw the conclusion that the defendant is guilty of the crime stated and can be found guilty.

In civil law, the burden of proof is "by a preponderance of the evidence." Florida recently changed this standard to be called "by a greater weight of the evidence." However, the two phrases mean the same thing. *Preponderance of the evidence* means "[t]he greater weight of the evidence; superior evidentiary weight that, though not sufficient to free the mind wholly from all reasonable doubt, is still sufficient to incline a fair and impartial mind to one side of the issue rather than the other. This is the burden of proof in a civil trial, in which the jury is instructed to find for the party that, on the whole, has the stronger evidence, however slight the edge may be."[5] The best way to describe this standard in understandable or quantifiable terms is to think of the lady justice, which demonstrates a blindfolded lady holding a scale that is equally distributed as demonstrated in **Figure 2-1**.

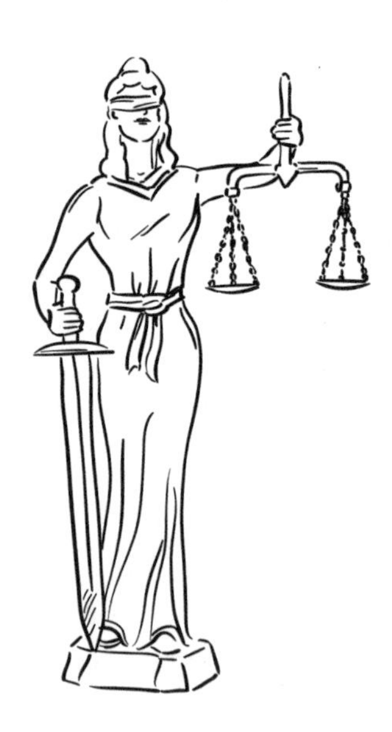

FIGURE 2-1 Scales of Justice

A preponderance of the evidence means that the scale tips toward one side or the other. The lady being blindfolded represents that the legal system accepts both parties as equal until such time as all the evidence has been presented and admitted into evidence. Then someone, usually a jury, determines on which side the scale tips. For civil law, it is merely the tipping of the scale; whereas, for criminal law the scale must tip greatly—to the point of beyond a reasonable doubt. Another way to quantitatively view this burden of persuasion is 51 percent compared to the other side at 49 percent. Under a preponderance of evidence standard, 51 percent tips the scale and that side wins.

Another burden of persuasion is called the clear and convincing standard. The *clear and convincing standard* is defined as "[e]vidence indicating that the thing to be proved is highly probable or reasonably certain. This is a greater burden than preponderance of the evidence, the standard applied in most civil trials, but less than evidence beyond a reasonable doubt, the norm for criminal trials."[6] Thus, again trying to assign some type of quantitative value, some people view this as approximately 75 percent. In some states, a claim for punitive damages, which will be discussed in detail in Chapter 5, requires a party to prove its party's claim or part of the lawsuit at the clear and convincing standard.

Hence, schematically the burdens of persuasion can be illustrated as shown in **Figure 2-2**.

Everyone is familiar with the crime of murder; thus, to explain various legal principles, the crime and prosecution of murder will be used as an example to demonstrate the concept of applying facts to the "elements of a cause of action." Remember, every crime will have its specific elements of the cause of action that must be proven as specified in a state's laws or statutes. Recall that in criminal law, the jury must find that each element of the crime (cause of action) has been proven beyond a reasonable doubt. In civil law, each element of the cause of action must be proven usually at the preponderance of the evidence standard.

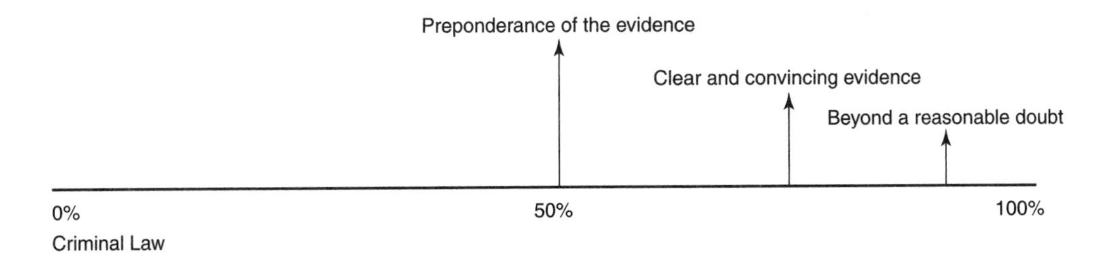

FIGURE 2-2 Preponderance of the Evidence

Generally speaking, the cause of action for the crime of murder is the killing of a human being with malice aforethought. At the outset it should be understood that this is the general criminal definition of the crime for murder. Each state will have specific language in its statutes (laws) that will define murder for that state. Usually each state will also have various degrees of murder such as first, second, and manslaughter. However, for illustration of legal concepts, this example will be kept simple with the use of this definition.

In order to convict someone for the crime of murder, the prosecutor must break down this crime into elements and prove each element beyond a reasonable doubt. This is how the breakdown into elements of the crime would appear:

1. The killing
2. Of a human being
3. With malice aforethought

This crime has three elements. If any one of the three elements is not proven beyond a reasonable doubt, then the jury must find that the defendant is innocent or not guilty of the crime.

An example of a crime a physical therapist, physical therapist assistant, or student might be prosecuted for is fraudulently billing Medicare for the provision of services. The general definition for this crime is "[a] knowing misrepresentation of the truth or concealment of a material fact to induce another to act to his or her detriment."[7] To break down the elements:

1. A knowing misrepresentation
2. Of the truth
3. Or concealment
4. Of a material fact
5. To induce another
6. To act
7. To his or her detriment

In order to be found guilty of fraudulent billing, the prosecutor must prove each of these elements beyond a reasonable doubt. Hence, if a physical therapist, physical therapist assistant, or student fraudulently billed Medicare for reimbursement of physical therapy services, the facts might be applied as explained in the next factual scenario.

A physical therapist, physical therapist assistant, or student treated a Medicare recipient for a balance and gait disorder. The modalities usually used included gait training, therapeutic exercises, neuromuscular reeducation, and sometimes therapeutic activities. However, when the physical therapist, physical therapist assistant, or student completes his or her charges for the patient, he or she also knowingly billed the patient for wheelchair mobility. The purpose of adding wheelchair mobility to the billing was to increase the number of modalities (CPT codes), which would increase the amount of money billed by the clinic. However, at no time did the patient receive wheelchair mobility. Thus, applying the facts of this scenario to the elements of the cause of action for fraud would be as follows:

1. A knowing misrepresentation—The physical therapist, physical therapist assistant, or student knowingly billed Medicare for wheelchair mobility when the services had not been provided to the Medicare recipient,
2. Of the truth—The physical therapist, physical therapist assistant, or student knew the wheelchair mobility modality had not been provided,
3. Or concealment—Not applicable,
4. Of a material fact—Whether a modality of service has been provided to a patient entitling the physical therapist, physical therapist assistant, or student to bill for those services would be material,
5. To induce another—Medicare,
6. To act—The physical therapist, physical therapist assistant, or student billed the wheelchair modality to Medicare to induce Medicare to pay for this additional modality of service,
7. To his or her detriment—It would be to Medicare's detriment and ultimately to taxpayers' detriment to pay for services that were not delivered.

Thus, the facts of a case are applied to the elements of a cause of action. Each element of the cause of action must be proven. The type of law or type of cause of action will dictate the burden of persuasion required or the burden of proof required for each element of the cause of action.

Likewise, in this example, the physical therapist or physical therapist assistant could also be sued in civil court by the patient for fraud. Each of the elements would need to be proven either at the preponderance of evidence or the clear and convincing standard of persuasion as established by a particular state for this cause of action. Additionally, the physical therapist or physical therapist assistant could have a complaint filed against his or her license in that state for fraudulent billing practices and could face sanctions against his or her license through administrative law.

As a real case example, in New York in 2006, three health care providers on Long Island were investigated for improper Medicaid billing practices (fraudulent billing practices). Medicaid, a national health insurance program that is funded by federal and state governments, essentially provides health insurance for the poor and is administered through state agencies.

On March 23, 2006, the New York Attorney General reported settlement agreements had been reached with the three health care providers: (1) Long Island Head Injury Association, Inc.; (2) Dr. Simon Zysman; and (3) Dr. Lewis Milhim.[8] Long Island Head Injury Association, Inc., agreed to pay $3 million to settle allegations it had billed Medicaid for treatments rendered by unqualified personnel. In addition to treatments being rendered by unqualified staff, the association also did not have documentation to substantiate treatments that had been billed to Medicaid to substantiate the care alleged in billing to have been provided had actually occurred. One of the motives to prosecute these claims was recovery of taxpayers' money that had been inappropriately spent.[9]

Dr. Simon Zysman agreed to pay $700,000 to resolve the investigation into his billing practices wherein he allegedly provided false cost reports that led to Medicaid overpayments for patient treatments. Dr. Milhim agreed to pay the state $145,000 to resolve allegations he failed to properly register his clinic with Medicaid, which resulted in billings to Medicaid that were ineligible for reimbursement.[10]

Physical therapists and physical therapist assistants should pay close attention to the rules and regulations promulgated not only for the practice of their profession, but also to any rules and regulations promulgated by the insurance carriers under which reimbursement for physical therapy services is sought. A failure to adhere to an insurance carrier's rules and regulations could be viewed and prosecuted as fraud. Further, an allegation of fraud could lead to an administrative complaint being filed against the physical therapist's or physical therapist assistant's license, which could lead to an administrative legal battle.

CIVIL LAW

Civil law deals with an attempt to compensate a victim monetarily for losses that should or could have been prevented. *Black's Law Dictionary* defines *civil law* as "an action brought to enforce, redress, or protect a private or civil right; a noncriminal litigation."[11] For physical therapists, physical therapist assistants, and students, the most likely civil cause of action they will face is medical malpractice or medical negligence. The elements for this cause of action generally will be:

1. The therapist owed a **duty** to someone, most likely the patient,
2. The physical therapist, physical therapist assistant, or student **breached the duty** that was owed,
3. The breach of the duty **caused** some type of harm,
4. Damages occurred as a result of the **harm** caused by the breach of the duty.

These elements and these types of actions will be discussed in much greater detail in Chapter 5. Suffice for this chapter to know that in civil actions, the goal of the plaintiff is remuneration for an alleged harm that was caused by the act(s) or omission(s) of the defendant. There are many types of civil actions a physical therapist, physical therapist assistant, or student could be involved with and the different types of actions will be discussed in Chapter 7.

However, an example will be presented here to assist with the explanation of these concepts. In *Patton v. Healthsouth of Houston, Inc.*, 2004 WL 253282 (Tex.App.-Hous. 1st Dist. 2004), a patient sued the rehabilitation hospital alleging he suffered burns as the result of heat applied during physical therapy. The case was ultimately dismissed on a technicality but the facts of the case are instructional for the purpose of this book.

The patient (plaintiff) in this type of case would have to assert that the physical therapist, physical therapist assistant, or student owed a duty to the patient to apply heat in a reasonable manner such that the patient would not suffer a burn. Then the patient would have to allege that the physical therapist, physical therapist assistant, or student breached that duty and did not apply the heat in a reasonable manner. The duty could be breached because the physical therapist, physical therapist assistant, or student did not test sensation immediately before application of the heat or inspect the area to observe for any new skin conditions.

Additionally, it should be foreseeable that a failure to test sensation before heat application and/or a failure to inspect the skin before heat application could lead to a patient suffering a burn from the application of heat. The next factual assertion would be the causal link between the duty owed and the failure to perform that duty that caused some harm to the patient.

In this example, the plaintiff would likely assert the physical therapist, physical therapist assistant, or student did not test sensation and/or observe the skin immediately before placement of the heat as being the causal link to harm. Because of this omission to act, assume hypothetically the physical therapist, physical therapist assistant, or student missed that the patient had a new sunburn. Hence, when the heat was applied to the patient, no additional precautions were taken and the applied heat caused an exacerbation of the preexisting thermal injury. Thus, the breach of duty—failure to test sensation and/or inspect the skin—caused an exacerbation of a thermal injury that resulted in pain and required medical treatment.

Accordingly, the patient would sue the physical therapist, physical therapist assistant, or student for medical malpractice seeking remuneration or "damages" for the medical expense of requiring treatment as well as remuneration for the subjective "pain and suffering." There could also be asserted damages for mental anguish and possibly even physical disfigurement.

To complicate the example even more, if the plaintiff also could assert that the thermal treatment was administered by an aide under the "supervision" of the physical therapist, physical therapist assistant, or student, the plaintiff may even have a cause of action for improper supervision of an employee and/or impropr delegation to a subordinate. Thus, it can be seen how a simple therapeutic modality can lead to a complicated lawsuit. This example and other cases will be discussed in much greater detail in subsequent chapters.

ADMINISTRATIVE LAW

Administrative law is "the law governing the organization and operation of the executive branch of government (including independent agencies) and the relations of the executive with the legislature, the judiciary, and the public."[12] For physical therapists, physical therapist assistants, and students the usual agency overseeing the practice of physical therapy is a state's department of health or similarly titled agency. The department of health has the authority to create some type of board that will oversee the practice of physical therapy in its particular state; a board of physical therapy practice. Hence, each state may vary under which state agency the board of physical therapy practice falls, but it is most likely going to be under the umbrella of a health agency. For example, in Florida, the Board of Physical Therapy Practice falls under the Department of Health.

The board of physical therapy is responsible for the interpretation and enforcement of the rules and regulations governing the profession of physical therapy for that state. At times the board may even promulgate new rules and/or regulations. The physical therapy state associations and/or the American Physical Therapy Association can suggest to a board of physical therapy practice how to interpret the rules and regulations of a particular state; however, the board is empowered and has the authority to determine, within reason, how to regulate physical therapists, physical therapist assistants, and students in its state.

Likewise, other boards governing physicians, chiropractors, and nurses are performing the same types of duties as the board of physical therapy practice. These boards are also ensuring someone within its state is not practicing outside the scope of his or her license or practicing without a license. An excellent example of administrative law and its potential penalties is the case of *Arkansas State Board of Chiropractic Examiners v. Teston*, 2005 WL 775805 (April 7, 2005). In this case, a physical therapist was accused of practicing outside the scope of physical therapy when he performed manipulations.

Hence, not only was the physical therapist accused of practicing outside the scope of his license, but concomitantly was accused of practicing chiropractic medicine without a license. Thus, one infraction has the potential for multiple causes of action.

The Arkansas Board of Chiropractic Examiners charged the physical therapist with performing treatments defined within the Chiropractic Practice Act and not being licensed to perform those treatments. After an administrative hearing before the Arkansas Board of Chiropractor Examiners, the physical therapist was fined $10,000 per violation (each and every incident of performing manipulation without a license that could be proven). The physical therapist appealed the decision of the Arkansas Board of Chiropractic Examiners to the Arkansas Circuit Court. On August 19, 2003, the Arkansas Circuit Court upheld the decision of the Board of Chiropractic Examiners. Thereafter, the physical therapist appealed the decision of the Arkansas Circuit Court to the Arkansas Supreme Court.

On April 12, 2005, the Arkansas Supreme Court upheld the decision of the Arkansas Circuit Court that had upheld the decision of the Arkansas Board of Chiropractic Examiners. Therefore, the physical therapist was found to have acted outside the scope of the Arkansas Physical Therapy Practice Act because he performed spinal manipulation that was not defined within the Arkansas Physical Therapy Practice Act. Further, it was practicing without a license because spinal manipulation was defined as being provided by chiropractors under the Arkansas Chiropractic Practice Act.

As can be seen from the dates alone, this particular case took over 2 years to come to a conclusion and cost a lot of money to defend. Further, in the end, the physical therapist lost the lawsuit (administrative complaint) and would have to pay the fine imposed by the Arkansas Board of Chiropractic Examiners. Additionally, the physical therapist had to pay his attorney fees and the costs associated with the litigation of the matter. The chiropractic board also could ask the court to award its attorney fees and costs, or, in layperson's terms, make the physical therapist pay for their fees and costs. Thus, every physical therapist, physical therapist assistant, and student should read and understand his or her particular state's practice act to know what may be performed and by omission what may not be performed. **Ignorance of the law will never be a defense!**

Another interesting administrative case that appears rather common deals with advertising services. In the case of *Pennsylvania Bureau of Professional and Occupational Affairs v. State Board of Physical Therapy*, the Bureau of Professional and Occupational Affairs charged a chiropractic group with violating the Pennsylvania Practice Act because the chiropractic group advertised in the newspaper that the group provided physical therapy,[13] yet the advertisement did not conspicuously identify that the group consisted of chiropractors and not physical therapists.[14] This charge was brought by the Board of Physical Therapy Practice because the allegation was that the physical therapy practice act had been violated and that Board investigates and punishes violators of its practice act.

A hearing examiner ruled that because the chiropractors were certified in "adjunctive procedures," the advertisements were allowed and charges were dropped.[15] On appeal to the Commonwealth Court, the decision was reversed; hence, the chiropractors' advertisements violated the Physical Therapy Practice Act.[16] The Supreme Court of Pennsylvania then granted review of the Commonwealth Court decision of interpretation of the Physical Therapy Practice Act.[17] The Supreme Court of Pennsylvania ruled that it was in the interest of the public to protect the public from chiropractors misleading the public as to the scope of the chiropractors' treatments.[18]

Accordingly, the Supreme Court of Pennsylvania upheld the Commonwealth Court's decision and as such the chiropractic group could not advertise it provided physical therapy services.[19] Of interest, two justices of the Supreme Court of Pennsylvania filed a dissenting opinion wherein both justices opined that chiropractors and physical therapists "perform some of the same services" and that the chiropractors had clearly identified themselves as chiropractors.[20] Thus, the dissenting opinion, if it had been the majority's opinion, would have changed the outcome of the case.

COURT SYSTEMS

Now that there is a basic understanding of the three general types of law, there will be discussion of the multitude of courts where those different types of law are practiced. Most everyone will be familiar with "the state" court or criminal justice center simply from watching television. However, the court systems are more than just the criminal justice system. Just as there are three different types of laws at work every day, there are also two legal systems at work every day where criminal, civil, or administrative law is practiced. These two court systems are divided into federal and state courts. The various courts within these two systems will be discussed later; however, understanding how a particular court is selected for filing a lawsuit will be discussed first.

SELECTING THE CORRECT COURT

Whether someone can be required to appear before a particular court depends generally on three issues:

1. Venue
2. Personal jurisdiction
3. The court's subject matter jurisdiction

These categories are very important and must be pled (alleged) in every complaint so that a court will know that the lawsuit has been filed in the proper court and the court can hear the matter being brought forth. Each of these categories will be discussed in further detail.

Venue

Venue is defined as "[t]he proper or a possible place for the trial of a lawsuit, usu[ally] because the place has some connection with the events that have given rise to the lawsuit. The county or other territory over which a trial court has jurisdiction."[21] Thus, for physical therapists, physical therapist assistants, or students, in relation to medical malpractice lawsuits, this will usually be the county where the physical therapist, physical therapist assistant, or student provided the physical therapy services being sued upon. If the physical therapist, physical therapist assistant, or student was providing home health services in different counties, the proper venue most likely will be the county where the physical therapist, physical therapist assistant, or student provided the physical therapy services that are the subject of the lawsuit.

Personal Jurisdiction

Personal jurisdiction is defined as "[a] court's power to bring a person into its adjudicative process; jurisdiction over a defendant's personal rights, rather than merely over property interests."[22] Thus, again for the physical therapist, physical therapist assistant, or student in a medical malpractice lawsuit, the court where the lawsuit is brought must be able to exercise jurisdiction authority over the physical therapist, physical therapist assistant, or student.

As an example, suppose a physical therapist, physical therapist assistant, or student was working for a traveling therapy company and worked in a particular state. During the course of working in that state, a patient alleges the physical therapist, physical therapist assistant, or student was negligent in the provision of care. However, the physical therapist, physical therapist assistant, or student does not permanently reside in that state, does not own property in that state, and has since moved to another traveling assignment in another state. In this scenario, the court might have difficulty asserting personal jurisdiction over the physical therapist, physical therapist assistant, or student who no longer works in that state and essentially has no ties to the state.

For this particular example, the plaintiff would likely not be without remedy because the plaintiff could file the lawsuit against the traveling therapy company for the act(s) and/or omission(s) of its employee. The therapist may or may not be able to be brought into court depending on the state's laws. The decision of whether a court can assert personal jurisdiction over someone usually revolves around whether the person could reasonably expect to be brought into that particular state's court and if the person has minimal contacts with the state.

Subject Matter Jurisdiction

Subject matter jurisdiction is defined as "[j]urisdiction over the nature of the case and the type of relief sought; the extent to which a court can rule on the conduct of persons or the status of things."[23] It is not uncommon for county courts to have subject matter jurisdiction over controversies that allege damages less than $15,000; whereas, lawsuits that allege greater than $15,000 in damages are referred to the county's circuit court system. Thus, every complaint must assert why the court has subject matter jurisdiction. As most of the courts can hear either criminal or civil cases, the court system generally posts dollar limits on its jurisdiction.

It is essential that these categories—venue, subject matter jurisdiction, and personal jurisdiction—be pled in a complaint, which will be discussed in greater detail in Chapter 14 when corporate structure is discussed. One way to ensure the location of where a physical therapist or physical therapist assistant and/or the physical therapist's or physical therapist assistant's business will litigate cases is through the selection of different corporate structures. Thus, the physical therapist, physical therapist assistant, or student may want to tab these pages for ease of reference when undertaking Chapter 14. These essential categories are consistent for both court systems, federal or state, which will be discussed in detail now.

FEDERAL COURT SYSTEM

Each state has at least one federal court where lawsuits may be filed to invoke the assistance of the federal courts. Federal courts have jurisdiction over federal agencies' rules and regulations as well as over the laws of the United States, which is called the United States Code (U.S.C.). Each state's federal court(s), known as district courts, are listed in Appendix 2A. Depending on the venue of the lawsuit in the district court, the appellate court that could potentially hear an appeal will be based on the location of the initiating court. The appellate court in the federal court system is called a circuit court of appeal.

Once a circuit court of appeal renders its appellate decision, a party may petition the U.S. Supreme Court for another chance. The U.S. Supreme Court selects the cases it will hear through a process of judicial discretion. In other words, no one has a "right" to have his or her matter heard before the U.S. Supreme Court; but rather it is the Supreme Court's discretionary judgment as to which cases it will hear.

The last distinction to understand in the federal court system is the labeling of parties throughout the litigation phases. At the district court level, which is the initiating court of the litigation, parties are called state or government and defendant in criminal cases; whereas in civil cases the parties are called plaintiff and defendant. However, at the circuit court of appeal level, the first level of appeal, the party bringing the appeal is called the appellant and the party defending the appeal is called the respondent. If the U.S. Supreme Court grants a petition for review of the circuit court of appeal's decision, then the party bringing the case to the Supreme Court is called the petitioner and the party defending the matter is called the respondent.

STATE COURT SYSTEM

Most states divide their court systems into county courts, circuit courts, district courts of appeal, and a state supreme court. However, there are states that have different systems, including but not limited to New York. Generally speaking, whether a case goes to county court or circuit court (sometimes called district court or superior court) depends on the court's subject matter jurisdiction as discussed previously. Each state's court system is provided in Appendix 2B. Hence, venue, personal jurisdiction, and subject matter jurisdiction, would dictate where someone would file any lawsuit.

OTHER COURTS

This chapter has discussed the basic court systems. However, it should be recognized there are other types of courts that have subject matter jurisdiction specialty areas like bankruptcy, municipal matters, traffic, or juvenile. A further itemized breakdown though is beyond the scope of this book.

APPEAL

The last legal division concept that should be considered is an appeal. An *appeal* is defined as, "[t]o seek review (from a lower court's decision) by a higher court."[24] Generally speaking, in every case the losing party will have the right of appeal. However, an appeal beyond the first level is usually discretionary of the court being appealed to. The cases discussed throughout this book are the result of cases decided at the appellate level.

SUMMARY

There are essentially three types of law (criminal, civil, and administrative) that are litigated in two separate court systems every day. The different court systems are divided into state and federal. The federal court system's jurisdiction is invoked when the matter being litigated involves federal laws, federal agencies, disputes between states, and sometimes when disputes involve citizens of different states. The state court system's jurisdiction is invoked when the matter involves state laws or matters arising out of conduct or property within the state. Once a matter is litigated, whether it involved a jury trial or bench trial (trial where the judge rather than a jury makes the decision), the losing party generally has the right to one appeal. The actual court the matter will be appealed to depends on the court in which the matter originated. Whether a matter can be appealed a second time generally will be a matter of court discretion.

DISCUSSION QUESTIONS

1. What are the different types of laws?
2. Explain the differences in the types of laws.
3. What is burden of persuasion?
4. What are the different levels of burden of persuasion?
5. Explain each level of burden of persuasion and when it would be applicable.

6. What are the two court systems?
7. How is the proper court selected for a lawsuit?
8. What is an appeal?
9. What are the courts available in your state?

NOTES

[1] *Black's Law Dictionary*, 538 (Bryan A. Garner, ed., 7th ed., West Group, 1999).
[2] *Id.* at 1038.
[3] *Id.* at 1234
[4] *Id.* at 1272.
[5] *Id.* at 1201.
[6] *Id.* at 577.
[7] *Id.* at 670.
[8] Andrews Litigation Reporter, *N.Y. Authorities Settle Medicaid Billing Cases for Nearly $4 Million*, page 11 (April 14, 2006).
[9] *Id.*
[10] *Id.*
[11] *Black's Law Dictionary*, 12 (Bryan A. Garner, ed., 7th ed., West Group, 1999).
[12] *Id.* at 17.
[13] *Pennsylvania Bureau of Professional & Occupational Affairs v. State Board of Physical Therapy*, 728 A.2d 240 (PA 1999).
[14] *Id.* at 270.
[15] *Id.*
[16] *Id.*
[17] *Id.*
[18] *Id.* at 276.
[19] *Id.*
[20] *Id.* at 277.
[21] *Black's Law Dictionary*, 1553 (Bryan A. Garner, ed., 7th ed., West Group, 1999).
[22] *Id.* at 857.
[23] *Id.*
[24] *Id.* at 1553.

Appendix 2A

STATE-BY-STATE LISTING OF FEDERAL COURTS

Alabama has three district courts: Northern, Middle, and Southern.

U.S. District Court for Northern District of Alabama
1729 Fifth Avenue North
Birmingham, Alabama 35203

U.S. District Court for the Middle District of Alabama has three locations.
Frank M. Johnson U.S. Courthouse Complex*
One Church Street
Montgomery, Alabama 36104-4018

GW Andrews Federal Building and U.S. Courthouse
701 Avenue A
Opelika, Alabama 36801-4977

Federal Building and U.S. Courthouse
100 West Troy Street
Dothan, Alabama 36303-4574

U.S. District Court for the Southern District of Alabama has two locations.

Mobile Division
113 Saint Joseph Street
Mobile, Alabama 36602

Selma Division
908 Alabama Avenue
Selma, Alabama 36701

* Location for documents to be mailed.

Alaska has five locations.

U.S. District Court–Anchorage
222 West 7th Avenue, 4
Anchorage, Alaska 99513

U.S. District Court–Fairbanks
101 12th Avenue, Room 332
Fairbanks, Alaska 99701

U.S. District Court–Juneau
P.O. Box 020349
Juneau, Alaska 99802
(Located in room 979 of the U.S. Federal Building at 709 West 9th Street)

U.S. District Court–Ketchikan
648 Mission Street
Ketchikan, Alaska 99901

U.S. District Court–Nome
P.O. Box 130
Nome, Alaska 99762
(Located on 2nd floor Post Office Building at 113 Front Street)

Arizona has two locations.

Sandra Day O'Connor U.S. Courthouse
401 West Washington Street, Suite 130, SPC1
Phoenix, Arizona 85003-2118

Evo A. DeConcini U.S. Courthouse
405 West Congress Street, Suite 1500
Tucson, Arizona 85701-5010

Arkansas is divided into two divisions: Eastern and Western.

Eastern Division has three locations.

Little Rock Main Office
600 West Capital Avenue, Suite 402
Little Rock, Arkansas 72201-3325

Jonesboro Divisional Office
615 South Main, Room 312
Jonesboro, Arkansas 72401

Pine Bluff Divisional Office
100 East 8th Street, Room 3103
Pine Bluff, Arkansas 71602

Western Division has six locations.

U.S. District Court–El Dorado
101 South Jackson Street, Room 205
P.O. Box 1566*
El Dorado, Arkansas 71731-1566

U.S. District Court–Fayetteville
John Paul Hammerschmidt Federal Building
35 East Mountain Street, Suite 510
Fayetteville, Arkansas 72701-5354

U.S. District Court–Fort Smith
Judge Isaac C. Parker Federal Building
South 6th Street and Rogers Avenue
P.O. Box 1547*
Fort Smith, Arkansas 72902-1547

U.S. District Court–Harrison
J. Smith Healey Federal Building
402 North Walnut Street, Room 238
Harrison, Arkansas 72601

U.S. District Court–Hot Springs
U.S. Courthouse
100 Reserve Street, Room 347
P.O. Box 6486*
Hot Springs, Arkansas 71902-6486

U.S. District Court–Texarkana
U.S. Courthouse and Post Office
500 State Line Avenue
P.O. Box 2746*
Texarkana, Arkansas 75504-2746

*Location for documents to be mailed.

California is divided into three districts: Northern, Central, and Southern.

U.S. Northern District has four locations.

U.S. District Court–Eureka
514 H Street
Eureka, California 95501-1038

U.S. District Court–Oakland
1301 Clay Street, Suite 400S
Oakland, California 94612-5212

U.S. District Court–San Francisco
450 Golden Gate Avenue
San Francisco, California 94102

U.S. District Court–San Jose
280 South 1st Street
San Jose, California 95113

U.S. Central District has four locations.

U.S. Eastern Division–Riverside Courthouse
3470 12th Street
Riverside, California 92501

U.S. Southern Division–Santa Ana Courthouse
411 West 4th Street, Room 1053
Santa Ana, California 92701-4516

U.S. Western Division–Roybal Federal Building
255 East Temple Street
Los Angles, California 90012

U.S. Western Division–Spring Street Courthouse
312 North Spring Street
Los Angles, California 90012

U.S. Southern District
800 Front Street, Suite 4290
San Diego, California 92101-8900

Colorado has one district court.

U.S. District Court for the District of Colorado
Alfred A. Arraj U.S. Courthouse
901 19th Street, Room A-105
Denver, Colorado 80294-3589

Connecticut has three district courts.

U.S. District Court of the District of Connecticut.

Hartford Division
450 Main Street
Hartford, Connecticut 06103

New Haven Division
141 Church Street
New Haven, Connecticut 06510

Bridgeport Division
915 Lafayette Boulevard
Bridgeport, Connecticut 06604

Delaware has one district court.

U.S. District Court for District of Delaware
J. Caleb Boggs Federal Building
844 North King Street
Wilmington, Delaware 19801

District of Columbia has one district court.

U.S. District Court for District of Columbia
333 Constitution Avenue, NW
Washington, D.C. 20001

Florida is divided into three districts: Northern, Middle, and Southern.

U.S. District Court for the Northern District of Florida has four locations.

Gainesville Division
U.S. Courthouse
401 SE 1st Avenue, Room 243
Gainesville, Florida 32601

Panama City Division
U.S. Courthouse
30 West Government Street
Panama City, Florida 32401

Pensacola Division
U.S. Courthouse
1 North Palafox Street
Pensacola, Florida 32502

Tallahassee Division
U.S. Courthouse
111 North Adams Street
Tallahassee, Florida 32301-7730

U.S. District Court for the Middle District of Florida has five locations.

Ft. Myers Division
U.S. Courthouse and Federal Building
2110 1st Street
Ft. Myers, Florida 33901

Jacksonville Division
U.S. Courthouse
300 North Hogan Street
Jacksonville, Florida 32202

Ocala Division
Golden-Collum Memorial Federal Building and U.S. Courthouse
207 N.W. 2nd Street
Ocala, Florida 34475

Orlando Division
George C. Young and U.S. Courthouse and Federal Building
80 North Hughey Avenue
Orlando, Florida 32801

Tampa Division
Sam M. Gibbons U.S. Courthouse
801 North Florida Avenue
Tampa, Florida 33602

U.S. District Court for the Southern District of Florida
301 North Miami Avenue
Miami, Florida 33128

Georgia is divided into three districts: Northern, Middle, and Southern.

U.S. District Court for the Northern District of Georgia has four locations.

Atlanta Division
Richard B. Russell Federal Building and Courthouse
75 Spring Street, SW, Room 2211
Atlanta, Georgia 30303-3361

Gainesville Division
Federal Building
121 Spring Street, SE, Room 201
Gainesville, Georgia 30501

Newman Division
18 Greenville Street
Newman, Georgia 30264

Rome Division
600 East 1st Street
Rome, Georgia 30161

U.S. District Court for the Middle District of Georgia has six locations.

Albany Division
L.B. King U.S. Courthouse
201 West Broad Avenue
Albany, Georgia 31701

Athens Division
U.S. Post Office and Courthouse
115 East Hancock Avenue
P.O. Box 1106
Athens, Georgia 30601

Columbus Division
U.S. Post Office and Court House
120 12th Street
P.O. Box 124
Columbus, Georgia 31902

Macon Division
William A. Bootle Federal Building and U.S. Courthouse
P.O. Box 128
475 Mulberry Street
Macon, Georgia 31202

Thomasville Division
U.S. Courthouse and Post Office
404 North Broad Street
Thomasville, Georgia 31792

Valdosta Division
U.S. Courthouse and Post Office
401 Patterson Street, Suite 212
Valdosta, Georgia 31601

Hawaii has one district court.

U.S. District Court for the District of Hawaii
300 Ala Moana Boulevard
Honolulu, Hawaii 96850

Idaho is divided into four districts: Northern, Central, Eastern, and Southern.

U.S. District Court for the Northern District of Idaho
205 North 4th Street, Room 202
Coeur d'Alene, Idaho 83814

U.S. District Court for the Central District of Idaho
220 East 57th Street, Room 304
Moscow, Idaho 83843

U.S. District Court for the Eastern District of Idaho
801 East Sherman Street
Polatello, Idaho 83201

U.S. District Court for the Southern District of Idaho
550 West Fort Street
Boise, Idaho 83724

Illinois is divided into three districts: Northern, Central, and Southern.

U.S. District Court for the Northern District of Illinois has two locations.

Eastern Division
Everett McKinley Dirksen Building
219 South Dearborn Street
Chicago, Illinois 60604

Western Division
U.S. Courthouse
211 South Court Street
Rockford, Illinois 61101

U.S. District Court for the Central District of Illinois has four locations.

Peoria Division
309 U.S. Courthouse
100 NE Monroe Street
Peoria, Illinois 61602

Rock Island Division
40 U.S. Courthouse
211 19th Street
Rock Island, Illinois 61201

Springfield Division
151 U.S. Courthouse
600 East Monroe Street
Springfield, Illinois 62701

Urbana Division
218 U.S. Courthouse
201 South Vine Street
Urbana, Illinois 61802

U.S. District Court for the Southern District of Illinois has two locations.

Benton Division
301 West Main Street
Benton, Illinois 62812

East St. Louis Division
750 Missouri Avenue
East St. Louis, Illinois 62201

Indiana is divided into two districts: Northern and Southern.

U.S. District Court for the Northern District of Indiana has four locations.

1108 East Ross Adain Federal Building
1300 South Harrison Street
Ft. Wayne, Indiana 46802

5400 Federal Plaza, Suite 2300
Hammond, Indiana 46320

102 Robert A. Grant Federal Building
204 South Main Street
South Bend, Indiana 46601

214 Charles Halleck Federal Building
230 North 4th Street
P.O. Box 1498
Lafayette, Indiana 47902

U.S. District Court for the Southern District of Indiana
46 East Ohio Street, Room 105
Indianapolis, Indiana 46204

Iowa is divided into two districts: Northern and Southern.

U.S. District Court for the Northern District of Iowa has three locations.

Fort Dodge Division
Post Office Building
205 South 8th Street
Fort Dodge, Iowa 50501

Sioux City Division
320 6th Street
Sioux City, Iowa 51101

Cedar Rapids Division
101 1st Street, SE
Cedar Rapids, Iowa 52401

U.S. District Court for the Southern District of Iowa has three locations.

Central Division
123 East Walnut Street, Room 300
P.O. Box 9344
Des Moines, Iowa 50306-9344

Davenport Division
131 East 4th Street
Davenport, Iowa 52801-1516

Western Division
6th and Broadway, Room 313
Council Bluffs, Iowa 51502

Kansas has three locations for its district courts.

U.S. District Court for the District of Kansas.

161 Robert J. Dole U.S. Courthouse
500 State Avenue
259 U.S. Courthouse
Kansas City, Kansas 66101

444 SE Quincy
490 U.S. Courthouse
Topeka, Kansas 66683

401 North Market
204 U.S. Courthouse
Wichita, Kansas 67202

Kentucky is divided into Western and Eastern divisions.

U.S. District Court for the Western District of Kentucky has four locations.

Bowling Green Division
241 East Main Street, Suite 120
Bowling Green, Kentucky 42101-2175

Louisville Division
Gene Snyder U.S. Courthouse
601 West Broadway, Room 106
Louisville, Kentucky 40202

Owensboro Division
423 Frederica Street, Suite 126
Owensboro, Kentucky 42301-3013

Paducah Division
501 Broadway, Suite 127
Paducah, Kentucky 42001-6801

U.S. District Court for the Eastern District of Kentucky has six locations.

Lexington Division
101 Barr Street, Room 206
Lexington, Kentucky 40588-3074

Ashland Division
336 Carl Perkins Federal Building
1405 Greenup Avenue
Ashland, Kentucky 41101

Frankfort Division
313 John C. Watts Federal Building
330 West Broadway
Frankfort, Kentucky 40601

Pikeville Division
110 Main Street, Suite 203
Pikeville, Kentucky 41501-1100

Covington Division
35 West 5th Street
P.O. Box 1073
Covington, Kentucky 41102-1073

London Division
310 South Main Street
P.O. Box 5121
London, Kentucky 40745-5121

Louisiana is divided into three districts: Western, Middle, and Eastern.

U.S. District Court for the Western District of Louisiana has five locations.

105 U.S. Post Office and Courthouse
515 Murray Street
Alexandria, Louisiana 71301

Lafayette Division
U.S. Courthouse, Suite 2100
800 Lafayette Street
Lafayette, Louisiana 70501

Lake Charles Division
Edwin F. Hunter, Jr.
U.S. Courthouse and Federal Building, Suite 188
611 Broad Street
Lake Charles, Louisiana 70601

Monroe Division
Federal Building, Suite 215
201 Jackson Street
Monroe, Louisiana 71201

Shreveport Division
U.S. Courthouse, Suite 1167
300 Fannin Street
Shreveport, Louisiana 71101

U.S. District Court for the Middle District of Louisiana
777 Florida Street, Suite 139
Baton Rouge, Louisiana 70801

U.S. District Court for the Eastern District of Louisiana
New Orleans Courthouse
500 Poydras Street
New Orleans, Louisiana 70130

Maine has one district court.

U.S. District Court for the District of Maine
156 Federal Street
Portland, Maine 04101

Maryland has two locations.

U.S. District Court for Maryland.

Baltimore Division
101 West Lombard Drive
Baltimore, Maryland 21201

Greenbelt Division
6500 Cherrywood Land
Greenbelt, Maryland 20770

Massachusetts has three locations.

U.S. District Court for Massachusetts.

Boston Division
1 Courthouse Way
Boston, Massachusetts 02210

Worcester Division
595 Main Street
Worcester, Massachusetts 01608

Springfield Division
1550 Main Street
Springfield, Massachusetts 01103

Michigan is divided into two districts: Western and Eastern.

U.S. District Court for the Western District of Michigan has four locations.

Grand Rapids Division, Headquarters
399 Federal Building
110 Michigan Street, NW
Grand Rapids, Michigan 49503

Kalamazoo Division
B-35 Federal Building
410 West Michigan Avenue
Kalamazoo, Michigan 49007

Lansing Division
113 Federal Building
315 West Allegan Street
Lansing, Michigan 48933

Marquette Division
P.O. Box 698
229 Federal Building
202 West Washington Street
Marquette, Michigan 49855

U.S. District Court for the Eastern District of Michigan has five locations.

U.S. District Courthouse
1000 Washington Avenue, Room 304
P.O. Box 913
Bay City, Michigan 48707

U.S. District Court Flint
600 Church Street
Flint, Michigan 48502

Detroit Division
Theodore Levin U.S. Courthouse
231 West Lafayette Boulevard
Detroit, Michigan 48226

Ann Arbor Division
U.S. District Courthouse
200 East Liberty Street
Ann Arbor, Michigan 48104

Port Huron Division
U.S. District Courthouse
526 Water Street
Port Huron, Michigan 48060

Minnesota has four districts.

U.S. District Court for the District of Minnesota has four locations.

Minneapolis Division
202 U.S. Courthouse
300 South 4th Street
Minneapolis, Minnesota 55415

St. Paul Division
700 Federal Building
316 North Robert Street
St. Paul, Minnesota 55101

Duluth Division
417 Federal Building
515 West 1st Street
Duluth, Minnesota 55802-1397

Fergus Fall Division
212 U.S. Post Office Building
118 South Mill Street
Fergus Fall, Minnesota 56537

Mississippi is divided into two districts: Northern and Southern.

U.S. District Court for Mississippi's Northern District has three locations.

Aberdeen Thomas G. Abernathy Federal Building
301 West Commerce Street
P.O. Box 704*
Aberdeen, Mississippi 38730

Greenville Division
U.S. District Court
305 Main Street, Room 329
Greenville, Mississippi 38701

Oxford Division
Room 369 Federal Building
911 Jackson Avenue
Oxford, Mississippi 38655

*Location for documents to be mailed.

United States District Court for Mississippi's Southern District has three locations.

U.S. District Court
245 East Capitol Street, Suite 316
Jackson, Mississippi 39201

Hattiesburg Division
U.S. District Court
701 Main Street, Suite 200
Hattiesburg, Mississippi 39401

Gulfport Division
U.S. District Court
2012 15th Street, Suite 403
Gulfport, Mississippi 39501

Missouri is divided into two districts: Western and Eastern.

U.S. District Court for Missouri's Western District has four locations.

Jefferson City
U.S. District Court
131 West High Street
Jefferson City, Missouri 65101

Joplin–SW Division
Jasper Center Courthouse
Courthouse Division II Courtroom
302 South Main Street
Carthage, Missouri 64836

Kansas City Division
Charles Evan S. Whittaker Courthouse
400 East 9th Street
Kansas City, Missouri 64106

St. Joseph Division
U.S. Court
8th and Edmond Street, 2nd Floor
St. Joseph, Missouri 64501-1727

U.S. District Court for Missouri's Eastern District has three locations.

St. Louis Division
111 South 10th Street, Suite 3.300
St. Louis, Missouri 63102

Cape Girardeau Division
339 Broadway
Cape Girardeau, Missouri 63701

Hannibal Division
801 Broadway
Hannibal, Missouri 63401

Montana has one district court.

U.S. District Court for District of Montana
James F. Battin Courthouse
316 North 26th Street
Billings, Montana 59101

Nebraska has two locations.

U.S. District Court for District of Nebraska
Omaha Division
111 South 18th Plaza
Omaha, Nebraska 68102

U.S. District Court for District of Nebraska
Lincoln Division
593 Federal Building
100 Centennial Mall
Lincoln, Nebraska 68508-3803

Nevada has two locations.

U.S. District Court for District of Nevada
Las Vegas Division
333 South Las Vegas
Las Vegas, Nevada 89101

U.S. District Court for District of Nevada
Reno Division
400 South Virginia Street
Reno, Nevada 89501

New Hampshire has one district court.

U.S. District Court for District of New Hampshire
Warren B. Rudman U.S. Courthouse
55 Pleasant Street, Room 110
Concord, New Hampshire 03301-3941

New Jersey has one district court.

U.S. District Court for District of New Jersey
50 Walnut Street, Room 4015
Newark, New Jersey 07101

New Mexico has four locations.

U.S. District Court for District of New Mexico has four locations.

Albuquerque Division
U.S. District Court
333 Lomas NW
Albuquerque, New Mexico 87102

Las Cruces Division
U.S. District Court
2009 Griggs, 2nd Floor
Las Cruces, New Mexico 88001

Roswell Division
U.S. District Court
Roswell, New Mexico 88201

Santa Fe Division
U.S. District Court
120 South Federal Plaza
Santa Fe, New Mexico 87501

New York is divided into four districts: Eastern, Northern, Southern, and Western.

U.S. District Court for New York's Eastern District has two locations.

Brooklyn–Main
Eastern Division of New York
225 Cadman Plaza East
Brooklyn, New York 11201

Long Island Courthouse
100 Federal Plaza
Central Islip, New York 11722-4438

U.S. District Court for New York's Northern District has seven locations.

Albany Division
James T. Foley—U.S. District Court
445 Broadway, Room 509
Albany, New York 12207-2924

Auburn Division
Old Post Office and Courthouse
157 Genesee Street, 2nd Floor
Auburn, New York 13021

Binghamton Division
U.S. Courthouse and Federal Building
15 Henry Street
Binghamton, New York 13902-2723

Fort Drum Division
U.S. Courthouse
Lewis Avenue
Fort Drum, New York 13602

Syracuse Division
U.S. District Court
100 South Clinton Street
P.O. Box 7367
Syracuse, New York 13261-7367

Utica Division
Alexander Pirnie Federal Building
10 Broad Street
Utica, New York 13501-1233

Watertown Division
Jefferson Center Courthouse
Dulles State Office Building
317 Washington Street, 10th Floor
Watertown, New York 13601

U.S. District Court for New York's Southern District
U.S. Courthouse
500 Pearl Street
New York, New York 10007-1312

U.S. District Court for New York's Western District
304 U.S. Courthouse
68 Court Street
Buffalo, New York 14202

North Carolina is divided into three districts: Eastern, Middle, and Western.

U.S. District Court for North Carolina's Eastern District has six locations.

Elizabeth City Division
306 East Main Street
Elizabeth City, North Carolina 27909

Fayetteville Division
U.S. Post Office and Courthouse
301 Greet Street, 3rd Floor
Fayetteville, North Carolina 28302

Greenville Division
U.S. Court
201 South Evans Street, Room 209
Greenville, North Carolina 27858-1137

New Bern Division
U.S. Courthouse
413 Middle Street
New Bern, North Carolina 28560

Raleigh Division
Terry Sanford Federal Building and Courthouse
310 New Bern Avenue
Raleigh, North Carolina 27601

Wilmington Division
Alton Lennon Federal Building
2 Princess Street
Wilmington, North Carolina 28401

U.S. District Court for North Carolina's Middle District has three locations.

Greensboro Division
U.S. District Court
324 West Market Street, Suite 401
Greensboro, North Carolina 27401

Winston-Salem Division
251 North Main Street
Winston-Salem, North Carolina 27101

Durham Division
323 East Chapel Hill Street
Durham, North Carolina 27702

U.S. District Court for North Carolina's Western District has three locations.

Charlotte Division
401 West Trade Street, Room 212
Charlotte, North Carolina 28202

Statesville Division
200 West Broad Street
Statesville, North Carolina 28677

Bryson City Division
Federal Building
306 Main Street
Bryson City, North Carolina 28713

North Dakota has four locations.

U.S. District Court for North Dakota has four locations.

Minot Division
100 1st Street, SW
Minot, North Dakota 58701

Grand Fork Division
102 North 4th Street
Grand Fork, North Dakota 58201

Fargo Division
655 1st Avenue North
Fargo, North Dakota 58102

Bismarck Division
220 East Rosser Avenue
P.O. Box 1193
Bismarck, North Dakota 58502

Ohio is divided into two districts: Northern and Southern.

U.S. District Court for Ohio's Northern District has four locations.

Toledo Division
114 U.S. Courthouse
1716 Spielbusch A
Toledo, Ohio 43604-1363

Cleveland Division
Carl B. Stokes U.S. Court House
801 West Superior Avenue
Cleveland, Ohio 44113-1830

Akron Division
568 U.S. Courthouse Federal Building
Two South Main Street
Akron, Ohio 44308-1813

Youngstown Division
337 U.S. Federal Building and Courthouse
125 Market Street
Youngstown, Ohio 44503-1780

U.S. District Court for Ohio's Southern District has three locations.

Cincinnati Division
Potter Stewart U.S. Courthouse
100 East 5th Street
Cincinnati, Ohio 45202

Columbus Division
Joseph P. Kinneary U.S. Courthouse, Room 260
85 Marconi Boulevard
Columbus, Ohio 43215

Dayton Division
Federal Building, Room 712
200 West 2nd Street
Dayton, Ohio 45402

Oklahoma is divided into three districts: Eastern, Northern, and Western.

U.S. District Court for Oklahoma's Eastern District
101 North 5th Street, Room 208
Muskogee, Oklahoma 74401

U.S. District Court for Oklahoma's Northern District
333 West 4th Street, Room 411
Tulsa, Oklahoma 74103

U.S. District Court for Oklahoma's Western District
200 NW 4th Street, Room 1210
Oklahoma City, Oklahoma 73102

Oregon has three locations.

U.S. District Court for Oregon has three locations.

Mark O. Hatfield U.S. Courthouse
1000 SW 3rd Avenue
Portland, Oregon 97204-2902

Wayne L. Morse U.S. Courthouse
405 East 8th Avenue, Room 2100
Eugene, Oregon 97401

James A. Redden, U.S. Courthouse
310 West 6th Street, Room 201
Medford, Oregon 97501

Pennsylvania is divided into three districts: Eastern, Middle, and Western.

U.S. District Court for Pennsylvania's Eastern District has four locations.

Allentown Division
504 Hamilton Street, Room 1601
Allentown, Pennsylvania 18101-1514

Easton Division
The Holmes Building, 4th Floor
101 Larry Holmes Drive
Easton, Pennsylvania 18042-7722

U.S. Courthouse
601 Market Street, Room 2609
Philadelphia, Pennsylvania 19106-1797

Reading Division
The Madison Building
400 Washington Street, Room 401
Reading, Pennsylvania 19601-3956

U.S. District Court for Pennsylvania's Middle District has four locations.

Scranton Headquarters
William J. Nealon Federal Building and U.S. Courthouse
235 North Washington Avenue
P.O. Box 1148
Scranton, Pennsylvania 18501

Harrisburg Division
Federal Building and Courthouse
228 Walnut Street
P.O. Box 983
Harrisburg, Pennsylvania 17108

Williamsport Division
U.S. Courthouse and Federal Office Building
240 West 3rd Street, Suite 218
Williamsport, Pennsylvania 17701

Wilkes-Barre Division
Max Rosean U.S. Courthouse, Suite 161
Wilkes-Barre, Pennsylvania 18701

U.S. District Court for Pennsylvania's Western District has three locations.

Erie Division
17 South Park Row
Erie, Pennsylvania 16501

Johnstown Division
Penn Traffic B
319 Washington Street
Johnstown, Pennsylvania 15901

Pittsburgh Division
829 U.S. Courthouse
7th and Grant Street
Pittsburgh, Pennsylvania 15219

Puerto Rico has one district court.

U.S. District Court for Puerto Rico
Clemente Ruiz-Nazaro U.S. Courthouse
Federico Degetan Federal Building
150 Carlos Chardon Street
Hato Rey, Puerto Rico 00918

Rhode Island has one district court.

U.S. District Court for Rhode Island
One Exchange Terrace
Federal Building and Courthouse
Providence, Rhode Island 02903

South Carolina has eight locations.

U.S. District Court for South Carolina has eight locations.

Aiken Division
Charles E. Simons, Jr. Federal Courthouse
223 Park Avenue, SW
Aiken, South Carolina 29801

Anderson Division
G. Ross Anderson Jr. Federal Building and U.S. Courthouse
315 South McDuffie Street, 2nd Floor
Anderson, South Carolina 29624

Beaufort Division
Beaufort Federal Courthouse
1501 Bay Street
Beaufort, South Carolina 29401

Charleston Division
Charleston Federal Courthouse
85 Broad Street
Charleston, South Carolina 29401

Columbia Division
Matthew J. Perry, Jr. Courthouse
901 Richland Street
Columbia, South Carolina 29201

Florence Division
McMillan Federal Building
401 West Evans Street
Florence, South Carolina 29501

Greenville Division
Clement F. Haynsworth Federal Building
300 East Washington Street
Greenville, South Carolina 29601

Spartanburg Division
Donald S. Russell Federal Building
201 Magnolia Street
Spartanburg, South Carolina 29301

South Dakota has one district court.

U.S. District Court for South Dakota
400 South Phillips Avenue
Sioux Falls, South Dakota 57104

Tennessee is divided into three districts: Eastern, Middle, and Western.

U.S. District Court for Tennessee's Eastern District has four locations.

Chattanooga–South Division
U.S. District Court
900 Georgia Avenue
Chattanooga, Tennessee 37402

Greenville–NE Division
U.S. District Court
220 West Depot Street, Suite 200
Greenville, Tennessee 37743

Knoxville–North Division
U.S. District Court
800 Market Street, Suite 130
Knoxville, Tennessee 37902

Winchester Division
U.S. District Court
200 South Jefferson Street
Winchester, Tennessee 37398

U.S. District Court for Tennessee's Middle District
Room 242, Federal Building
167 North Main Street
Memphis, Tennessee 38103

U.S. District Court for Tennessee's Western District
Room 262, U.S. Courthouse
111 South Highland Avenue
Jackson, Tennessee 38301

Texas is divided into four districts: Eastern, Northern, Western, and Southern.

U.S. District Court for Texas' Eastern District has six locations.

Beaumont Division
300 Willow Street, Suite 104
Beaumont, Texas 77701

Lufkin Division
104 North 3rd Street
Lufkin, Texas 75901

Marshall Division
100 East Houston, Room 125
Marshall, Texas 75670

Sherman Division
101 East Pecan, Room 216
Sherman, Texas 75090

Texarkana Division
500 State Line Avenue
Texarkana, Texas 75501

Tyler (Headquarters) Division
211 West Ferguson Street, Room 106
Tyler, Texas 75702

U.S. District Court for Texas' Northern District has seven locations.

Abilene Division
341 Pine Street, 2008
Abilene, Texas 79601

Amarillo Division
205 East 5th Street, 133
Amarillo, Texas 79101-1559

Dallas Division
1100 Commerce Street, Room 1452
Dallas, Texas 75242

Ft. Worth Division
501 West 10th Street, Room 310
Ft. Worth, Texas 76102-3673

Lubbock Division
1205 Texas Avenue, Room 209
Lubbock, Texas 79401-4091

San Angelo Division
33 East Twohig Street, 202
San Angelo, Texas 76903-6451

Wichita Falls
1000 Lamar Street, 203
Wichita Falls, Texas 76301

U.S. District Court for Texas' Western District has 10 locations.

Austin Division
2000 West 8th Street, Room 130
Austin, Texas 78701

Del Rio Division
111 East Broadway, Room L100
Del Rio, Texas 78840

El Paso Division
511 East San Antonio Avenue, Room 219
El Paso, Texas 79901

Midland-Odessa Division
200 East Wall, Room 107
Midland, Texas 79701

Pecos Division
410 South Cedar
Pecos, Texas 79772

Alpine Division
803 Fighting Buck Avenue
Alpine, Texas 79830

San Antonio Division
655 East Durango Boulevard, Room G65
San Antonio, Texas 78206

Waco Division
800 Franklin Avenue, Room 380
Waco, Texas 768701

Fort Hood Division
MG Williams Individual Center
Building 5794, Tank Destroyer Boulevard
P.O. Box 5507
Fort Hood, Texas 76544-0507

Temple Division
U.S. Probation Office
1005 Marlandwood Road, Suite 119
Temple, Texas 76502

U.S. District Court for Texas' Southern District has seven locations.

Brownsville Division
Reynaldo G. Garza-Filemon B. Vela
U.S. Courthouse
600 East Harrison Street
Brownsville, Texas 78520

Houston Division
U.S. Courthouse
515 Rusk Avenue
Houston, Texas 77002

Victoria Division
Martin Luther King, Jr. Federal Building
312 South Main, Room 406
Victoria, Texas 77901

Corpus Christi Division
U.S. Courthouse
1133 North Shoreline Boulevard
Corpus Christi, Texas 78401

Laredo Division
U.S. Courthouse
1300 Victoria Street
Laredo, Texas 78040

Galveston Division
U.S. Post Office and Courthouse
601 Rosenberg, Room 411
Galveston, Texas 77550

McAllen Division
Bentsen Tower
1701 West Business Highway 83, Suite 1011
McAllen, Texas 78501

Utah has one district court.

U.S. District Court for Utah
350 South Main Street, Room 150
Salt Lake City, Utah 84101

Vermont has three locations.

U.S. District Court for Vermont's three locations.

Brattleboro Division
204 Main Street, Room 201
Brattleboro, Vermont 05301

Burlington Division
11 Elmwood A, Room 506
Burlington, Vermont 05401

Rutland Division
151 West Street, Room 204
Rutland, Vermont 05701

Virginia is divided into two districts: Eastern and Western.

U.S. District Court for Virginia's Eastern District has four locations.

Alexandria Division
Albert V. Bryan U.S. Courthouse
401 Courthouse Square
Alexandria, Virginia 22314

Newport News Division
U.S. Post Office and Courthouse B
101 25th Street
P.O. Box 494
Newport News, Virginia 23607

Norfolk Division
Walter E. Hoffman U.S. Courthouse
600 Granby Street
Norfolk, Virginia 22510

Richmond Division
U.S. Courthouse
1000 East Main Street
Richmond, Virginia 23219

U.S. District Court for Virginia's Western District has seven locations.

Abingdon Division
180 West Main Street, Room 104
Abingdon, Virginia 24210

Big Stone Gap Division
322 East Wood Avenue, Room 204
Big Stone Gap, Virginia 24219

Charlottesville Division
255 West Main Street, Room 304
Charlottesville, Virginia 22904

Lynchburg Division
1101 Court Street, Suite A66
Lynchburg, Virginia 24504

Danville Division
700 Main Street, Room 202
Danville, Virginia 24541

Harrisonburg Division
116 North Main Street, Room 314
Harrisonburg, Virginia 22802

Roanoke Division
210 Franklin Road, Room 308
Roanoke, Virginia 24011

Virgin Islands has two locations.

U.S. District Court for Virgin Islands.

St. Croix Division
3013 Estate Golden Rock, Suite 219
St. Croix, Virgin Islands 00820

St. Thomas/St. John Division
5500 Veterans Drive, Room 310
St. Thomas, Virgin Island 00802

Washington is divided into two districts: Eastern and Western.

U.S. District Court for Washington's Eastern District has three locations.

Thomas S. Foley U.S. Courthouse
920 West Riverside Avenue
Spokane, Washington 99201

William O. Douglas Courthouse
255 3rd Street
Yakima, Washington 98907

U.S. Courthouse and Federal Building
825 Jadwin Avenue
Richland, Washington 99352

U.S. District Court for Washington's Western District has two locations.

Tacoma Division
Union Station Courthouse
1717 Pacific Avenue
Tacoma, Washington 98402

Seattle Division
U.S. Courthouse
700 Stewart Street
Seattle, Washington 98101

West Virginia is divided into two districts: Northern and Southern.

U.S. District Court for West Virginia's Northern District has four locations.

Martinsburg Division
217 West King Street
Martinsburg, West Virginia 25401-3286

Wheeling Division
1125 Chaplin Street
Wheeling, West Virginia 26003-2976

Clarksburg Division
500 West Pike Street
Clarksburg, West Virginia 26301-2664

Elkins Division
300 3rd Street
Elkins, West Virginia 26241-3898

U.S. District Court for West Virginia's Southern District has five locations.

Bluefield–Division 1
601 Federal Street, Room 2303
Bluefield, West Virginia 24701

Charleston–Division 2
Robert C. Byrd U.S. Courthouse
300 Virginia Street East, Suite 2400
Charleston, West Virginia 25301

Huntington–Division 3
Sidney L. Christie 713
845 5th Avenue, Room 101
Huntington, West Virginia 25716

Beckley–Division 4
110 North Heber Street, Room 119
Beckley, West Virginia 25801

Parkersburg–Division 5
425 Juliana Street, Room 5102
Parkersburg, West Virginia 26101

Wisconsin is divided into two districts: Eastern and Western.

U.S. District Court for Wisconsin's Eastern District has two locations.

Milwaukee Division
362 U.S. Courthouse
517 East Wisconsin Avenue
Milwaukee, Wisconsin 53202

Green Bay Division
125 South Jefferson Street
P.O. Box 22490
Green Bay, Wisconsin 54305-2490

U.S. District Court for Wisconsin's Western District
120 North Henry Street, Room 320
P.O. Box 432
Madison, Wisconsin 53701-0432

Wyoming has two locations.

U.S. District Court for Wyoming has two locations.

Cheyenne Division
2120 Capitol Avenue
Cheyenne, Wyoming 82001

Casper Division
111 South Wolcott, Room 121
Casper, Wyoming 82601

There are 11 circuit courts of appeal, which are divided geographically around the states, from which appeals are taken. The distribution is listed here:

U.S. Court of Appeals for the First Circuit
1 Courthouse Way
Boston, Massachusetts 02210

The First Circuit Court of Appeals receives appeals from federal district courts representing Maine, New Hampshire, Massachusetts, Rhode Island, and Puerto Rico.

U.S. Court of Appeals for the Second Circuit
500 Pearl Street
New York, New York 10007

The Second Circuit Court of Appeals receives appeals from federal district courts representing Vermont, New York, and Connecticut.

U.S. Court of Appeals for the Third Circuit
James A. Byrne Courthouse
601 Market Street
Philadelphia, Pennsylvania 19106

The Third Circuit Court of Appeals receives appeals from federal district courts representing Pennsylvania, New Jersey, Delaware, and the Virgin Islands.

U.S. Court of Appeals for the Fourth Circuit
Lewis F. Powell, Jr. U.S. Courthouse
1100 East Main Street
Richmond, Virginia 23219

The Fourth Circuit Court of Appeals receives appeals from federal district courts representing Maryland, West Virginia, Virginia, North Carolina, and South Carolina.

U.S. Court of Appeals for the Fifth Circuit
600 South Maestri Place
New Orleans, Louisiana 70130-3408

The Fifth Circuit Court of Appeals receives appeals from federal district courts representing Mississippi, Louisiana, and Texas.

U.S. Court of Appeals for the Six Circuit
100 East 5th Street
540 Potter Stewart U.S. Courthouse
Cincinnati, Ohio 45202

The Sixth Circuit Court of Appeals receives appeals from federal district courts representing Michigan, Ohio, Kentucky, and Tennessee.

U.S. Court of Appeals for the Seventh Circuit
Room 2722
219 South Dearborn Street
Chicago, Illinois 60604

The Seventh Circuit Court of Appeals receives appeals from federal district courts representing Wisconsin, Illinois, and Indiana.

U.S. Court of Appeals for the Eighth Circuit
Thomas F. Eagleton U.S. Courthouse
111 South 10th Street
St. Louis, Missouri 63102

The Eighth Circuit Court of appeals receives appeals from federal district courts representing North Dakota, South Dakota, Nebraska, Minnesota, Iowa, Missouri, and Arkansas.

U.S. Court of Appeals for the Ninth Circuit
95 7th Street
San Francisco, California 94103

The Ninth Circuit Court of Appeals receives appeals from federal districts courts representing Washington, Oregon, Idaho, Montana, Nevada, California, Arizona, Arizona, Hawaii, and Guam.

U.S. Court of Appeals for the Tenth Circuit
The Bryon White U.S. Courthouse
1823 Stout Street
Denver, Colorado 80257

The Tenth Circuit Court of Appeals receives appeals from federal districts courts representing Wyoming, Utah, New Mexico, Colorado, Kansas, and Oklahoma.

U.S. Court of Appeals for the Eleventh Circuit
Elbert P. Tuttle U.S. Court of Appeals Building
56 Forsyth Street, NW
Atlanta, Georgia 30303

The Eleventh Circuit Court of Appeals receives appeals from federal districts courts representing Alabama, Georgia, and Florida.

U.S. Court of Appeals for Federal Circuit
717 Madison Place, NW
Washington, DC 20439

U.S. Court of Appeals for District of Columbia Circuit
E. Barrett U.S. Courthouse
333 Constitution Avenue, NW
Washington, DC 20001

Appendix 2B

STATE-BY-STATE LISTING OF COURT SYSTEMS

Alabama

The highest ranking state court in Alabama is the Alabama Supreme Court, which reviews cases decided at the Alabama Court of Civil Appeal or Alabama Court of Criminal Appeal. The Alabama Courts of Appeal (civil and criminal) hear cases brought forth on appeal from the Alabama Circuit Courts. There are 40 Alabama circuit courts, which have general subject matter jurisdiction over felonies, civil action for greater than $3,000, and domestic relations, and concurrent jurisdiction with district courts over issues related to juveniles. Alabama also has 68 probate courts, 67 district courts, and 257 municipal courts.

Alaska

The highest ranking state court in Alaska is the Alaska Supreme Court, which reviews cases decided by the Alaska Court of Appeals. The Alaska Court of Appeals hears cases on appeal from the trial courts, called superior courts, and some cases from the district courts. Alaska has divided the state into four judicial districts. Each judicial district has a superior court and a district court. The superior court has general jurisdiction over subject matters while the district court has limited jurisdiction over misdemeanors, civil cases up to $100,000, and small claims not exceeding $10,000.

Arizona

The highest ranking state court in Arizona is the Arizona Supreme Court, which reviews cases decided by the Arizona Courts of Appeals. There are two Arizona courts of appeal: Division One and Division Two. The Arizona Courts of Appeal hear cases brought forth on appeal from the trial courts, called superior courts. There are also administrative tribunal courts and city courts.

Arkansas

The highest ranking state court in Arkansas is the Arkansas Supreme Court, which reviews cases decided by the Arkansas Court of Appeals. The Arkansas Court of Appeals hears cases on appeal from the circuit courts and sometimes the district courts. There are also city courts. The circuit courts are of general jurisdiction and hear cases of five different subject matter jurisdictions: criminal, civil, probate, domestic relations, and juvenile. District courts' subject matter jurisdiction are misdemeanor, preliminary felony, and civil cases less than $5,000.

California

The highest ranking court in California is the California Supreme Court, which reviews cases decided by the California Courts of Appeal. There are six California courts of appeal that are divided by districts: District 1 is in San Francisco; District 2 is in Los Angles; District 3 is in Sacramento; District 4 is in San Diego; District 5 is in Fresno; and District 6 is in San Jose. The California Courts of Appeal review cases decided at the trial courts, which in California are also called superior courts. There are 58 trial courts in California, one in each county.

Colorado

The highest ranking court in Colorado is the Colorado Supreme Court, which reviews cases decided by the Colorado Court of Appeals. The Colorado Court of Appeals hears cases of appeal from Colorado's district courts and sometimes county courts. The district courts have subject matter jurisdiction over any civil action, domestic relations, criminal, juvenile, probate, and mental health. The county courts have limited jurisdiction over civil cases less than $15,000 in damages, misdemeanors, traffic, felony complaints and small claims. There are also water courts and the Denver Court System because Denver is both a city and a county.

Connecticut

The highest ranking court in Connecticut is the Connecticut Supreme Court, which hears appeals from the Connecticut Appellate Court. The Connecticut Appellate Court hears appeals taken from superior courts, which have subject matter jurisdiction over civil, criminal, family, and juvenile. There are also judicial district courts, geographical area courts, and juvenile matters courts.

Delaware

The highest ranking court in Delaware is the Delaware Supreme Court, which hears appeals from Delaware's superior courts and courts of chancery. It occasionally hears appeals from family courts. The superior courts have general subject matter jurisdiction over criminal, civil, and felonies. The courts of chancery have subject matter jurisdiction over matters in equity. The other courts in Delaware are alderman's courts, justice of the peace courts, court of common pleas, and family court.

District of Columbia

The District of Columbia is not a state; therefore, it does not have a state court system.

Florida

The highest ranking court in Florida is the Florida Supreme Court, which hears appeals from Florida district courts of appeal. Florida has five district courts of appeal, which hear appeals from trial courts, called circuit courts. Florida has 20 circuit courts. There are also county courts.

Georgia

The highest ranking court in Georgia is the Georgia Supreme Court, which hears appeals from the Georgia District Court of Appeal. Georgia's District Court of Appeal hears appeals from Georgia's superior courts, which are the trial courts in Georgia. The superior courts have general subject matter jurisdiction over felonies, divorce, and equity. There are 10 judicial districts with 49 judicial circuits. Each county has its own superior court. There are also state courts that have limited subject matter jurisdiction over misdemeanors and civil. There are also magistrate courts, juvenile courts, probate courts, and municipal courts.

Hawaii

The highest ranking court in Hawaii is the Hawaii Supreme Court, which hears appeals from the Hawaii Intermediate Court of Appeal. Hawaii's Intermediate Court of Appeal hears appeals from the circuit courts, which have general subject matter jurisdiction over civil actions alleging damages in excess of $20,000, as well as criminal, probate, and felonies. There are also district courts of limited jurisdiction and family courts.

Idaho

The highest ranking court in Idaho is the Idaho Supreme Court, which hears appeals from the Idaho Court of Appeal. The Idaho Court of Appeal hears appeals from trial courts (district courts). There are also drug courts, family courts, and youth courts.

Illinois

The highest ranking court in Illinois is the Illinois Supreme Court, which hears appeals from the Illinois Appellate Court. The Illinois Appellate Court hears appeals from trial courts, called circuit courts.

Indiana

The highest ranking court in Indiana is the Indiana Supreme Court, which hears appeals from Indiana District Courts of Appeal. Indiana has five district courts of appeal, which hear appeals from trial courts. There are also tax courts.

Iowa

The highest ranking court in Iowa is the Iowa Supreme Court, which hears appeals from Iowa's Court of Appeal. Iowa's Court of Appeal hears appeals from trial courts, called district courts.

Kansas

The highest ranking court in Kansas is the Kansas Supreme Court, which hears appeals from the Kansas Court of Appeal. Kansas' Court of Appeal hears appeals from trial courts, called district courts. There are also municipal courts.

Kentucky

The highest ranking court in Kentucky is the Kentucky Supreme Court. There is a Kentucky Court of Appeal that hears appeals from circuit courts. There are also district courts that have limited subject matter jurisdiction, including civil matters of less than $4,000 in damages. There are also family courts.

Louisiana

The highest ranking court in Louisiana is the Louisiana Supreme Court, which hears appeals from the five district courts of appeal. The district courts of appeal hear appeals from the district courts, which are divided by parishes. There are also city and parish courts.

Maine

The highest ranking court in Maine is the Maine Supreme Court, which hears appeals from the superior courts. There are 17 superior courts in the state. There are also 31 district courts that sit without a jury and hear small claims of less than $4,500.

Maryland

The highest ranking court in Maryland is the Court of Appeals, which hears appeals from the Court of Special Appeals. The Court of Special Appeals is the intermediate court of appeals for Maryland. The trial courts are called circuit courts and district courts, with the circuit courts having general jurisdiction and district courts having limited jurisdiction.

Massachusetts

The highest ranking court in Massachusetts is the Supreme Judicial Court, which hears appeals from the Massachusetts Appeal Court. The Massachusetts Appeal Court hears appeals from a multitude of courts, some of which include Boston Municipal Court Department, the Housing Court Department, the Land Court Department, the Superior Court Department, the District Court Department, the Juvenile Court Department, and Probate and Family Court Department.

Michigan

The highest ranking court in Michigan is the Michigan Supreme Court, which hears appeals from the Michigan Court of Appeals. The Michigan Court of Appeals hears appeals from the trial courts.

Minnesota

The highest ranking court in Minnesota is Minnesota's supreme court, which hears appeals from the Minnesota Court of Appeals. The Minnesota Court of Appeals hears appeals from the 10 district courts that are divided by judicial districts. There are also problem-solving courts.

Mississippi

The highest ranking court in Mississippi is the Mississippi Supreme Court, which hears appeals from the Mississippi Court of Appeals. The Mississippi Court of Appeals hears appeals from the circuit courts and chancery court. There are also county courts, justice courts, and municipal courts.

Missouri

The highest ranking court in Missouri is the Missouri Supreme Court, which hears appeals from Missouri's three courts of appeals. The courts of appeals hear matters originating in the 45 circuit courts. There are also 473 municipal courts.

Montana

The highest ranking court in Montana is the Montana Supreme Court. Of note there is not a Montana appellate court. There are district courts in 56 counties. There are also four water courts, a worker's compensation court, 66 courts for justice of the peace, 5 municipal courts, and 81 city courts.

Nebraska

The highest ranking court in Nebraska is the Nebraska Supreme Court, which hears appeals from the Nebraska Court of Appeal. It should be noted that Nebraska did not have a court of appeal until September 6, 1991. There are 12 districts courts as well as separate juvenile courts, 93 county courts, and 1 worker's compensation court.

Nevada

The highest ranking court in Nevada is the Nevada Supreme Court, which hears appeals from the nine district courts. There is no intermediate appellate court. There are also justice courts in 55 towns and 118 municipal courts in incorporated cities and towns.

New Hampshire

The highest ranking court in New Hampshire is the New Hampshire Supreme Court, which hears appeals from the 11 superior courts. There is no intermediate appellate court. There are probate courts in 10 counties and 37 district courts.

New Jersey

The highest ranking court in New Jersey is the New Jersey Supreme Court, which hears appeals from the appellate division of the superior court. The court of general jurisdiction is the superior court, which subject matter jurisdiction includes civil, family, general, equity, and criminal. There are 15 vicinages in 21 counties. There are also tax courts and 544 municipal courts.

New Mexico

The highest ranking court in New Mexico is the New Mexico Supreme Court, which hears appeals from the New Mexico Court of Appeal. The next ranking court are the 13 district courts. There are also 54 magistrate courts, 83 municipal courts, probate courts in 33 counties, and a Bernalillo County Metropolitan Court, which handles tort, contract, real property of less than $10,000, and misdemeanors.

New York

The highest ranking court in New York is the Court of Appeal, which hears appeals from the intermediate courts of appeal. The intermediate courts of appeal are called appellate terms of supreme court and appellate divisions of supreme court. There are four appellate divisions of supreme court. The intermediate appellate courts hear appeals from the trial courts, which are called supreme courts. There are supreme courts in 12 districts. There are also 57 county courts outside New York City. Other courts include Criminal Court of the City of New York, 14,878 town and village courts, one court of claims, 62 counties with surrogates courts, 62 counties with family courts, the District Court for Nassau and Suffolk, 79 city courts, and the Civil Court of the City of New York.

North Carolina

The highest ranking court for North Carolina is the North Carolina Supreme Court, which hears appeals from the North Carolina Court of Appeals. The North Carolina Court of Appeals hears appeals from the trial courts, which are called superior courts. There are 146 superior courts of general subject matter jurisdiction. There are also district courts of limited jurisdiction.

North Dakota

The highest ranking court in North Dakota is the North Dakota Supreme Court. There is no intermediate court of appeal. The courts of general jurisdiction are called district courts and are divided into seven districts. There are also 80 municipal courts, which have limited jurisdiction.

Ohio

The highest ranking court in Ohio is the Ohio Supreme Court, which hears appeal from the state's 12 courts of appeals. The Ohio courts of appeals hear cases from the 88 courts of common pleas, which are the courts of general jurisdiction. The other types of courts in Ohio are 122 municipal courts, 44 county courts, 1 court of claims, and 428 mayor's courts.

Oklahoma

The highest ranking courts in Oklahoma are the Oklahoma Supreme Court and the Oklahoma Court of Criminal Appeal. The Oklahoma Supreme Court hears appeals from the Oklahoma Court of Civil Appeals, while the Oklahoma Court of Criminal

Appeal hears appeals from the criminal courts. There are 26 district courts of general jurisdiction. There are also 340 municipal courts not of record, 2 municipal criminal courts of record, and 1 court of tax review.

Oregon

The highest ranking court in Oregon is the Oregon Supreme Court, which hears appeals from the Oregon Court of Appeals. The Oregon Court of Appeals hears appeals from the tax court and the 27 circuit courts. There are also 7 county courts, 30 justice courts, and 135 municipal courts.

Pennsylvania

The highest ranking court in Pennsylvania is the Pennsylvania Supreme Court, which hears appeals from the intermediate appellate courts, called commonwealth courts, and superior courts. The intermediate appellate courts hear appeals from the 60 courts of common pleas, which are the courts of general jurisdiction. There are also 551 district justice courts, Philadelphia Municipal Court 1st District, Philadelphia Traffic Court 1st District, and Pittsburgh City Magistrate 5th District.

Puerto Rico

The highest ranking court in Puerto Rico is the Puerto Rico Supreme Court, which hears appeals from the circuit court of appeals. The circuit court of appeals hears appeals from the court of first instance, which is the court of general jurisdiction. Other courts with limited jurisdiction are superior division and municipal division.

Rhode Island

The highest ranking court in Rhode Island is the Rhode Island Supreme Court, which hears appeals from the four divisions of superior courts. There is no intermediate appellate court. The superior courts are courts of general subject matter jurisdiction. There are a worker's compensation court, 4 divisions of district courts, 4 divisions of family courts, traffic tribunal, 16 municipal courts, and 39 probate courts in towns and cities.

South Carolina

The highest ranking court in South Carolina is the South Carolina Supreme Court, which hears appeals from the South Carolina Court of Appeal. The South Carolina Court of Appeal hears appeals from the 16 circuit courts. There are also 16 circuits of family courts, 286 magistrate courts, 46 probate courts, and 200 municipal courts.

South Dakota

The highest ranking court in South Dakota is the South Dakota Supreme Court, which hears appeals from the seven circuit courts. There is no intermediate appellate court.

Tennessee

The highest ranking court in Tennessee is the Tennessee Supreme Court, which hears appeals from either the three divisions of the courts of appeals or the three divisions of the courts of criminal appeals. The courts of appeal hear matters on appeal from judicial districts, which include circuit courts, chancery courts, and criminal courts representing 95 counties. There is also one probate court. The courts of limited jurisdiction include 98 juvenile courts, 300 municipal courts, and general session courts in the 98 counties.

Texas

The highest ranking courts in Texas are the Texas Supreme Court and the Texas Court of Criminal Appeals. These courts hear appeals from the 14 Texas courts of appeal. There are 418 district courts, which have general subject matter jurisdiction. There are also 472 courts of limited jurisdiction including county-level courts hearing matters of constitutional county court, probate court, county court at law, municipal court, and justice of the peace court.

Utah

The highest ranking court in Utah is the Utah Supreme Court, which hears appeals from Utah's court of appeals. Utah's court of appeals hears appeals from the 40 district courts, which are the courts of general subject matter jurisdiction. There are also 20 juvenile courts and 139 justice courts.

Vermont

The highest ranking court in Vermont is Vermont Supreme Court, which hears appeals from Vermont's family courts, superior courts, and district courts in each of the 14 counties. There are also environmental courts, probate courts, and Vermont's judicial bureau.

Virginia

The highest ranking court in Virginia is the Virginia Supreme Court, which hears appeals from the Virginia Court of Appeals. Virginia's Court of Appeals hears appeals from the courts of general subject matter jurisdiction that include 31 circuit courts in 120 counties. There are also 130 courts of limited jurisdiction called districts courts.

Virgin Islands

The highest ranking court in the Virgin Islands is the Appellate Division of the District Court of the Virgin Islands. Appeals from the Appellate Division of the District Court of the Virgin Islands go to the U.S. Court of Appeals for the Third Circuit and then to the U.S. Supreme Court (federal). The court of general jurisdiction is the Superior Court of the Virgin Islands.

Washington

The highest ranking court in Washington is the Washington Supreme Court, which hears appeals from Washington's three courts of appeals. Washington's three courts of appeals hear appeals from the superior courts that are in 31 districts. There are also 121 municipal courts and 49 district courts.

West Virginia

The highest ranking court in West Virginia is the West Virginia Supreme Court, which hears appeals from the 55 circuit courts. There is no intermediate court of appeal. The circuit courts are courts of general jurisdiction. There are also courts of limited jurisdiction that include magistrate courts in 55 counties, 122 municipal courts, and family courts in 26 circuits.

Wisconsin

The highest ranking court in Wisconsin is the Wisconsin Supreme Court, which hears appeals from the four district courts of appeals. The courts of appeals hear appeals from the circuit courts that cover 69 circuits. There are also 224 municipal courts.

Wyoming

The highest ranking court in Wyoming is the Wyoming Supreme Court, which hears appeals from the nine district courts. There is no intermediate appellate court. The district courts have general subject matter jurisdiction. There are also courts of limited subject matter jurisdiction including 7 justice of the peace courts, 79 municipal courts, and 16 circuit courts.

CHAPTER 3

Understanding Tort Reform

This chapter will explain the dynamic forces working between reimbursement and liability. As this book is written, several states and the federal government are debating the necessity of tort reform in order to bring insurance carriers back into a state to insure high-risk health care providers. The most affected professions, which have led to exorbitantly priced insurance premiums with less insurance coverage, are obstetrics, cardiology, vascular surgery, and, in some states, nursing home care. Plaintiffs' lawyers have sued for enormous dollars, which allegedly has led to the destruction of the insurance industry in these areas. The remainder of this chapter will discuss the interplay between insurance and lawsuits as well as the benefits and detriments associated with tort reform.

KEY CONCEPTS

What is tort reform?
Why has tort reform become a national issue?
What are some of the pros and cons of tort reform?
Insurance industry
Insurance terms

WHAT IS TORT REFORM?

Tort reform is a philosophy that there needs to be change in the civil law system, ostensibly to manage the uncontrolled effects of litigation on the U.S. economy, especially as it relates to the insurance industry. In the last 10 years, the issue of tort reform has been high profile in both state and federal forums. Remember, state and federal governments are separated; therefore, the issue of tort reform is being addressed on both fronts. Some states are ahead of the federal movement on the issue and already have passed legislation pertaining to that particular state.

In 1996, a joint economic committee examined three potential tort reform proposals that were being discussed in the U.S. Congress.[1] The accepted foundation necessitating the tort reform proposal was a belief that the American tort (civil actions) system was too costly and inefficient.[2] Actuarials from Tillinghast-Towers Perrin documented tort costs rose "from $67 billion in 1984 to $152 billion in 1994, an increase of 125 percent."[3] The increased litigation costs resulted in higher insurance premiums that burdened businesses and families, which also lead to higher costs for health businesses.[4] Thus, from a business perspective, especially as it relates to medical practices, increased frequency of litigation leads to an increase in litigation costs. An increase in litigation costs requires an increase in medical costs of services to cover the increased costs associated with litigation because revenues must exceed expenses to stay in business. For the health company there are also, at the same time, increased costs associated with increasing insurance rates (premiums) as a result of the increased litigation expenses. The simple formula to remember for business is that to stay in business, revenues must exceed costs of doing the business.

As of 2005, the majority of states had some form of medical liability laws with most states having a 2-year statute of limitations*.[5] Further, over one half of the states had some form of limitation on damage awards for medical malpractice claims.[6] In 2005 alone, 48 states' legislatures introduced over 400 different bills in an attempt to provide some relief to the problem.[7] Additionally, "during the 2005 legislative session, 32 states enacted over 60 bills, and two more states had Supreme Court rulings related to medical liability lawsuit statutes."[8]

The issue of tort reform found an audience at the federal level with the issue "a centerpiece" in the 2004 presidential election.[9] This creates an interesting potential complication. If federal enactments are stronger than state enactments, which will ultimately rule? Usually if there is a federal law and state law on the same issue, as long as the state law minimally requires the same thing as the federal law, then there is no conflict—but if the state law is not as strong as the federal law, then will the state have to change its law? "Traditional supporters of federalism** have turned their back on

---

* A statute of limitations is defined as "[a] statute establishing a time limit for suing in a civil case, based on the date when the claim accrued (as when the injury occurred or was discovered). The purpose of such a statute is to require diligent prosecution of known claims, thereby providing finality and predictability in legal affairs and ensuring that claims will be resolved while evidence is reasonably available and fresh." Black's Law Dictionary, 1422 (Bryan A. Garner, ed., 7th ed., West 1999).

** *Federalism* is defined as "[t]he relationship and distribution of power between the national and regional governments within a federal system of government." Black's Law Dictionary, 627 (Bryan A. Garner, ed., 7th ed., West 1999). Generally, traditional federalist's individuals fight to promote a state's authority over the intrusion of the federal government's authority.

their states in favor of intrusive legislation that will nullify the work of their state legislatures executed over the last three years."[10]

From the state and federal level, there is a movement to change the way the current civil law deals with medical malpractice. The unknowns are what will be the limits and which will triumph, the state tort reform or the federal tort reform? Hence, the debate over tort reform will continue in the years ahead. Physical therapists, physical therapist assistants, and students will now enter the debate not just as consumers, but also as health care providers being affected when there is no tort reform. Some of the state-specific tort reform and the 2005 federal platform for tort reform is provided in Appendix 3A.

INSURANCE INDUSTRY

Currently, the American Physical Therapy Association has endorsed a liability insurance program for physical therapists, physical therapist assistants, and students through the CNA insurance company. The insurance plan is administered through Healthcare Providers Service Organization (HPSO). HPSO is CNA's marketing and administration program agent for this product line.[11] (The product is professional malpractice insurance for physical therapists, physical therapist assistants, and students.)

Premium rates vary depending on geographic location, whether the primary practice is in a hospital or a freestanding clinic, whether the therapist works full time or less than 24 hours a week, whether the therapist is a physical therapist or physical therapist assistant, and whether the physical therapist or physical therapist assistant is a recent graduate, meaning within the last 12 months. The insurance coverage provided is generally $1,000,000 per occurrence with a $3,000,000 aggregate per year. What every physical therapist and physical therapist assistant should understand is that these insurance premiums are considered inexpensive—yet, if the number and severity of claims against physical therapists, physical therapist assistants, or students rises, there will be no recourse but for the insurance premiums to increase and possibly for the insurance coverage to decrease.

One of the example professions where the escalating numbers and severity of claims rose dramatically is obstetrics. The profession of delivering babies is fraught with high risk for bad outcomes. Generally, if a baby is born with any kind of a problem, there is much sympathy for the parents, which translates in a court of law as pain and suffering damages for the mother and father as well as medical expenses for the impaired child for the remainder of that child's life. Because the risk of costly settlements or jury awards are high and the cost of defending such claims is very expensive, this scenario has led to extremely costly premiums for obstetricians to obtain insurance coverage. The reason it is so costly is because the insurance carrier is almost 100 percent at risk of having to pay out the policy's aggregate limit.

Thus, the insurance carrier is almost guaranteed it will have to defend and pay policy limits for each obstetrician it insures. Accordingly, because the insurance carriers are in the business to make money, the insurance carrier realizes it must receive more money in premiums than it pays out in policy coverage; otherwise, no insurance carrier will operate a business. As such, because obstetricians are such a high-risk profession for lawsuits, the premiums to purchase minimal insurance coverage are astronomical. Many states have enacted statutory protections for obstetricians in an attempt to limit potential jury verdicts, thus, providing insurance carriers with identifiable and quantifiable risks. Once the insurance carrier knows a given risk, it can calculate and project appropriate premiums for the insurance provided.

INSURANCE TERMS

A *claim limit* is the maximum amount of money that the insurance carrier will pay for a covered claim. It should be noted that many professional malpractice insurance policies' claim limits are depleted based on the costs of defense. In other words, the fees that are paid to the defense lawyer come from the total amount of money that is allocated to pay the covered claim. Thus, if the insurance policy is for $1,000,000 for a covered claim, the defense lawyer's costs will deplete the $1,000,000 with payment of his or her fees. Additionally, costs associated with the defense of the covered claim will also likely deplete the maximum allowable claim limit. Hence, after several years of litigation, the maximum amount of money left to pay a claim will likely be far less than $1,000,000.

This concept is important for physical therapists, physical therapist assistants, and students because if a jury awarded damages in excess of the remaining insurance policy money, and the physical therapist, physical therapist assistant, or student had no excess liability insurance coverage, then the physical therapist, physical therapist assistant, or student could be held personally liable for the outstanding amount. However, before any physical therapist, physical therapist assistant, or student buys excess professional liability insurance it would be recommended to seek the advice of a lawyer to understand the benefits and risks of additional layers of insurance coverage.

An *aggregate limit* is the total amount of money the insurance policy will pay out during the policy period to cover all claims. Generally spaeking, the current most popular malpractice insurance policy for physical therapists, physical therapist assistants, and students is the $1,000,000 per claim and $3,000,000 aggregate policy. Thus, if a physical therapist, physical therapist assistant, or student had three malpractice claims against him or her during a given year, the maximum amount of money that will be paid for any one of the three claims would be $1,000,000. Further, the maximum amount of money that will be paid out for that insurance policy, irregardless of the number of claims, will be $3,000,000. If the physical therapist, physical therapist assistant, or student had another claim brought forward during that policy year, then there would be no funds left to pay toward that fourth, or subsequent, claim. However, if the three earlier claims had only paid out a total of $1,500,000, then there would still be the $1,000,000 available for the fourth occurrence and a total of $1,500,000 remaining in aggregate—or, if the earlier three claims had paid out $2,500,000, then there would only be $500,000 left available for the fourth claim.

Additionally, physical therapists, physical therapist assistants, and students should understand what the insurance policy considers covered practice and what, if any, exclusions apply to that particular insurance policy. As an example, an insurance policy for malpractice might exclude acts outside the physical therapist's or physical therapist assistant's state practice act. Suppose a physical therapist was practicing in the state of Arkansas and performed a spinal mobilization that the patient interprets as a spinal manipulation. The patient then sues alleging an injury from what the patient interprets as spinal manipulation. The insurance carrier may deny coverage of the claim, or reserve its rights to deny coverage, because spinal manipulation is prohibited under the Arkansas Physical Therapy Practice Act as described in the case of *Teston v. Arkansas State Board of Chiropractic Examiners*, 2005 WL 775805 (April 7, 2005). Thus, the insurance carrier may deny coverage, asserting that the physical therapist, physical therapist assistant, or student acted outside the scope of the Physical Therapy Practice Act for a given state and therefore the alleged claim is outside the coverage of the insurance policy.

Other terms that should be understood are the number of claims or frequency of claims, severity of claim, and average costs per claim. An insurance company is not unlike any other business; it is in the business to make money. Therefore, if it pays out more money on policies without taking in more money through premiums, it will go out of business. When an insurance company studies actuarials, it studies historical perspectives of claims paid for a particular insured group like physical therapy. An *actuary* is "[a] statistician who determines the present effects of future contingent events; especially: one who calculates insurance and pension rates on the basis of empirically based tables."[12] These historical perspectives include the number of claims paid, the geographical areas of claim occurrence, and the number of claims paid for a particular category of insured. These types of studies assist the insurance carrier with how many claims it may expect for an insured group and the likely severity of each claim.

Therefore, insurance carriers must make a decision as to whether the insured is worth the risk, and if the insured is worth the risk, how much the insurance carrier should charge in premiums for the amount of coverage being provided. As a result, some insurance companies are electing not to provide insurance coverage for some high-risk professions and/or businesses—or, to offset cost, the insurance companies are charging more for the insurance in premiums as a way to offset costs for the claims they anticipate they will have to pay out. However, if the return on the investment is not reasonable, many insurance carriers can and do choose to insure other product lines with a greater return on the investment.

One of the best examples of this insurance dilemma is homeowners' insurance for property for the Gulf of Mexico residents. Due to the recent destruction of homes and properties in and around the Gulf of Mexico coastline, many insurance companies have elected not to provide insurance coverage for homeowners living in those regions of the county. Why? The answer is simple; the insurance company cannot take in enough money through insurance premiums to cover the losses suffered during the recent hurricanes and predicted storms. Thus, the risks associated with insuring that particular product line do not make "good business sense" when there are other product lines that can have a greater return on their investment.

In contrast to high-risk geographical zones, physical therapists, physical therapist assistants, and students are generally thought to not perform high-risk procedures. However, that belief could, and probably will, change as physical therapists become entry-level health care practitioners pursuant to the APTA's Vision 2020. With the evolution of the physical therapy profession, physical therapists, physical therapist assistants, and students will have to diagnostically rule out other disease processes before implementing a physical therapy plan of treatment, or the patient will need to be referred for diagnostic testing to rule out other causes for the patient's symptoms. The failure to diagnose and/or refer for appropriate follow-up could lead to the physical therapist, physical therapist assistant, or student being sued for a misdiagnosis.

When the physical therapist, physical therapist assistant, or student is treating pursuant to a physician's referral (order or prescription), the general presumption is the physician has ruled out other disease processes as the cause of the patient's complaint. Hence, the physician remains what the legal community calls "the captain of the ship." Legally, when the physician is the captain of the ship, then the physician remains liable for any omission or failure to diagnose. However, with physical therapists becoming entry-level health care practitioners, the umbrella of protection where the physician will possibly be at fault, will be eliminated. As a result, as an entry-level health care practitioner, physical therapists will take on the responsibility to thoroughly rule out or refer patients presenting with nonphysical therapy treatment diagnoses to the appropriate health care provider. Hence, the responsibility associated with evaluating and treating patients will rise, which will have the unintentional affect of increasing liability risk exposure.

BENEFITS OF TORT REFORM

Tort reform benefits are many and may have an impact on capping noneconomic damages. Other benefits include changes to the statute of limitations, changes in the quality of expert witnesses required to prove a case, control over insurance rates, and a reduction in the plaintiff's attorney fees. As will be explained in Chapter 5, noneconomic damages include damages (money) for alleged pain and suffering. Obviously there is no mathematical formula to calculate or determine what someone's pain and suffering is for any particular set of circumstances. At trial, one jury might award $100,000 for pain and suffering damages for a plaintiff with a back injury from a car accident, while another jury might award $200,000.

The variable in these two examples is not the plaintiff, the injury, or the factual circumstances, but rather the makeup of the jury. Much research has been and continues to be done on how to select jurors, but that discussion is beyond the scope of this book. Nonetheless, physical therapists, physical therapist assistants, and students should understand when a lawsuit is tried before a jury, one of the most difficult variables to control at trial is the composition of the jury pool and ultimately the seating of the jury panel, which can result in unpredictable outcomes.

However, when there has been tort reform and there is a cap on noneconomic damages, insurance carriers can better predict potential claim losses, which allows more precise predictions of money paid out for claims. This then allows better decisions as to premiums to charge for a particular policy of insurance. Thus, insurance carriers are more available to provide insurance protection for covered health care practitioners.

Other alleged benefits of tort reform are fewer frivolous claims. However, there are also studies that hold there is no relationship between premiums for medical malpractice insurance and tort-reform measures.[13] A study conducted by a professor of economics at Dartmouth College and an assistant professor of economics at the Kennedy School of Government at Harvard University drew the conclusion that there was "no relationship between the level of malpractice premiums and the presence of traditional tort-reform measures such as damage caps."[14] Another conclusion from the study was that there was "little evidence that malpractice payments are driving the dramatic increase in overall health care expenditures."[15] Nonetheless, promoters of tort reform still believe in its benefits despite this study.

DETRIMENTS OF TORT REFORM

The other side of tort reform is capping of noneconomic damages on cases that are severe and catastrophic. If a loved one were severely injured as the result of a health care provider's negligence, the likelihood you would want that claim to be capped for noneconomic pain and suffering is very slim. In fact, you would probably want to obtain the highest possible verdict as some type of remuneration for the loss the loved one suffered. However, under tort reform, there would likely be some limit or cap to those damages.

Another possible negative effect of tort reform is the potential to "chill" lawyers from bringing these types of claims. Most plaintiff lawyers work on a contingency fee arrangement with their clients. A *contingency fee arrangement* is defined as "[a] fee charged for a lawyer's services only if the lawsuit is successful or is favorably settled out of court. Contingency fees are usu[ally] calculated as a percentage of the client's net recovery (such as 25% of the recovery if the case is settled, and 33% if the case is won at trial)."[16] Thus, if the potential for a high recovery is gone, some of these highly skilled lawyers may not be willing to bring these types of claims because their skills will be more fruitful for another type of claim. As it is, these claims are very time consuming and costly.

Additionally, the reduction in the statute of limitations could prohibit some claims from being brought. Although many argue that 2 years is plenty of time to know if a medical mistake was made, it may not be enough time for some people to deal with the loss and then find the time to seek and retain a lawyer to fight for their rights. Thus, the potential downside to tort reform is that victims of medical malpractice may not have their claims adequately compensated.

SUMMARY

Tort reform is one of the hottest issues currently facing the United States. One of the most prominent suggestions for tort reform is to cap the amount of money a plaintiff can recover for noneconomic damages such as pain and suffering. A converse argument to caps is that a limit on those dollars that can be awarded for medical malpractice may relax health care providers' astuteness to changes in medicine. There is also the concern as to whether caps can adequately compensate someone who has suffered a horrendous loss. While physical therapists, physical therapist assistants, and students have predominately not been concerned about these issues, with the evolution of the practice in response to APTA's Vision 2020, it is likely physical therapists, physical therapist assistants, and students will become a greater part of the health care providers affected by increasing insurance premiums and escalating litigation frequency and costs.

DISCUSSION QUESTIONS

1. Discuss tort reform.
2. How will tort reform, or the lack of tort reform, affect physical therapists, physical therapist assistants, and students?
3. Discuss the effects of tort reform from a consumer's standpoint.
4. Discuss the effects of tort reform from a physical therapist's, physical therapist assistant's, and student's standpoint.
5. What is meant by occurrence limit and aggregate limit?
6. What could cause an insurance carrier to deny coverage of a claim?
7. Discuss whether liability exposure may be rising for physical therapy professionals.
8. What are some of the alleged benefits of tort reform?
9. What are some of the alleged detriments of tort reform?
10. Discuss reasons you would support or fight tort reform.

Appendix 3A

STATE AND FEDERAL TORT REFORM MEASURES

Arizona

Arizona had five bills presented in the legislature with two bills being passed. Nothing of significance was passed related to tort reform. However, Senate Bill (SB) 1102, which modified public disclosure of medical malpractice, was passed and signed by the governor on April 6, 2006.[17] This legislation provided that "pending complaints are not posted on public website but may be released to a member of the public via phone or written request."[18]

California

Although California has not passed tort reform legislation, there are two bills of significance that may pass. Bill AB 28 provided civil liability protection to health care providers that offered quality free medical services to individuals who were receiving Medicaid or were uninsured.[19] Additionally AB 2342 empowered a study, which is to be reported to the legislature before January 1, 2008, of the state providing medical malpractice insurance for those physicians who provide unpaid medical services.[20]

Colorado

One of Colorado's bills, SJR 11, died as the legislature adjourned sine die on May 10, 2006.[21] SJR 11 simply requested "that Congressional delegation support medical malpractice liability reform."[22] The other legislation that was passed and signed by the governor on June 1, 2006, was HB 1330, which "[r]epeals existing provisions allowing medical malpractice insurers to use loss experiences from other states and nationwide experiences in certain situations when setting rates; specific information factors not to be included."[23]

Connecticut

Legislation was signed by the governor on June 2, 2006, that "[e]liminates requirements that medical professional liability insurance policies issued on a claims-made basis provide prior acts coverage without additional charge to insured; extended reporting coverage liability insurers must provide under certain circumstance."[24]

District of Columbia

Although not passed, two bills were under consideration with one bill going forth with a public hearing on March 20, 2006. B16-0334 had the public hearing and the bill was designed to require approval before an insurance carrier could raise medical malpractice rates over 7 percent.[25] B16-0418 required "Mayor to dedicate number of full-time employees within Department of Health to assist in improving performance of Board of Medicine; creation of centralized database for analysis of adverse medical events'; also database for closed claims against obstetricians for analysis in improving health care delivery; notice requirements for filing lawsuits alleging medical malpractice; required mediation for medical malpractice litigation; expression of sympathy or apology by health care provider not admissible as evidence of admission of liability; medical malpractice insurance rates, rate changes, and payment to be made public."[26]

Florida

All of the Florida bills died in committee, however, the bills that were brought forth are indicative of the tort reform changes being debated in the Florida legislature. Senate Bill (SB) 272 and House Bill (HB) 565 dealt with "[r]ules for 'financial responsibility requirements' for physicians relating to liability insurance, submission of documentation to Department of Health relating to insurance coverage or other alternative financial arrangements, related suspension of medical license in certain circumstance."[27] SB. 614 was to create a Florida medical malpractice insurance fund to provide medical malpractice insurance policies to any physician and would be operated by the Office of Insurance Regulation.[28] SB 2160 and HB 1293 actually gave some limitations as "[m]edical malpractice insurers may issue insurance coverage to exclude medical negligence within a specified hospital or trauma center; noneconomic damages limited to $500,000 for hospital complying with certain patient-safety measures; requirements, examinations, and approval process for certification as patient-safety facility; reporting requirements for patient-safety certified facilities but records will not be admissible as evidence in legal proceedings."[29] Lastly SB 2212 and HB 1111 directly specify that nurse practitioners would not be required to carry medical malpractice insurance; however, in cases of medical malpractice, certain cases to be specified, the nurse practitioners would be required to pay a specified sum and some cases would warrant license suspension.[30]

Hawaii

Hawaii had six different bills introduced in 2005 and carried over to the 2006 legislative session; however, none were passed at the adjournment of the legislature. SB 2284 and HB 2321 specifically dealt with tort reform and limitations of damages.[31] "Noneconomic damages in medical tort actions limited to $250,000; plaintiff attorney fees for medical tort actions limited on sliding scale, 15% of any award over $600,000; periodic payments and attorney fees based on life expectancy of plaintiff; court to assess percentage of negligence upon request of non-settling healthcare provider, used to base amount of economic damages allocated to each defendant; joint and several liability to apply if healthcare provider's degree of negligence is 25% or more, noneconomic damages recoverable in proportion to degree of negligence if less than 25%."[32] SB 3279 dealt with any statement or conduct to the patient or family wherein a health care provider apologized, took responsibility for the mistake or accepted liability for the mistake regarding the pain, injury or death was to be "inadmissible as evidence of an admission of liability or against interest."[33] SCR 152 empowered the legislative reference bureau to conduct a study regarding the regulation of the insurance industry specific to medical malpractice and propose reforms with a report to the 2008 legislative session.[34] HB 1845 proposed a $250,000 limit on noneconomic damages when a lawsuit was brought against a health care provider professional who was acting through emergency services or a hospital's emergency department.[35] Lastly, HB 2025 was for "[n]oneconomic damages in medical tort lawsuit limited to $250,000; jury not to be informed of noneconomic limit; multiple defendants severally liable with separate judgments against each for damages; attorney fees limited on sliding scale from 40 percent of first $50,000 to 15 percent of award or settlement over $600,000; collateral benefits may be introduced into evidence; punitive damages only awarded if actual malice proven; periodic payments for any award over $50,000; statute of limitations set at 1 year, 3 years or age 8 for minors."[36]

Indiana

Indiana's HB 1112 was passed and signed by the governor on March 17, 2006. The bill specifically differentiated between a "statement of sympathy" and a "statement of fault" such that a statement of sympathy was not admissible as evidence at trial; whereas a statement of fault was admissible as evidence.[37] Two other bills were referred to the judiciary committee. These bills were HB 1260 and HB 1277. HB 1260 provided that "[a]ny statement or conduct expressing apology, fault or sympathy made by health care provider to patient or family member relating to pain, injury or death is inadmissible as evidence of admission of liability or against interests," and HB 1277 provided "[i]n all civil actions, attorney fees shall be awarded to the prevailing party."[38]

Iowa

Although SF 2218 did not pass, it attempted tort reform with a $500,000 cap on noneconomic damages in any medical malpractice lawsuit.[39] However, HF 2716 did pass and was signed by the governor on May 24, 2006. It provided "[i]n any civil action against medical professional or health care facility, any statement or conduct expressing sympathy or condolence regarding injury or death as result of alleged breach of standard of care is inadmissible as evidence of admission of liability or against interest."[40] There were also another six bills that were created during the legislative period, but did not pass. These additional bills dealt with requiring certificate that the lawsuit brought against the health care provider had merit, expert witness in medical malpractice matter must be of the same specialty, pretrial medical review panel may be requested by either side and its report would subsequently be admissible at trial, and expert witnesses in medical malpractice action must be actively practicing within same specialty for the previous three years.[41]

Kansas

Kansas had three bills brought forth during the legislative period, but none were passed. One bill, SB 335, would have allowed collateral benefits to be considered when awarding damages in personal injury cases.[42] HB 2547 would have allowed the judge to instruct the jury regarding the $250,000 cap on noneconomic damages.[43] Lastly HB 2563 would have raised the cap on noneconomic damages from $250,000 to $750,000.[44]

Kentucky

Kentucky had six different bills brought forth during the legislative period, but none passed. SB 1 would have allowed a cap on noneconomic damages and/or punitive damages at $250,000; changed the statute of limitations for medical malpractice actions; and required some type of alternative dispute resolution be attempted prior to trial.[45] Additional items contained in the proposed legislation included certificate of merit of the medical malpractice claim, certificate from medical expert as to the alleged deviation from the applicable standard of care, a request for a "medical malpractice liability reform," and other bills specifically dealing with the insurance carriers and rates.[46]

Louisiana

Louisiana had eight bills brought forth during its legislative period, but only one passed with the governor signing it into law on June 29, 2006. HB 412 was implemented and called for "[e]xpanded definitions for patient, malpractice, and heath care under Malpractice Liability Law."[47] The other proposed legislation dealt with an award of attorney fees and court costs if a medical malpractice claim was determined to be frivolous and one bill that called for separate definitions of noneconomic and economic damages in medical malpractice claims.[48] Lastly, one bill, SB 406, called for an "[e]xpedited process for review panel prior to medical liability lawsuit being filed, with agreement of all parties; opinion of panel not permitted as evidence in court, panel members may not be called by either party as witnesses."[49]

Maine

Maine passed LD 1378 and it was signed by the governor on June 10, 2005. LD 1378 implemented "[c]omparative negligence of plaintiff to reduce award in personal injury or wrongful death cases; jury to specify amount of damages award to be paid by each defendant in multiple-defendant medical malpractice complaint; noneconomic damages limited to $250,000; punitive damages limited to $75,000; statement or conduct acknowledging sympathy, apology or fault made by health care provider to patient or patient's representative relating to injury or death as result of unanticipated medical outcome not admissible as evidence of admission of liability."[50] Otherwise, Maine had two other bills that were not passed dealing with insurance rates and the revocation of health care provider's license when adjudicated with three professional negligence claims.[51]

Maryland

Maryland had seven bills introduced during the legislative period but none passed. These bills dealt with a committee to addresses issues relating to birth-related neurological injuries, expert witnesses' certificates for medical malpractice claims, cap on noneconomic damages at $500,000, medical malpractice claims must be submitted to medical malpractice administrative review board, the chief judge of appeals to consider establishment of medical malpractice court division, and tax credit against state income tax liability for medical malpractice insurance premiums.[52]

Massachusetts

Massachusetts had one bill introduced in 2006 that would set the interest rate for medical malpractice lawsuits when damages were awarded, but it was not passed during its legislative period.[53]

Michigan

Michigan in 2006 introduced five bills, however, none passed during the legislative period. The bills included methods for the parties to challenge the merits of the opposing parties' affidavit in support of medical malpractice claims, expert witness must be licensed in the state and provisions would be made to grant out-of-state expert witness limited license for purpose of testifying in medical malpractice action, and some revisions to the expert witness standards.[54]

Minnesota

Although no action was taken, Minnesota proposed through HF 2832: "Commerce Commissioner to provide annual report to legislature about status of medical malpractice insurance market based on annual statements filed by insurance providers; insurance providers required to file reports with certain data to Commerce Commissioner, including specific coverage for individual emergency and obstetrics physicians, medical facilities and nursing homes."[55]

Mississippi

Mississippi in 2006 introduced five bills regarding tort reform and SB 2056 was passed and signed by the governor on April 24, 2006.[56] SB 2056 provided a "temporary market of last resort to make medical malpractice insurance available for hospitals, institutions for the aged or infirm, or other licensed health care facilities; also for physicians, nurses, and any other personnel licensed to practice in any health care facility including hospitals."[57] Other bills were attempts to have congressional support for medical malpractice liability reform, track judgments against physicians in the state, and create a medical review panel.[58]

Missouri

Missouri had 12 bills introduced during the session and only one passed. HB 1837 passed and was signed by the governor on July 1, 2006, and provided "[m]edical malpractice insurers required to submit annual report to Department of Insurance, specific information required; Director of Insurance required to submit annual report on medical malpractice insurance to Governor and state legislature, specific information required; all information submitted held confidential and not subject to disclosure; notification requirements when insurer pays judgment or settlement in medical malpractice claims to appropriate licensing board of health care provider; base rates regulation for medical malpractice insurance."[59]

Nebraska

Nebraska introduced but it did not pass legislation for caps. LB 1260 provided "[d]amages limited to $500,000 when good faith effort has been made to resolve or settle medical liability case for incident on or before 12/31/84; $1 million for incident between 12/31/84 and 12/31/92; $1,250,000 for incident between 12/31/92 and 12/31/03; and $1,750,000 for incident after 12/31/03; no damages limits if no good faith effort to settle; payment may be made from Excess Liability Fund."[60]

New Hampshire

New Hampshire introduced four bills, however, none passed. The bills introduced dealt with a grant program to subsidize medical liability insurance premiums, medical malpractice insurance study commission, a temporary freeze on medical malpractice insurance rates, and a feasibility study on forming self-insurance groups for medical malpractice coverage.[61]

New Jersey

New Jersey was probably the most active and introduced 19 bills having something to do with tort reform, none of which passed. The bills had to do with caps on noneconomic damages at $100,000 or three times the economic damages or at $500,000 or $750,000 depending on the circumstances surrounding the injury and future disability; creation of a medical malpractice court; caps of $250,000 on noneconomic damages for claims arising out of emergency services; revisions to the statute of limitations; caps on damages to extent of medical malpractice insurance coverage; reports from state boards on complaints and disciplinary actions; reporting of professionals whose conduct had been called into question; some restrictions on expert witnesses; creation of a special medical malpractice part of law division of the state superior court; toll discovery limit of 4 years; notice requirements before the filing of a medical malpractice lawsuit; establishment of a medical malpractice liability insurance premium assistance fund; and establishment of a medical malpractice liability insurance premium increase review panel as part of the department of banking.[62]

New Mexico

New Mexico had three bills during the legislation that died. The contents of the bills called for a task force to study medical malpractice insurance issues, support for congressional malpractice reform, and the creation of a medical malpractice joint underwriting association to provide professional liability insurance.[63]

New York

New York also was very active and had at least 20 bills dealing with some type of tort reform. None of the specific bills passed. However, the contents of the bills included creation of an impaired infant compensation fund; personal liability caps for obstetricians and midwives at $250,000; and the creation of birth-related neurological injury compensation fund.[64]

North Carolina

North Carolina introduced five bills, but none passed. The bills addressed issues of rates for professional liability insurance; reporting of settlements in medical malpractice claims; bifurcation of issues of liability and damages in medical malpractice cases; and payment of future expense in medical malpractice cases with periodic payments.[65]

Oklahoma

The state adopted SB 192, however, there was no indication it was executed by the governor. SB 1928 called for "[p]eriodic payments allowed in medical malpractice judgments over $100,000; joint and several liability allowed for multiple defendants unless over 50% at fault; no prejudgment interest awarded in any case; collateral source payments reported from plaintiff to court; statute of repose in any medical malpractice case limited to 8 years."[66] The other bills that were not adopted included provisions for a medical malpractice premium fund to offset portions of medical malpractice insurance premiums and to request congressional support for medical malpractice reform.[67]

Pennsylvania

Pennsylvania had one bill that was not passed. The bill proposed was related to reporting by the insurance carriers of loss and expenses so a determination could be made whether rates were fair.[68]

Rhode Island

Rhode Island had 11 bills dealing with some form of tort reform but none passed. The bills included reports to the legislature on medical malpractice losses; lowering of the interest rate on civil judgments from 12 percent to 6 percent; changes to the statute of limitations; caps on noneconomic damages of $250,000; substantive disclosure of information on expert witnesses; increased regulation on insurance carriers; limits on plaintiff's attorney fees; and the creation of a comprehensive study for reporting back to the 2008 general assembly.[69]

South Carolina

South Carolina had two bills brought forth and SB 1059 was passed with execution by the governor on May 9, 2006.[70] SB 1059 provided that "any conduct or statements constitution voluntary offers of assistance or expressions of regret, mistake, error, sympathy or apology between parties or potential parties to a medical care civil action should be encouraged and not considered admission of liability; medical malpractice defendant can waive inadmissibility of any statements."[71] The other bill that did not pass dealt with mandatory alternative dispute resolution before trial of a medical malpractice matter.[72]

South Dakota

South Dakota had one bill, but it did not pass. The bill dealt with requiring an affidavit from a medical expert that the medical malpractice allegation had been evaluated.[73]

Tennessee

Tennessee had 11 bills brought forth, but none passed. These bills dealt with removal of the governmental tort liability limits for civil medical malpractice against facilities and employees protected under the government umbrella; capped noneconomic damages at $250,000; provided for period payments of future damages if the damages exceeded $75,000; new requirements for expert witnesses; and a request for congressional delegation to support medical malpractice reform.[74]

Utah

Utah passed SB 41, which was signed by the governor on March 17, 2006. SB 41 provided that "[i]n any civil action or arbitration proceeding relating to unanticipated outcome of medical care, any statement, gesture, or conduct expressing apology, sympathy or describing event leading to outcome to patient by defendant is inadmissible as evidence of admission of liability or against interest."[75]

Vermont

Vermont brought forth five bills and SB 198 passed with the governor executing on May 15, 2006. SB 198 provided that "[e]xpression of regret or apology by health care provider inadmissible in any civil or administrative proceeding when made within 14 days of when provider knew or should have known consequences of error; health care providers required to report medical errors to patients; Sorry Works program established on voluntary basis, providers who choose to participate required to report unexpected injuries to patient and provider's safety officer; program maintains confidential database of incidents; grants awarded to heath care providers to offset costs of participation."[76] The other bills dealt with minimal standards for reporting medical malpractice incidents; changes to statute of limitations; changes in collateral source evidence; caps on noneconomic damages of $250,000; establish a screening panel for medical injury claims; and approval of premium rate increase by the insurance commissioner.[77]

Virginia

Virginia introduced seven bills and had three pass. The governor executed SB 338 on April 5, 2006, and SJR 90 and HJR 183 on April 4, 2006. SB 610 was adopted on March 23, 2006. SB 338 provided that "[c]ertain professionals including health care practitioners not permitted to disclose confidential information communicated in professional capacity when testifying in civil maters; exceptions for consent of client."[78] SJR 90 and HJR 183 provided "[c]ontinued work of Joint Subcommittee to Study Risk Management Plans for Physicians and Hospitals examining medical malpractice issues and feasibility of creation of health courts."[79] SB 601 provided "[r]isk management plan allowing certain physicians and community hospitals to purchase malpractice insurance extended from 2006 to 2008; *only effective if funding is provided in budget bill*."[80] The other bills dealt with caps for punitive damages at $350,000, which would be deposited into state fund and there would be no plaintiff attorney awards for punitive damages; changes to notices required by insurers when changing rates; and commissioning a study on the establishment of health courts.[81]

Washington

Washington had multiple bills, some of which had carried over from the previous year. These bills also dealt with a statement of apology and whether the statements would be admissible in court; physicians providing care to the indigent could not be held liable for medical malpractice; and issues revolving around insurance premiums.[82]

Wisconsin

Wisconsin introduced four bills regarding tort reform and AB 1072 passed and was executed by the governor on March 22, 2006. AB 1072 provided that "[c]ollateral source payments allowed into evidence in medical malpractice cases, amount of payments, amount claimant is obligated to reimburse, reduction of amount of damages awarded by that amount."[83] Of note two bills passed congress but were vetoed by the governor. These included AB 960 and AB 1073. AB 906 provided "[n]oneconomic damages for medical malpractice occurrence limited to $750,000, plus $5,000 for each year that insured's life expectancy, adjusted annually for inflation; Injured Patients and Families Compensation Fund to adopt life expectancy table; separate limit on noneconomic damages equal to 25% of injury's damages for certain relative; financial maintenance regulations of Fund by Board of Directors and Insurance Commissioner that could affect amount of noneconomic damages limit in certain circumstance."[84] AB 1073 provided that "[n]oneconomic damages for medical malpractice limited to $750,000; Board of Injured Patients and Families Compensation Fund to report to legislature every 2 years any suggested changes to damages limit."[85] The other bill dealt with attorney fees.[86]

Wyoming

Wyoming had two bills, one of which was passed and signed by the governor. HB 81 became law on March 24, 2006, and provided that "Department of Health program to provide loans to physicians for medical malpractice insurance premiums assistance extended until March 2007."[87] The other bill dealt with additional assistance to physicians for payment of malpractice insurance.[88]

Adapted with permission by National Conference of State Legislatures.

FEDERAL

At the federal level, the 2005 proposed legislation was:

- "Limits on noneconomic (pain and suffering) damages at $250,000;
- A 3-year statute of limitations to initiate lawsuits, or one year from discovery; statute of limitations for children until age 8;
- Limits on attorneys' fees in settlement or judgment;
- Collateral source benefits may be introduced into evidence in court;
- Periodic payments ordered for future damages exceeding $50,000;
- Standard guidelines for awarding punitive damages and limitations on the amount awarded;
- Prohibitions on instructing a jury about any limitations to damage awards;
- Punitive damages may not be awarded against the manufacturer or distributor of a medical product approved by the Food and Drug Administration;
- A specific statement that the provisions would preempt all state laws not in conformance with the standards presented."[89]

NOTES

[1] Joint Economic Committee Study, *Improving the American Legal System: The Economic Benefits of Torts Reform* (March 1996), www.house.gov/jec/tort/tort/tort/htm

[2] *Id.*

[3] *Id.*
[4] *Id.*
[5] National Conference of State Legislature, Medical Malpractice Tort Reform (May 1, 2006), www.ncsl.org/standcomm/sclaw/medmaloverview.htm
[6] *Id.*
[7] *Id.*
[8] *Id.*
[9] *Id.*
[10] *Id.*
[11] CNA Insurance web page, www.cna.com, *CNA Study Analyzes Professional Liability Claims, Offers Risk Management Solutions for Physical Therapists* (December 4, 2006).
[12] *Black's Law Dictionary,* 37 (Bryan A. Gardner, ed., 7th ed., West Group, 1999).
[13] Andrews Litigation Reporter, *Study: Tort Reform Has Little Effect on Med-Mal Insurance Rates,* page 10, February 17, 2006.
[14] *Id.*
[15] *Id.* at 11.
[16] *Black's Law Dictionary,* 315 (Bryan A. Gardner, ed., 7th ed., West Group, 1999).
[17–89] National Conference of State Legislature, Medical Malpractice Tort Reform (May 1, 2006), www.ncsl.org/standcomm/sclaw/medmaloverview.htm

CHAPTER 4

The Laws Governing Physical Therapy

This chapter will explain the laws, rules, and regulations governing the practice of physical therapy. These laws should not be confused with the American Physical Therapy Association's policies or practice guidelines. As an organization, the APTA promulgates principles, policies, and position statements for the practice of physical therapy. Principles, policies, and position statements do not require mandatory compliance, whereas, laws require mandatory compliance or the physical therapist, physical therapist assistant, or student could face prosecution (criminal, civil, or administrative) for violation of the law. Recall from Chapter 2 that a violation of a criminal statute subjects someone to criminal prosecution; a violation of a civil right law can subject someone to a lawsuit for liability associated with the violation whereby remuneration has to be paid. Additionally, violation of the law could subject the physical therapist, physical therapist assistant, or student to disciplinary actions against his or her license or prevent a student from obtaining his or her license to practice.

Conversely, violation or lack of adherence to a policy or guideline of the APTA could be used as evidence in a criminal or civil lawsuit or could lead to a member of the association being barred from membership. Thus, this chapter will specifically look at the laws governing physical therapy as well as the rules and regulations governing physical therapy. This chapter will also review other laws that physical therapists, physical therapist assistants, and students must comply with but are not necessarily specific to the profession of physical therapy. These include ordinances, county laws, business laws, and federal regulations.

KEY CONCEPTS

State practice acts
State boards of physical therapy practice

Each state's rules and regulations governing physical therapy
City ordinances
County ordinances
Business laws
Federal regulations
Federation of Physical Therapy State Boards
Medicare regulations
Licensure complaints
Administrative cases

GOVERNMENT ORGANIZATION

The United States' federal government system was established within the Constitution of the United States. In the U.S. Constitution, the government system was divided into a legislative branch, an executive branch, and a judicial branch. However, the federal government for the most part does not control states' actions. In fact, when a state feels that the federal government is overreaching its authority, this is generally called *federalism*. (Refer to Chapter 2 for greater discussion.) Each state's government organization is generally the same but can be a little different.

Just as the president of the United States is the leader for the country of the United States, the governor of a state is the leader and decision maker for his or her state. As with the federal government, the state government has two branches of government so that power is balanced: the house of representatives and the senate. Laws for the state must be approved through both the state's house of representatives and the senate before being signed by the governor. Thus, the laws governing physical therapy for a particular state would have been drafted and promulgated through that state's house and senate and ultimately signed by the state's governor.

As such, states can have different practice and licensure laws. Thus, it is critical before any physical therapist, physical therapist assistant, or student practices in a state that he or she read and understand the laws governing the practice of physical therapy in that state. Recall, ignorance of the law will never be an excuse. The laws governing the practice of physical therapy in that state are referred to as that state's practice act.

Additionally, it should be noted that there is currently a recommendation from the Federation of Physical Therapy State Boards that every state implement a mandatory test for new licensees of that state's laws, rules, and regulations governing the practice of physical therapy in that state. Further, there is some discussion ongoing about making the laws, rules, and regulations exam a mandatory test for all licensees to obtain licensure renewal.

Likewise, it should be recognized that laws can be difficult to understand, change through the legislative and judicial processes, and sometimes are interpreted by decisions rendered through litigation. The rules and regulations promulgated through each state's board of physical therapy practice can also change. Consequently, physical therapists, physical therapist assistants, and students should be active in not only knowing the laws that govern his or her profession, but also active in the process of revising those laws, rules, and regulations as the need arise.

STATE PRACTICE ACTS

Each state has legislatively (house of representatives, senate, and governor) promulgated laws (statutes) that govern the practice of physical therapy in its state. Each state's practice act defines the scope of practice for physical therapists, physical therapist assistants, and students in its state. Most states then delegate the responsibility of further interpretation and rule making for the regulation of the physical therapy profession to that state's board of physical therapy practice. Hence, if a particular law was broad and not well-defined, then the board of physical therapy practice might take that law and develop rules that further define what that particular law means. One example is the definition of supervision. While most states' physical therapy practice acts require ancillary staff to be supervised, there has been much debate on exactly what supervision means and entails. Accordingly, some states' boards of physical therapy practice have defined supervision for their states. Additionally, the APTA has drafted position statements on the issue. Each state's specific practice act is listed in Appendix 4A.

STATE BOARDS OF PHYSICAL THERAPY PRACTICE

Generally, each state has a board of physical therapy practice that is responsible for the rules and regulations governing the profession of physical therapy in its state as well as overseeing the state licensure of physical therapists and physical therapist assistants. The rules and regulations are different than the state's practice act. The state's practice act contains laws or statutes and the board of physical therapy promulgates rules and regulations that expand or define the particular state's laws. These rules and regulations usually can be found in a particular state's administrative code. Some states also define the rules and regulations through the particular agency assigned to license physical therapists and physical therapist assistants.

Thus, the state law might require "appropriate supervision" of nonlicensed personnel, whereas the board of physical therapy practice for that state may further define what "appropriate supervision" means. The physical therapist, the physical therapist assistant, or student should be familiar with his or her state practice act as well as the rules and regulations of his or her board of physical therapy practice.

The state's board of physical therapy practice should not be confused with the state's physical therapy association, which is a component (formerly known as "a chapter") of the APTA. The contact information for each state's board of physical therapy practice as well as the reference for each state's physical therapy rules and regulations, if in existence, are listed in Appendix 4B.

LICENSURE COMPLAINTS

Generally speaking, the boards of physical therapy practice are responsible for reviewing complaints brought against physical therapists, physical therapist assistants, or students for the violation(s) of its rules and regulations or unlawful practice. Usually a consumer or another health care provider will report a violation of the practice act to the state's board of physical therapy practice or a similar department or agency. Each state will have a mechanism for investigating complaints and once the investigation is completed, recommending whether there is probable cause to bring charges against the physical therapist, physical therapist assistant, or student. This is called a *probable cause hearing*.

At a probable cause hearing, the evidence against the physical therapist, physical therapist assistant, or student, usually collected by an investigator for the state, is presented and a panel appointed by the board of physical therapy practice determines whether grounds exist to prosecute the physical therapist, physical therapist assistant, or student for an alleged violation of the practice act. As a note, the laws, rules, and regulations are established generally to ensure public safety. At the probable cause hearing, the physical therapist, physical therapist assistant, or student can also present evidence and has the right to representation by counsel. Because some of the sanctions for violations can be severe, including revocation of the physical therapist's or physical therapist assistant's license or prohibition from obtaining a license, it is recommended to have legal representation.

Once the probable cause panel makes its determination, the complaint is either over and the complaining party is notified so that he or she can appeal the decision, or the panel determines there was probable cause and the physical therapist, physical therapist assistant, or student is prosecuted for the alleged violation of the practice act. Once the probable cause panel finds in the affirmative (there was probable cause to believe there was a violation of the physical therapy practice act), then the matter becomes public record. Prior to that, the matter is usually confidential and not available for public viewing. Thereafter, a hearing will be scheduled and a decision rendered whether there was a violation, and if there was, what, if any, sanction (punishment) should be applied. Available sanctions include monetary fines, suspension, mandatory continuing education, remedial education, revocation of license, or any combination of those sanctions. The sanction is usually discretionary but guidelines usually are found in the rules and regulations for physical therapy for that state.

To further understand this process, a review of the Florida system will be presented. In Florida, the Board of Physical Therapy Practice is an agency within the state's Department of Health. A *complainant* (person making a complaint) would either in written correspondence, E-mail correspondence, or telephonically report to the Board of Physical Therapy Practice or the Department of Health a complaint against a physical therapist or physical therapist assistant licensee or a student of either. The complaint then would be referred to a medical investigator within the Department of Health. The medical investigator would contact both the complainant and the physical therapist, physical therapist assistant, student, or entity against whom the complaint had been registered.

The recipient physical therapist, physical therapist assistant, student, or entity would be given an opportunity to respond to the medical investigator, but is not required to do so. Once the medical investigator completes his or her investigation, the information is turned over to an attorney for the Department of Health who reviews and makes a determination of whether to recommend to the Florida Board of Physical Therapy Practice's probable cause panel that probable cause exists to pursue the complaint, or recommend that probable cause does not exist and the complaint should be dismissed. Ultimately, the Florida Board of Physical Therapy Practice's panel on probable cause makes the decision, but generally relies on the recommendation from the Department of Health's attorney.

If no probable cause exists, then the complainant is notified and he or she can either drop the matter or continue to pursue the matter through civil litigation. Additionally, the recipient physical therapist, physical therapist assistant, or student is also notified in writing of the decision that no probable cause was found to substantiate the complaint; therefore, the matter will not be pursued and remains confidential.

If there was probable cause, then the matter is referred to the Florida Board of Physical Therapy for a hearing. At the hearing both parties (the attorney for the department of health and the recipient physical therapist, physical therapist assistant, or student of the complaint) are allowed to present evidence. At the conclusion, the board of physical therapy practice will make a determination on the merits of the complaint and if the complaint is affirmed, then what type of sanction and the severity of sanctions that should be given. Once the sanction(s) is/are determined, then the board of physical therapy practice will also oversee and verify completion of the sanction. The physical therapist, physical therapist assistant, or student could also petition for review of the decision of the Florida Board of Physical Therapy Practice to Florida's 1st District Court of Appeal.

Lastly, the physical therapist, physical therapist assistant, or student should understand what each potential sanction entails. Some of the potential sanctions (punishment) against licensees include a reprimand, remedial work, revocation, fines, or suspension. A *reprimand* is "a form of discipline—imposed after trial or formal charges—that declares the [physical therapist's, physical therapist assistant's or student's] conduct [was] improper but does not limit his or her right to practice [physical therapy].[1] This written reprimand will be maintained in the physical therapist's, physical therapist assistant's, or student's licensure file and will be available for review as public record. Hence, in litigation, an attorney may request a copy of the licensee's licensure file that could contain this information. This information could then possibly be used in a court of law as evidence to help prove liability. The lawyer attempting to use this information might say to a jury that the physical therapist, physical therapist assistant, or student had been reprimanded or had completed remedial work and yet required additional remedial work; therefore, this therapist or student is clearly incompetent.

Remedial work is a mandate that the physical therapist, physical therapist assistant, or student take a certain number of hours of continuing education or a mandate that the physical therapist, physical therapist assistant, or student take a certain number or type of course within a specified time frame. *Fines* are monetary in nature and are discretionary with guidance from the rules and regulations as to the amount. It should be noted and understood that fines could be adjudicated for each instance of conduct in violation of the physical therapy practice act.

Suspension means the physical therapist, physical therapist assistant, or student is prohibited from practicing physical therapy for a specified amount of time. This again is made a part of the physical therapist's, physical therapist assistant's, or student's licensure file and is available to the public for review.

Revocation is the permanent cancellation of the physical therapist's or physical therapist assistant's license to practice physical therapy in that state. Thus, if the physical therapist's or physical therapist assistant's license is revoked, that therapist will not be allowed to practice physical therapy in that state from that date forward. It is also unlikely the physical therapist, physical therapist assistant, or student could obtain a license to practice physical therapy in any other state.

THE FEDERATION OF STATE BOARDS OF PHYSICAL THERAPY

The Federation of State Boards of Physical Therapy (FSBPT) is composed of a representative from each of the states' boards of physical therapy practice. The FSBPT is responsible for the development and administration of the licensure examination for physical therapists and physical therapist assistants. The examination for physical therapists' and physical therapist assistants' licensure is called the National Physical Therapy Examination (NPTE) and is administered in all 50 states as well as three other jurisdictions.[2]

The FSBPT also has developed a jurisprudence examination for physical therapists, physical therapist assistants, or students to test their knowledge of the laws, rules, and regulations governing physical therapy. As of 2007, the jurisprudence examination currently is being administered in Alabama, Arizona, the District of Columbia, California, Georgia, Florida, and Nebraska. There is discussion and promotion by the FSBPT to require this examination as part of the licensure process in all states. Further, there is some discussion about making the jurisprudence examination and achieving a passing score as a requirement for renewal of the physical therapist's and physical therapist assistant's license.

ADMINISTRATIVE CASE

Now to look at a case that is about violations of the physical therapy practice acts, rules, or regulations of a state. In *Sibley v. The North Carolina Board of Therapy Examiners*, 566 S.E.2d 486 (N.C. App. 2002), a physical therapist was accused of having relationships, including sexual relations, with patients who were on active caseload. The physical therapist denied that there were ever any relations, including sexual relations, with either patient while they were on active caseload.[3]

After a 2-day hearing before the North Carolina Board of Physical Therapy Practice, the board suspended the physical therapist's license.[4] Thereafter, the physical therapist petitioned for a review of the decision before the superior court in

Buncombe County.[5] The trial court remanded the decision back to the North Carolina Board of Physical Therapy Practice for a determination of whether the physical therapist "knew or should have known whether [the] behavior constituted grounds for disciplinary actions."[6]

The North Carolina Board of Physical Therapy Practice responded back in the affirmative that the physical therapist knew or should have known his conduct would be a matter for disciplinary action.[7] Thus, the North Carolina Board of Physical Therapy Practice upheld its prior decision and told the superior court that the physical therapist knew or should have known his conduct could be subjected to disciplinary action. The physical therapist again appealed the decision to the superior court in Buncombe County.[8] The trial court (Superior Court in Buncombe County) affirmed the North Carolina Board of Physical Therapy Practice's decision.[9] Thereafter, the physical therapist appealed to the North Carolina Court of Appeal.[10]

Before the North Carolina Court of Appeal, the physical therapist first argued the case against him was barred because of *laches* (statute of limitations expiration).[11] In that regard, the physical therapist pointed out that the alleged violations (conduct) occurred in 1990 and 1991.[12] The first time the physical therapist received notification from the North Carolina Board of Physical Therapy Practice that there was a complaint was in August 1996, which would be approximately 5 to 6 years after the alleged misconduct had occurred,[13] then the hearing before the North Carolina Board of Physical Therapy Practice did not occur for another 2 years, in August 1998.[14]

The physical therapist argued the ability to recall events and details had faded with time and irreparably impaired his ability to defend the action, which would be akin to a violation of the physical therapist's due-process rights.[15] The appellate court disagreed and essentially stated there was no "case where the defense of laches had been applied to an administrative hearing concerning the revocation of a professional license."[16] Further, the appellate court reminded the physical therapist that one of the alleged victims had filed a civil lawsuit against the physical therapist for this conduct in 1993.[17]

The physical therapist answered interrogatories for the civil lawsuit and was therefore very well aware of the allegations in 1993.[18] Additionally, the physical therapist identified no witness who demonstrated difficulty recalling events, no witness was unavailable, and the physical therapist was not demonstrating difficulty recalling the events.[19] Thus, the physical therapist failed to establish any due-process violation and no real prejudice could be established.[20] Hence, the argument of laches, expiration of the statute of limitations, failed.

The second argument the physical therapist made to the appellate court in an effort to have the appellate court overturn the superior court's affirmation of the North

Carolina Board of Physical Therapy Practice's decision was that the laws being applied to the physical therapist's conduct were unconstitutionally vague.[21] Again the appellate court disagreed.[22] For North Carolina law at the time, the test (standard) as to whether a law that set out standards for professional conduct was unconstitutionally vague was "whether a reasonably intelligent member of the profession would understand that the conduct in question [was] forbidden."[23] The particular laws, North Carolina General Statute § 90-270.36 (7) and North Carolina General Statute § 90-270.36 (9), stated the following:[24]

> N.C. Gen. Stat. § 90-270.37 (7)—The commission of an act or acts of malpractice, gross negligence or incompetence in the practice of physical therapy; and N.C. Gen. Stat. § 90-270.36 (9)—Engaging in conduct that could result in harm or injury to the public.

Accordingly, the question with regard to whether these laws were constitutionally vague was going to be answered on the basis of whether a reasonably intelligent member of the physical therapy profession would understand that the conduct in question was forbidden.

The appellate court looked at the question as to whether having a sexual relationship with a physical therapy patient "could result in harm or injury to the public."[25] The appellate court concluded that the North Carolina laws' language was adequate "to provide the North Carolina Board of Physical Therapy Practice with the authority to determine that [the physical therapist's] actions violated acceptable standards of practice in the physical therapy field."[26]

As with any appeal, the party filing the appeal usually asserts several arguments of error that occurred in the court below the appellate court. As such, in this case, the third argument the physical therapist used in an attempt to get the North Carolina Board of Physical Therapy Practice's ruling overturned was that the members of North Carolina Board of Physical Therapy Practice improperly used their own beliefs as physical therapists to determine whether the physical therapist knew or should have known the conduct would violate professional standards of conduct.[27] Based on prior decisions from cases, the appellate court again disagreed and this argument also failed.[28]

Another argument the physical therapist used in an attempt to get the decision overturned was that there was insufficient evidence for the North Carolina Board of Physical Therapy Practice to make its decision.[29] For North Carolina, the test to determine if there was sufficient evidence in the record was called the whole-record test.[30] The whole record test was defined as:

> If, after all of the record has been reviewed, substantial competent evidence is found which would support the agency ruling, the ruling must stand. In this context substantial evidence has been held to mean 'such relevant evidence as a reasonable mind might accept as adequate to support a conclusion.' Therefore, in reaching its decision, the reviewing court is prohibited from replacing the Agency's findings of fact with its own judgment of how credible, or incredible the testimony appears to them to be, so long as substantial evidence of those findings exists in the whole record.[31]

Thus, the appellate court enumerated the North Carolina Board of Physical Therapy Practice's factual findings as follows:

1. "A physical attraction confuses the relationship between the patient and the therapist, particularly in cranial sacral therapy, which can induce a somato emotional release that requires a very strong level of trust between the physical therapist and the patient";
2. [T]he therapist "knew it would be wrong to take advantage of a patient during somato emotional release";
3. [T]he therapist "knew that an attraction between himself and a patient would interfere with physical therapy treatment";
4. [T]he therapist "knew in 1991 that it was not permissible for a licensed physical therapist to have a sexual relationship with a patient outside the office";
5. "[D]uring physical therapy education, [the therapist] was taught not to have sex with a patient"; and
6. "Licensees, including [the therapist], should have known that it was a violation of the Physical Therapy Practice Act in 1991 to engage in full body hugs with a patient, kiss a patient on the lips or have sexual intercourse with a patient."[32]

Thus, based on these findings of fact, the North Carolina Board of Physical Therapy determined the physical therapist had violated the North Carolina Physical Therapy Practice Act.[33] The physical therapist argued against the North Carolina Board of Physical Therapy Practice's conclusion, stating that nothing "specifically prohibit[ed] sexual relations with a patient."[34]

However, the court reasoned the North Carolina Board of Physical Therapy Practice determined the physical therapist knew or should have known the conduct was improper; expert testimony supported the physical therapist knew or should have known the conduct was improper; and the physical therapist acknowledged he knew there should not have been a sexual relationship with a patient.[35] The physical therapist's testimony that during the time of the sexual relationship, treatment was not occurring, was not supported in the evidence.[36] Thus, after reviewing the whole record before the appellate court, the appellate court determined there was enough evidence to support the North Carolina Board of Physical Therapy Practice's ruling.[37]

One of the last arguments the physical therapist made was that there was a lack of evidence in the record to sustain the North Carolina Board of Physical Therapy Practice and trial court's determination of facts and conclusions.[38] The physical therapist argued that because the sexual conduct was consensual, it was not a violation of North Carolina laws.[39] Again the court used the whole-record test and determined that the physical therapist knew or should have known even consensual sexual activity with a patient, even if done outside the office, was prohibited.[40]

As a final attempt for leniency, the physical therapist argued the sanctions of the North Carolina Board of Physical Therapy Practice were "excessively severe and therefore arbitrary and capricious in nature and in violation" of another North Carolina law.[41] The other North Carolina law specifically stated:

> The arbitrary and capricious standard is a difficult one to meet. Administrative agency decisions may be reversed as arbitrary or capricious if they are patently in bad faith or whimsical in the sense that they indicate a lack of fair and careful consideration or fail to indicate any course of reasoning and the exercise of judgment.[42]

The appellate court reasoned the North Carolina Board of Physical Therapy Practice factually found the physical therapist had sexual relations with one patient and engaged in physical touching with another; therefore, the punishment of license suspension for 3 years with active suspension for 9 months did not violate this North Carolina law.[43] Thus, after all the physical therapist's arguments that the North Carolina Board of Physical Therapy Practice erred in its decision, and the trial court's upholding of the North Carolina Board of Physical Therapy Practice's decision, the appellate court determined no errors occurred and upheld the North Carolina Board of Physical Therapy Practice's decision.

The *Sibley* case demonstrates the process undertaken when a complaint is filed against a physical therapist's or physical therapist assistant's license. It should be recognized that the law the physical therapist was prosecuted under did not specifically state that physical therapists or physical therapist assistants could not engage in physical touching or sexual relations with a patient. Further, the physical therapist made this specific argument to the appellate court without success. Thus, not only do physical therapists, physical therapist assistants, and students need to know the laws, rules, and regulations of his or her state, the physical therapist, physical therapist assistant, and student also need to consider whether his or her conduct could be construed to be of potential harm to the public.

In the *Sibley* case, it appears the North Carolina Board of Physical Therapy Practice was concerned with physical therapists or physical therapist assistants performing treatments that could lead to a patient having an emotional release such that intimate relations with that patient might be the result of taking advantage of the patient because the provider just performed a treatment that led to emotional vulnerability. Thus, the concern or potential public harm could be that physical therapists or physical therapist assistants could use this technique to take advantage of some patients. Consequently, because the North Carolina Board of Physical Therapy Practice and each state's board of physical therapy practice is charged with protecting the public from such type of harm, the North Carolina Board of Physical Therapy Practice's decision was upheld by the superior court of Buncombe County and the subsequent appellate court. Consequently, the decision was that the physical therapist violated the North Carolina Physical Therapy Practice Act.

CITY AND COUNTY LAWS (ORDINANCES)

Depending on where the physical therapist, physical therapist assistant, or student practices, the clinic wherein the physical therapy services are being provided may also be subject to city and/or county ordinances related to the operation of the clinic. An *ordinance* is defined as "[a]n authoritative law or decree; esp[ecially] a municipal regulation. Municipal governments can pass ordinances on matters that the state government allows to be regulated at the local level."[44] Some of the typical city and county laws include occupational licenses, city taxes, county taxes, and infection control.

OTHER RULES AND REGULATIONS IMPACTING PHYSICAL THERAPY

Besides the state's physical therapy practice act, the state's board of physical therapy practice rules and regulations, and city and county ordinances, the physical therapist, physical therapist assistant, and student also should be aware of different rules and regulations promulgated by third parties involved in general business operation, including other rules and regulations contained within administrative codes, insurance companies, Medicare, and Medicaid. The best way to understand these additional laws, rules, and regulations—some of which are mandatory for insurance reimbursement—is to attend a course on continuing education or contact the agency for insurance and have your specific questions answered.

SUMMARY

Physical therapy services are governed by the laws, rules, and regulations of each individual state. States can vary in the particular laws, rules, and regulations governing the practice of physical therapy in its state. Each state's board of physical therapy practice promulgates rules and regulations that define the state's practice act in greater detail. Violations of a law, rule, or regulation can subject a licensee to sanctions by the state's board of physical therapy practice.

DISCUSSION QUESTIONS

1. What is a practice act?
2. What is the difference between a state's practice act and the state's board of physical therapy practice rules and regulations?
3. Explain a licensure complaint.
4. What are the stages in a licensure complaint?
5. What is probable cause as it relates to a licensure complaint?
6. Discuss some of the possible sanctions that can be given to a licensee for violation of the state's practice act.
7. What is FSBPT?
8. Discuss the *Sibley* case and its importance.
9. What are ordinances?

Appendix 4A

STATE-BY-STATE PRACTICE ACT REFERENCE

Alabama

Code of Alabama § 34–24–190, et. seq.—Physical Therapy Practice Act

Alaska

Alaska Statutes 08.04—Physical Therapy Practice Act

Alaska Centralized Licensing Statutes 08.01–08.03 (apply to all professions)

Arizona

Arizona Statutes Title 32

Chapter 19—Physical Therapy Practice Act

Arkansas

Arkansas Statutes Title 17

Subtitle 3

Chapter 93—Physical Therapy Practice Act

California

California Statutes

Business and Profession Code

Chapter 5.7—Physical Therapy Practice Act

§§ 2600–2696

Colorado

Colorado Statutes

Title 12

Article 41—Physical Therapy Practice Act

§§ 101–130

Connecticut*

Connecticut General Statutes

Chapter 376—Physical Therapy Practice Act

§ 83 of Public Act 06–195

Delaware

Delaware Code

Title 24

Chapter 26—Physical Therapy Practice Act

District of Columbia

District of Columbia Municipal Regulations

Title 17

Chapter 67—Physical Therapy Practice Act

Florida

Florida statutes

Chapter 486—Physical Therapy Practice Act

Chapter 456—applicable to health professional and occupations

Georgia

Georgia Statutes

Title 43

Chapter 33—Physical Therapy Practice Act

*__Mandatory professional liability insurance__ effective October 1, 2006

Hawaii

Hawaii Revised Statutes
Chapter 461J—Physical Therapy Practice Act
Chapter 436B—professional and vocational licensing

Idaho

Idaho Statutes
Title 54
Chapter 22—Physical Therapy Practice Act

Illinois

Illinois Compiled Statutes
Professions and Occupations
225 ILCS 90—Physical Therapy Practice Act

Indiana

Indiana Code
Title 25
Article 27—Physical Therapy Practice Act

Iowa

Iowa Statutes
Title IV—Public Health
Subtitle 3
Chapter 148A—Physical Therapy Practice Act

Kansas

Kansas Statutes
Chapter 65
Article 29—Physical Therapy Practice Act

Kentucky

Kentucky Statutes
Chapter 327—Physical Therapy Practice Act

Louisiana

Louisiana Revised Statutes
Title 37
§§ 2401–2421—Physical Therapy Practice Act

Maine

Maine Statutes
Title 32
Chapter 45A, §§ 3111–3119—Physical Therapy Practice Act

Maryland

Maryland Annotated Code
Title 13—Physical Therapy Practice Act

Massachusetts

Massachusetts General Laws
Part I
Chapter 112, §§ 23A–23Q and §§ 61–65

Michigan

Michigan Compiled Laws
Act 368 of 1978
Article 15
Part 178
Chapter 333, § 333.17801—Physical Therapy Act

Minnesota

Minnesota Statutes
Chapter 148, §§ 148.65–148.78—Physical Therapy Practice Act

Mississippi

Mississippi Code
Title 73
Chapter 23—Physical Therapy Practice Act

Missouri

Missouri Revised Statutes
Title XXII
Chapter 334—Physical Therapy Practice Act

Montana

Montana Code
Title 37
Chapter 11—Physical Therapy Practice Act

Nebraska

Nebraska Revised Statutes
Chapter 71, §§ 1-376–1-1.389

Nevada

Nevada Revised Statutes
Chapter 640—Physical Therapy Practice Act

New Hampshire

New Hampshire Revised Statutes
Title XXX
Chapter 328–A—Physical Therapy Practice Act

New Jersey

New Jersey Statutes
Title 45
Chapter 9—Physical Therapy Practice Act

New Mexico

New Mexico Statutes
Chapter 61
Article 12—Physical Therapy Practice Act

New York

New York Statutes
Title VII
Article 136—Physical Therapy Practice Act

North Carolina

North Carolina Statutes 90–270.24 through 90–270.39

North Dakota

North Dakota Statutes
Chapter 43
Subsection 26—Physical Therapy Practice Act

Ohio

Ohio Revised Code
Chapter 4755—Physical Therapy Practice Act

Oklahoma

Oklahoma Statutes
Title 59
§§ 887.1 through 887.18

Oregon

Oregon Revised Statutes
Volume 15
Chapter 688

Pennsylvania

Pennsylvania Statutes
Act 92

Rhode Island

General Law of Rhode Island
Title 5
Chapter 40

South Carolina

South Carolina Code of Laws
Title 40
Chapter 45

South Dakota

South Dakota Code
Title 36
Chapter 10

Tennessee

Tennessee Statutes
Title 63
Chapter 13
Part 3

Texas

Texas Statutes
Occupation Codes
Title 3
Chapter 453

Utah

Utah Code
Title 58
Chapter 24a

Vermont

Vermont Statutes
Title 26
Chapter 38

Virginia

Virginia Statutes
Title 54.1
Chapter 34.1

Washington

Revised Code of Washington
Chapter 18.74

West Virginia

West Virginia Code
Chapter 30
Article 20

Wisconsin

Wisconsin Statutes
Chapter 448
Subchapter III

Wyoming

Wyoming Statutes
Title 33
Chapter 25

Appendix 4B

STATE BOARDS OF PHYSICAL THERAPY PRACTICE

Alabama

Alabama Board of Physical Therapy
100 North Union Street, Suite 724
Montgomery, Alabama 36130-5040

Alabama Administrative Code
Chapter 700–x–1

Alaska

State Physical Therapy and Occupational Therapy Board
Department of Community and Economic Development
333 Willoughby Avenue, 9th Floor
Juneau, Alaska 99811

Alaska Administrative Code
12 AAC 54
12 AAC 02—applies to all professions

Arizona

Arizona State Board of Physical Therapy
1400 West Washington, Suite 240
Phoenix, Arizona 85007

Arizona Administrative Code
Title 4
Chapter 24

Arkansas

Arkansas State Board of Physical Therapy
9 Shackleford Plaza, Suite 3
Little Rock, Arkansas 72211

Arkansas Administrative Code
Rules and Regulations of Arkansas State Board of Physical Therapy

California

Physical Therapy Board of California
1418 Howe Avenue, Suite 16
Sacramento, California 95825

California Code of Regulations
Title 16
Division 13.2

Colorado

Colorado Physical Therapy Licensure
Division of Registrations
1560 Broadway, Suite 1340
Denver, Colorado 80202-5146

Colorado Code of Regulation
Colorado Physical Therapy Licensure Rule 1–9

Connecticut

Office of Practitioner Licensing and Certification
410 Capital Avenue, MS 12APP
Hartford, Connecticut 06134-0308

Connecticut Administrative Rules and Regulations for Licensure

Delaware

Division of Professional Regulation
Cannon Building
861 Silver Lake Boulevard, Suite 203
Dover, Delaware 19904-2467

Delaware Administrative Code
Title 24
§ 2600

District of Columbia

District of Columbia Board of Physical Therapy
Health Professional Licensing Administration
717 14th Street, NW, Suite 600
Washington, DC 20005

No specific rules and regulations per administrative code

Florida

MQA/Board of Physical Therapy Practice
Bin C–05
4052 Bald Cypress Way
Tallahassee, Florida 32399-3255

Florida Administrative Code
Chapter 64B-17

Georgia

Georgia Board of Physical Therapy
237 Coliseum Drive
Macon, Georgia 31217-3858

Rules of Georgia State Physical Therapy Board of Physical Therapy
Chapter 490

Hawaii

Hawaii Department of Commerce and Consumer Affairs
P.O. Box 3496
Honolulu, Hawaii 96801

Hawaii Administrative Rules
Chapter 110

Idaho

Idaho State Board of Medicine
P.O. Box 83720
Boise, Idaho 83720-0058

Idaho Administrative Code
24.13.01

Illinois

Department of Professional Regulation
Attn: Health Services Section
320 West Washington Street, 3rd Floor
Springfield, Illinois 62786

Illinois Administrative Code
Title 68

Chapter VII
Part 1340

Indiana

Indiana Physical Therapy Committee
402 East Washington Street, Room W041
Indianapolis, Indiana 46204

Indiana Administrative Code
Title 844
Article 6

Iowa

Iowa Department of Public Health
Lucas State Office Building
321 East 12th Street, 5th Floor
Des Moines, Iowa 50319-0075

Human Services Department—Professional Licensure Regulation and Practice
Chapter 200

Kansas

Kansas State Board of Healing Arts
Physical Therapy Examining Committee
235 South Topeka Boulevard
Topeka, Kansas 66614

Kansas State Board of Healing Arts
Article 29

Kentucky

Kentucky Board of Physical Therapy
9110 Leesgate Road, 6
Louisville, Kentucky 40222-5159

Kentucky Administrative Regulations
Chapter 22

Louisiana

Louisiana State Board of Physical Therapy Examiners
104 Fairland Drive
Lafayette, Louisiana 70507

Louisiana Administrative Code
Part LIV
Subpart 1
Chapter 1 and Subchapter A

Maine

Board of Examiners in Physical Therapy
35 State House Station
Augusta, Maine 04333-0035

Rules of the Department of Professional and Finance Regulation
02 393
Chapter 1–7

Maryland

Maryland Board of Physical Therapy Examiners
4201 Patterson Avenue, 223
Baltimore, Maryland 21215-2299

Code of Maryland Regulations
Title 10
Subtitle 38

Massachusetts

Massachusetts Board of Allied Health Professionals
Division of Registration
239 Causeway Street, Suite 500
Boston, Massachusetts 02114

Allied Health Professional
259 Code of Massachusetts Regulation
§§ 2.00–6.00

Michigan

Michigan Department of Community Health
611 West Ottawa, 1st Floor
Lansing, Michigan 48909-7518

Michigan Administrative Rules
Department Community Health
Bureau of Health Profession
Board of Physical Therapy

Minnesota

Minnesota Board of Physical Therapy
2829 University Avenue, SE, Suite 420
Minneapolis, Minnesota 55414-3245

Minnesota Physical Therapy Rules
Chapter 5601

Mississippi

Mississippi State Board of PT
P.O. Box 55707
Jackson, Mississippi 39296-5707

Mississippi Agencies
Department of Health
Regulation and Licensure

Missouri

Missouri Advisory Commission for Professional Physical Therapists and Physical Therapist Assistants
P.O. Box 4
Jefferson, Missouri 65102

Department of Insurance, Finance
Title 20
Division 2150
Chapter 3

Montana

Montana Board of Physical Therapy
301 South Park, 4th Floor
P.O. Box 200513
Helena, Montana 59620

Montana Administrative Rules
Title 2
Chapter 15
Part 172D
8.42.101, et. seq.

Nebraska

Nebraska Board of Physical Therapy
Department of Regulation and Licensure
301 Centennial Mall
P.O. Box 94986
Lincoln, Nebraska 68509-4986

Nebraska Health and Human Services Department
Chapter 137

Nevada

Nevada State Board of Physical Therapy Examiners
810 South Durango Drive, Suite 109
Las Vegas, Nevada 89145

Nevada Administrative Code
Chapter 640

New Hampshire

Physical Therapy Governing Board of New Hampshire
Office of Allied Health Professionals
2 Industrial Park Drive
Concord, New Hampshire 03301

Governing Board of Physical Therapy
Med 800 rules—Chapter Med 100

New Jersey

New Jersey State Board of Physical Therapy
P.O. Box 45014
Newark, New Jersey 07101

Professional Boards and Advisory Committee
Health Related Professional Boards
Board of Physical Therapy

New Mexico

New Mexico Physical Therapy Board
P.O. Box 25101
Santa Fe, New Mexico 87505

New Mexico Administrative Code
Title 16
Chapter 20

New York

New York Physical Therapy, Podiatry and Ophthalmic Dispensing
Office of the Professions
New York Education Department
89 Washington Avenue
Albany, New York 12234

77 Regulation of the Community Health
Part 29 Rules of Board of Regents

North Carolina

North Carolina Board of Physical Therapy Examiners
18 West Colony Place, 140
Durham, North Carolina 27705

North Dakota

North Dakota State Examining Committee for PT
Box 69
Grafton, North Dakota 58237

North Dakota Administrative Code
Title 61.5

Ohio

Ohio Occupational Therapy, Physical Therapy, and Athletic Trainers Board
77 South High Street, 16th Floor
Columbus, Ohio 43215-6108

Ohio Administrative Code
Chapter 4755-21 through 4755-29

Oklahoma

Oklahoma Board of Medical Licensure and Supervision
Physical Therapy Advisory Committee
5104 North Francis, Suite C
Oklahoma, Oklahoma 73118-0256

Oklahoma Administrative Code
Title 435
Chapter 20

Oregon

Oregon Physical Therapy Licensing Board
800 NE Oregon Street, Suite 407
Portland, Oregon 97232-2187

Oregon Administrative Code
Chapter 848

Pennsylvania

Pennsylvania State Board of Physical Therapy
P.O. Box 2649
Harrisburg, Pennsylvania 17105-2649

Pennsylvania Administrative Code
Chapter 40
Subchapter A—physical therapists
Subchapter C—physical therapist assistants

Puerto Rico

Puerto Rico Office of Regulation and Certification
Call Box 10200
Santurce, Puerto Rico 00908

Rhode Island

Rhode Island Department of Health
3 Capitol Hill, Room 104
Providence, Rhode Island 02908-5097

Department of Health
Professional Regulation
Rules and Regulations for Licensing Physical Therapists and Physical Therapist Assistants

South Carolina

South Carolina Board of Physical Therapy Examiners
110 Centerview Drive
P.O. Box 11329
Columbia, South Carolina 29211

South Carolina Code of Regulations
Chapter 101

South Dakota

South Dakota Board of Medical Examiners
1323 South Minnesota Avenue
Sioux Falls, South Dakota 57105

South Dakota Administrative Rules
Rule 20:66

Tennessee

Tennessee Division of Health Related Boards
Board of Occupational and Physical Therapy
426 5th Avenue North, 1st Floor
Nashville, Tennessee 37247-1010

Tennessee Rules and Regulations
1150

Texas

Texas Board of Physical Therapy Examiners
333 Guadalupe, Suite 2–510
Austin, Texas 78701-3942

Texas Administrative Code
Title 22
Part 16
Chapters 321 through 347

Utah

Utah Division of Occupational and Professional Licensing
160 E 300 South
P.O. Box 146741
Salt Lake City, Utah 84114

Utah Administrative Code
Commerce
Rules 156–24a

Vermont

Vermont Physical Therapy Advisors
Office of Professional Regulation
26 Terrace Street
Drawer 09
Montpelier, Vermont 05609-1106

Vermont Secretary of State
Office of Professional Regulation
Administrative Rules for Physical Therapists and Physical Therapist Assistants

Virginia

Virginia Board of Physical Therapy
Department of Health Professions
6603 West Broad Street
Richmond, Virginia 23230

Virginia Administrative Code
Title 18
Agency 112
18 VAC 112020-10 et. seq.

Virgin Islands

Virgin Islands Boards of Physical Therapy Examiners
Department of Health—Department of Commissioner
48 Sugar Estate
St. Thomas, Virgin Islands 00802

Washington

Washington Board of Physical Therapy
P.O. Box 47867
Olympia, Washington 98504-7867

Washington Administrative Code
Title 246
Chapter 246–915

West Virginia

West Virginia Board of Physical Therapy
210 Oak Drive, Suite A
Clarksburg, West Virginia 26301

Regulatory Law—General Provision
Title 16
Series 1

Wisconsin

Wisconsin Department of Regulation and Licensing
1400 East Washington Avenue, Room 178
P.O. Box 8935
Madison, Wisconsin 53708-8935

Wisconsin Administrative Code
Physical Therapist Affiliated Credentialing Board
PT 1–PT 9

Wyoming

Wyoming Board of Physical Therapy
2020 Carey Avenue, Suite 201
Cheyenne, Wyoming 82002

Wyoming Professional Licensing Boards
PT Board

NOTES

[1] *Black's Law Dictionary*, page 1305 (Bryan A. Garner, ed., 7th ed., West Group, 1999).
[2] The Federation for Boards of Physical Therapy Practice webpage, www.fsbpt.org.
[3] *Sibley v. The North Carolina Board of Therapy Examiners*, 566 S.E.2d 486, 487 (N.C. App. 2002).
[4] *Id.*
[5] *Id.*
[6] *Id.*
[7] *Id.*
[8] *Id.*
[9] *Id.*
[10] *Id.*
[11] *Id.*
[12] *Id.*
[13] *Id.*
[14] *Id.*
[15] *Id.*
[16] *Id.*

[17] *Id.*
[18] *Id.*
[19] *Id.*
[20] *Id.*
[21] *Id.* at 489.
[22] *Id.*
[23] *Id.*
[24] *Id.*
[25] *Id.*
[26] *Id.*
[27] *Id.*
[28] *Id.*
[29] *Id.*
[30] *Id.*
[31] *Id.*
[32] *Id.*
[33] *Id.*
[34] *Id.*
[35] *Id.*
[36] *Id.*
[37] *Id.*
[38] *Id.* at 491.
[39] *Id.*
[40] *Id.*
[41] *Id.*
[42] North Carolina General Statute § 150B-51(b)(6).
[43] *Id.*
[44] *Black's Law Dictionary,* 1125 (Bryan A. Garner, ed., 7th ed., West Group, 1999).

CHAPTER 5

Negligence or Medical Malpractice Claims

In the world of law, lawsuits (civil) or criminal charges are brought based on certain causes of action. A *cause of action* is defined as "[a] group of operative facts giving rise to one or more bases for suing; a factual situation that entitles one person to obtain a remedy in court from another person. A legal theory of a lawsuit."[1] The most common cause of action a physical therapist, physical therapist assistant, or student will face is a claim of negligence. In some states, this cause of action, *negligence*, will actually be called *medical malpractice*. For this book's purpose, the two terms will be synonymous.

Each cause of action has specific elements that must be proven in order for a party to prevail. An *element* is defined as "[a] constituent part of a claim that must be proved for the claim to succeed."[2] Further, depending on the type of claim, different standards of proof are required. As previously discussed in Chapter 2, in criminal law, the standard of proof is beyond a reasonable doubt. In civil law, which is where a negligence claim would be brought, the standard of proof is by a preponderance of the evidence, or, as some states call it, the greater weight of the evidence. Lastly, some states have elevated the standard of proof for a claim of punitive damages and for some civil causes of action to the clear-and-convincing level. Thus, the most common lawsuit a physical therapist, physical therapist assistant, or student will confront is a claim asserting negligence that must have each element proven by a preponderance of the evidence, which is also known as by a greater weight of the evidence, in order for a plaintiff to prevail at trial.

The remainder of this chapter will further define these elements and actual cases of negligence will be discussed. Most of the cases used as illustration will usually involve physical therapists or physical therapist assistants.

KEY CONCEPTS

Elements for a cause of action in negligence (medical malpractice)
Duty
Breach of duty
Causation
Damages
Cause of action
Medical malpractice or negligence
Guide to Physical Therapy Practice

ELEMENTS FOR A CAUSE OF ACTION FOR MEDICAL NEGLIGENCE

As previously discussed, a cause of action has enumerated elements that must be proved at the different levels of burdens of persuasion depending on the type of action. For a cause of action of medical negligence, the elements are:

1. Duty
2. Breach of the duty
3. Causation to include actual and proximate
4. Damages

Each of these elements must be proven by a preponderance of the evidence or a greater weight of the evidence. Thus, a plaintiff must first establish the duty a physical therapist, physical therapist assistant, or student owed the plaintiff. The duty owed in the treatment of the patient will be different than the duty owed regarding the maintenance of the premises where the patient may be receiving the physical therapy services.

The *Guide to Physical Therapy Practice*, published by the American Physical Therapy Association, is now in its second edition and generally establishes guidelines for how a physical therapist, physical therapist assistant, or student should perform his or her duties and what should be considered in the determination of a plan of a care. While this is a guide, the physical therapist, physical therapist assistant, and student is now put into a position of defending and establishing that the guidance pursuant to this document has been considered and/or followed or the rationale for why it was not followed.

Regardless of whether it was intended to establish a physical therapist's, physical therapist assistant's, or student's duty, the *Guide to Physical Therapy Practice* can be argued as establishing his or her duty. Another phrase used to describe duty is the *standard of care*. In other words, what is the standard of care that the patient should expect to receive from the physical therapist, physical therapist assistant, or student?

A physical therapist, physical therapist assistant, and/or student generally should be expected to act as a reasonable or similarly situated physical therapist, physical therapist assistant, or student would act in like circumstances. Consequently, one document that could be used to establish this duty is the *Guide to Physical Therapy Practice*.

WHAT IS DUTY?

Duty is probably one of the most difficult concepts in law to define and is further complicated because, depending on the situation, a different level or type of duty might be applicable. *Black's Law Dictionary* defines *duty* as "[a] legal obligation that is owed or due to another and that needs to be satisfied; for every duty somebody else has a corresponding right."[3] There are multiple types of duty in the delivery of physical therapy services as well as duties created by various practice settings. This chapter will examine several duties related to the practice of physical therapy and Chapter 9 will discuss various duties created related to various practice settings. For the physical therapists, physical therapist assistants, and students, some of the duties that will be applicable to the practice of physical therapy include affirmative duty, contractual duty, duty to act, duty to speak, legal duty, nondelegable duty, duty of loyalty, and fiduciary duty.

Affirmative Duty

An *affirmative duty* is defined as "[a] duty to take a positive step to do something."[4] During the course of a physical therapist's, physical therapist assistant's, or student's practice, it is likely that the therapist will treat a patient who has signs or symptoms of physical, mental, or verbal abuse. The physical therapist, physical therapist assistant, or student is under an affirmative duty to take a step of action and report the suspected abuse to the proper authority. Thus, the physical therapist, physical therapist assistant, or student is under a duty to do something: report.

This situation is probably most observed with physical therapists or physical therapist assistants who work in acute care hospitals, pediatrics, or home health. In hospitals, the physical therapists, physical therapist assistants, and students may see patients following physical trauma and the description of how the trauma occurred raises suspicion that abuse (physical) may have occurred. The physical therapists, physical therapist assistants, or students have an affirmative duty to report their suspicions and the rationale for their suspicions, but should not be the individuals who undertake the investigation. The investigation should be left to the individuals who are trained for such an investigation.

In home health, physical therapists, physical therapist assistants, or students may encounter the same types of observations. There may be a bruise that was not there the previous treatment and the patient cannot explain how it occurred. Additionally, the patient's family may seem nervous or overly helpful with explaining how the bruise occurred, or there may be repetitive injuries without explanation. Thus, the physical therapist, physical therapist assistant, or student has a duty to report his or her observations, but again there is not a duty to investigate. Accordingly, the physical therapist, physical therapist assistant, or student should understand he or she is under a duty to report.

Likewise, physical therapists, physical therapist assistants, or students who are working in nursing homes or assisted-living facilities where the population is elderly may observe some of the same types of injuries. Every health care provider in facilities that care for the elderly are under an affirmative obligation (duty) to report any suspicion of any type of abuse to the proper authorities. Failure to report can be viewed as a breach of duty and could lead to a complaint being filed against a physical therapist's or physical therapist assistant's license. It should also be noted that not every observation or repetitive injury that cannot be explained is the result of some type of abuse. However, the duty is not to determine whether there is actual abuse, but rather the duty is to report what is out of the ordinary.

Contractual Duty

A *contractual duty* is defined as "[a] duty arising under a particular contract."[5] For physical therapists, physical therapist assistants, and students, it should be fairly easy to understand this particular type of duty that arises because of the existence of a contract between the therapist and someone else. The contract could be between the physical therapist and/or the physical therapist assistant and/or the student and his or her respective college or employer.

The contract could also exist after graduation between the physical therapist and/or physical therapist assistant and his or her subsequent employer. Another example might be the student physical therapist or physical therapist assistant who might sign a contract with a potential employer for hire after graduation. The potential employer has agreed to reimburse the student's college fees in exchange for the graduate physical therapist or graduate physical therapist assistant to work for the employer for a certain period of time after graduation. Thus, there exists between the two parties a contract for which each respective party has a duty to the other.

Another example of a contractual duty is an employment contract. However, the nuances of employment contracts will be discussed in greater detail in Chapter 6.

Duty to Act

The *duty to act* is defined as "[a] duty to take some action to prevent harm to another, and for the failure of which one may be liable depending on the relationship of the parties and the circumstances."[6] This is a difficult duty and will often place physical therapists, physical therapist assistants, or students in an awkward situation; however, they must remember they are under a duty to act.

As an example of the duty to act, suppose the physical therapist, physical therapist assistant, or student is working in an outpatient clinic where elderly patients are treated. One of the elderly patients being treated has a neurological insult. The physical therapist, physical therapist assistant, or student notices that the elderly neurologically impaired patient drove him- or herself to the clinic and parked in the parking lot. Now the physical therapist, physical therapist assistant, or student knows this patient should not be driving. The physical therapist, physical therapist assistant, or student nicely discusses with the patient that he or she should not be driving because the patient is unable to react quickly to changing driving conditions or may have visual problems. In other words, the patient is presenting a hazard on the road.

The patient shrugs off the physical therapist's, physical therapist assistant's, or student's concerns and essentially states he or she knows they should not drive any long distances, but only drives to and from physical therapy sessions and believes that is acceptable. Now the physical therapist, physical therapist assistant, or student is in an awkward position. If the physical therapist, physical therapist assistant, or student does nothing and the patient has an accident that causes injuries to the patient or someone else, the physical therapist, physical therapist assistant, or student could be held liable for a failure to act to prevent the impaired patient from driving. In the legal sense, there would be arguments on both sides as to whether the physical therapist, physical therapist assistant, or student failed to act.

The argument for yes would be that the physical therapist, physical therapist assistant, or student had some liability because he or she knew the patient was impaired and affirmatively acted when he or she discussed the problem with the patient in an attempt to have the patient voluntarily stop driving. Therefore, the physical therapist, physical therapist assistant, or student could foresee the potential problem, but in the end, allowed the patient to leave the clinic and drive without further reporting. The dilemma is that the physical therapist, physical therapist assistant, or student who does report this patient will probably lose the patient because the patient will be angry if he or she determines it was the physical therapist, physical therapist assistant, or student who reported the unsafe driving.

However, despite the potential to lose a patient, all physical therapists, physical therapist assistants, and students must understand their duty to act. In defense of not reporting the unsafe patient, the physical therapist, physical therapist assistant, or student might argue the patient was competent and had a right to make his or her own decisions. The physical therapist, physical therapist assistant, or student would further assert he or she explained the risks of driving and the rationale of why the patient was not safe to drive. After that, the patient still had the right to choose. This explanation should have been documented and made a part of the patient's medical record. Nonetheless, the patient continued to drive and ultimately was involved in a motor vehicle accident. This factual scenario would make for a very interesting case and there is no way to know how a jury might respond. However, a jury would likely feel or find business reasons were not a sufficient reason not to report the unsafe driver.

Duty to Speak

The *duty to speak* is defined as "[a] duty to say something to correct another's false impression."[7] This will be especially important for a physical therapist assistant when a patient misinterprets him or her to be the physical therapist versus being the assistant in the delivery of care. This also will be especially important as the profession of physical therapy evolves to a doctoring profession. There likely will be occasions when patients misperceive that the physical therapist is a medical doctor and not a doctor of physical therapy. Patients often may have difficulty keeping track of the different health care professionals and what the differences are for each service.

Thus, a patient may confide in the physical therapist under a belief that the physical therapist is a medical doctor in hopes that the physical therapist would be able to prescribe something for relief. Under the duty to speak, the physical therapist is obligated to tell the patient he or she is a doctor of physical therapy and is not a medical doctor. Additionally, the physical therapist, physical therapist assistant, or student is under the duty to refer the patient to a medical doctor or more appropriate health care provider if necessary.

Some states, out of concern about the potential for misleading the public with regard to identification of what the health care practitioner is and what the health care practitioner is not, have enacted legislation (laws) mandating that health care providers wear name tags that not only identify who they are, but also what discipline of service they provide. Florida enacted such a law in 2006 under HB 587. HB 587 related to health care practitioners or licensees ensuring patients did not misperceive who practitioners were. Accordingly, Florida Statute 456.072 now states, in part, "[t]he following acts shall constitute grounds for which disciplinary actions specified in section (2) may be taken: (a) [m]aking misleading, deceptive, or fraudulent representations in or related to the practice of the licensee's profession."[8]

Legal Duty

The next duty is probably one of the most critical duties for the physical therapist, physical therapist assistant, and student to understand and that is the therapist's legal duty. A *legal duty* "aris[es] by contract or by operation of law; an obligation the breach of which would be a legal wrong."[9] This describes the duty physical therapists, physical therapist assistants, and students will operate under in the delivery of physical therapy services to their patients.

Generally speaking, a physical therapist, physical therapist assistant, or student should expect this legal duty to be utilized in a negligence or medical malpractice claim and be referred to as *that which a similarly situated physical therapist or physical therapist assistant would do or not do in a like situation*. In some states, this duty may be statutorily (law) defined. In states that do not specifically define the duty a physical therapist, physical therapist assistant, or student owes a patient, the duty may be defined through common law (case law) for that particular jurisdiction or through expert testimony.

Another phrase that is commonly used to discuss or evaluate duty is *standard of care*. In other words, when trying to determine what duty a physical therapist or physical therapist assistant owed a patient, it may be easier to think in terms of what standard of care was required of the physical therapist or physical therapist assistant when treating that patient. An example may be helpful to illustrate this concept.

When a physical therapist or physical therapist assistant determines that a hot pack would be of therapeutic benefit to his or her patient, before application of the hot pack the physical therapist or physical therapist assistant must evaluate that patient's sensory perception in the area to be treated. Physical therapist assistants are included in this example because many times the physical therapist may simply prescribe in the plan of treatment to do therapeutic modalities without specifying what therapeutic modality. (Inclusion in the example does not necessarily condone the practice.)

The determination of whether the patient's senses are intact to the area to be treated may seem simplistic, but hot-pack burns are one of the leading negligence claims against physical therapists and physical therapist assistants. In fact, burns are the second most common injury alleged in lawsuits against physical therapists and physical therapist assistants.[10] The standard of care or duty is that before application of a hot pack a physical therapist or physical therapist assistant evaluates and determines that the patient's sensory reception is intact.

This is critical because if the patient's sensory reception is impaired or absent, the patient will not be able to report when he or she "feels" burning from the hot pack. Accordingly, failure to evaluate a patient's sensory reception to the area to be treated could be deemed a failure or breach of duty or breach in the standard of care. In other words, a physical therapist or physical therapist assistant who does not test sensation before application of a hot pack could arguably not be performing his or her duty or performing the delivery of physical therapy services as a similarly situated physical therapist or physical therapist assistant would.

For the majority of negligence actions against a physical therapist or physical therapist assistant, an expert witness will be necessary in order to establish what the applicable standard of care or duty was with respect to what the physical therapist or physical therapist assistant did or did not do. Additionally, the *Guide to Physical Therapy Practice* could also be used to establish the duty a physical therapist or physical therapist assistant owed a patient. There is the likelihood that this book (guide) will be used with greater frequency in the future to define or help establish the physical therapist's and/or physical therapist assistant's duty.

As an example, return to the hot-pack scenario. The *Guide to Physical Therapy Practice* states hot packs (physical agents and mechanical modalities) are a procedural intervention for the reduction of pain.[11] However, along with the use of the modality hot pack, there are many factors to consider in the physical therapist's evaluation process, including pathology, pathophysiology, various systems impairments, and functional limitations, as well as some others.[12] Included with the systems impairments are the assessment of "neuromotor development and sensory integration" as well as "sensory integrity."[13] Thus, the *Guide to Physical Therapy Practice* provided guidelines of the areas to consider when choosing to use hot packs as an intervention for the treatment of some patients' conditions.

This example will be taken even further to illustrate the duty owed by the physical therapist or physical therapist assistant. Prior to its publication, the *Guide to Physical Therapy Practice* could obviously not be used to support the applicable standard of care or duty owed by a physical therapist, physical therapist assistant, or student, but rather a physical therapist deemed as an expert in the field of physical therapy would testify as to the duty or standard of care that should have been followed. However, because in the example, the physical therapist or physical therapist assistant did not document the area being treated with the hot pack was tested for sensory integrity and found to be intact, and the patient ultimately suffered a burn from the hot pack; the plaintiff's case would be made simpler because there would be little or no evidence of compliance with the standard of care. The lack of documentation will be discussed later in Chapter 8.

Consequently, for this example, a physical therapist's or physical therapist assistant's duty before applying a hot pack to a patient, amongst other things, is to test for sensory deficits to the area being treated. The next logical question should be: Does sensory reception need to be tested every time before a hot pack is applied? The answer is not a simple "yes" or "no." The legal answer is, if it is always tested (and documented), then a plaintiff's lawyer will have a difficult time arguing to a jury that sensation was not tested. Understand that hot pack burns can occur in a patient with intact sensation. Thus, if the patient gets burned and the physical therapist, physical therapist assistant, or student did not assess the patient's sensation before applying the hot pack, he or she may have breached the community standard of care to evaluate for sensation before application of a hot pack.

After the physical therapist completes an evaluation and establishes a plan of treatment, that plan is an evolving treatment plan and must change as the patient's symptoms and/or signs of dysfunction change. Thus, a patient could enter the clinic for his or her second treatment and have developed a sunburn since his or her last treatment. If that patient's sensation is not once again evaluated before the application of the hot pack, the likelihood is the patient will receive a burn from the hot-pack application because the skin in the area being treated has changed. Hence, the additional heat may be enough to exacerbate the sunburn. For readers who at this point want to scream that the patient should also have a duty to tell about the sunburn, don't worry; a defense lawyer might argue this to assist in mitigation of damages.

However, when a patient is in the physical therapy clinic, the patient is under no duty other than to follow the directions of the physical therapist, physical therapist assistant, or student and act as a reasonable physical therapy patient would act in like circumstances. Hence, the physical therapist, physical therapist assistant, or student has the control and should always be reassessing for changes that could affect the established plan of care. To try and shift that burden to the patient is not wise and in a court of law likely will result in failure. The physical therapist, physical therapist assistant, or student has the legal duty to ensure that the use of the hot pack is clinically appropriate for the patient to treat the problem for which the patient has sought the physical therapy services, and to ensure the treatment is safe every time the patient receives treatment.

Nondelegable Duty

The next duty to discuss is *nondelegable duty*, which is defined as "[a] duty that cannot be delegated by a contracting party to a third party; or [a] duty that may be delegated to an independent contractor by a principal, who retrains primary (as opposed to vicarious) responsibility if the duty is not properly performed."[14] In order to understand this definition, additional definitions are necessary.

Principal is defined as "[o]ne who authorizes another to act on his or her behalf as an agent."[15] Thus, although a physical therapist may delegate portions of a patient's treatment to a physical therapist assistant who is not employed by the physical therapist, the physical therapist will still be liable for any act(s) and/or omission(s) of the physical therapist assistant with regard to delegated treatments to the patient. The same holds true even for students. The physical therapist or physical therapist assistant supervising a student will always remain responsible (liable) for the student's actions or omissions.

In the previous example, if the physical therapist was also the physical therapist assistant's employer, then the physical therapist would be liable under both duties, nondelegable duty and vicarious liability. *Vicarious liability* is defined as "[l]iability that a supervisory party (such as an employer) bears for the actionable conduct of a subordinate or associate (such as an employee) because of the relationship between the two parties."[16] This is also known as *respondeat superior*.[17]

Respondeat Superior

Respondeat superior is defined as "[t]he doctrine holding an employer or principal liable for the employee's or agent's wrongful acts committed within the scope of the employment or agency."[18] Thus, the physical therapist is going to be held liable for the act(s) and/or omission(s) of any subordinate providing care to any patient that is under the ultimate care and treatment of the physical therapist. Further, whomever or whatever is the employer of the physical therapist or the physical therapist assistant will also be responsible (held liable) for the act(s) and/or omission(s) of the physical therapist or physical therapist assistant in the treatment of that particular patient. This concept will be discussed further in Chapter 6 and ways to mitigate liability exposure for these situations will be discussed in Chapter 13.

Duty of Loyalty

The next duty to be discussed is the duty of *loyalty*. This duty is defined as "[a] person's duty not to engage in self-dealing or otherwise use his or her position to further personal interests rather than those of the beneficiary."[19] When physical therapists and physical therapist assistants begin to participate in various organizations and associations, they must be cognizant of this duty. Once the physical therapist or physical therapist assistant is elected to any type of officer position within an organization or association, he or she has a duty of loyalty to the organization.

An as example, a physical therapist or physical therapist assistant consents to run for the office of secretary of a state's physical therapy association. The physical therapist or physical therapist assistant is elected. During the course of serving the association as the secretary, the individual has the opportunity to call various vendors seeking sponsorships for various activities of the components of the organization. During the phone calls to the various vendors, the secretary not only solicits sponsorships for the association, but also markets and explains his or her personal clinic and what it has to offer in an attempt to solicit patients. Hence, the secretary is essentially accomplishing two goals with each phone call: soliciting sponsorships for the organization and marketing his or her personal clinic. Some individuals would see nothing wrong with this action; however, it is actually breaching the duty of loyalty to the association.

Another example of breaching the duty of loyalty (which is unfortunately not an uncommon situation) is when a physical therapist or physical therapist assistant works for a hospital that provides outpatient physical therapy services, while a friend, who is also a therapist, works for a freestanding outpatient clinic. While the hospital physical therapist or physical therapist assistant treats a patient at the hospital, the physical therapist or physical therapist assistant identifies that the patient will need additional therapy after discharge from the hospital.

However, instead of the hospital physical therapist or physical therapist assistant suggesting the patient return to the hospital's outpatient physical therapy clinic, the physical therapist or physical therapist assistant suggests to the patient that he or she should go to the friend's outpatient clinic. Thus, the physical therapist or physical therapist assistant actually generated business for the friend and lost business for the hospital.

There are many arguments that could support the hospital physical therapist's or physical therapist assistant's action, including that the freestanding outpatient physical therapy clinic had better physical therapists or physical therapist assistants, better equipment, or was easier to access. However, purely looking at the duty of loyalty, the hospital-based physical therapist or physical therapist assistant had a duty to the beneficiary, which in this example was the hospital that employed the therapist, to not engage in or exert influence to send business elsewhere to the harm of the hospital.

Fiduciary Duty

The last duty to be discussed in this chapter is the fiduciary duty. *Fiduciary duty* is defined as "[a] duty of utmost good faith, trust, confidence, and candor owed by a fiduciary (such as a lawyer or corporate officer) to the beneficiary (such as a lawyer's client or a shareholder); a duty to act with the highest degree of honesty and loyalty toward another person and in the best interests of the other person."[20] Thus, it should be easy to see that every relationship between a patient and a physical therapist or physical therapist assistant could involve a fiduciary duty.

When a patient arrives for physical therapy, regardless of the setting, the patient is at a disadvantage from the beginning because the patient does not generally have the knowledge necessary to determine whether the physical therapist or physical therapist assistant is being trustworthy with the information provided in relation to the evaluation and recommended plan of treatment. The physical therapist or physical therapist assistant sits in a position of trust and the patient usually has confidence in that physical therapist's or physical therapist assistant's evaluation and plan of treatment. This duty is even further complicated and heightened when the physical therapist or physical therapist assistant is treating a child and the parents are relying on the physical therapist or physical therapist assistant for not only evaluation and treatment but also for prognosis.

The duties discussed will be further addressed as the book continues through the breach of these duties and damages that could flow from the breach. For medical negligence, it is generally well accepted that there will be testimony required from an expert witness to establish the duty owed to the plaintiff and how the health care provider breached the prevailing standard of care (duty).

CASE EXAMPLE

A case example wherein an expert was used is *Lyons v. Biloxi, H.M.A., Inc.* In this case out of Mississippi, the appellate court upheld a lower court's ruling that whether a physical therapist breached the prevailing standard of care when ambulating a patient 1 day postoperation for a total hip replacement required expert testimony.[21] Thus, the court determined the applicable standard of care (duty) could not be elicited or determined through layperson testimony and such testimony required that of an expert.[22]

In the *Lyons* case, the morning after surgery, the physical therapist arrived and applied a gait belt to the waist of the patient.[23] Thereafter, the physical therapist ambulated the patient to the bathroom holding onto the gait belt.[24] Upon ambulating from the bathroom, the patient fell at the doorway, which the physical therapist called a "controlled descent."[25]

From that fall, the patient dislocated the new prosthetic hip.[26] During an attempted closed reduction of the dislocated hip, the patient suffered an avulsion fracture of the right greater trochanter,[27] and the patient underwent an open reduction surgery to fix the avulsed fracture.[28] The plaintiff argued the physical therapist breached the prevailing standard of care in the delivery of physical therapy services.

The plaintiff argued that the breach in the physical therapist's duty was that the physical therapist ambulated the patient to the bathroom too soon after surgery or that because the bathroom was so small, only one physical therapist could be in the bathroom assisting as the patient walked out of the bathroom when the patient needed the assistance of two persons. Thus, had there been two people assisting the patient, the patient would not have fallen or even had a controlled descent to the floor and therefore would not have dislocated her hip.

Accordingly, the breach in the standard of care caused additional injuries, including a dislocated hip and an avulsion fracture to the greater trochanter when a closed reduction was attempted on the dislocated hip. Additional damages alleged would be for the pain and suffering and further disability of the hip.[29] However, the appellate court upheld the trial court's decision on the grounds that expert testimony was necessary to establish what the prevailing standard of care was for the physical therapist. Further, expert testimony was required to determine whether the physical therapist had breached the prevailing standard of care.[30]

As with most medical negligence cases, expert testimony is going to be required to not only establish what the community's standard of care was for the physical therapist, physical therapist assistant, and/or student, but also whether the act(s) and/or omission(s) of the physical therapist, physical therapist assistant, or student breached the prevailing standard of care and were the legal cause of harm to the patient. Today there is also the addition of the APTA's *Guide to Physical Therapy Practice* that could assist an expert in reaching his or her opinions.

USING THE *GUIDE TO PHYSICAL THERAPY PRACTICE* TO ESTABLISH DUTY

The *Guide to Physical Therapy Practice*[31] can be utilized as a tool in litigation to establish or form the basis for expert opinions as to the duty or standard of care owed a physical therapy patient. As previously discussed, in medical malpractice cases, a patient sues one or more health care providers for some alleged negligence regarding the care and/or treatment the patient received or failed to receive.

Thus, the first element the plaintiff must assert and prove in a negligence (medical malpractice) case is the duty that was owed the patient. For the physical therapy patient, one tool experts testifying against physical therapists, physical therapist assistants, or students are using to form opinions about the duty a physical therapist, physical therapist assistant, or student owed a patient is the *Guide to Physical Therapy Practice*, 2nd Edition.

The authors and contributors of the *Guide* clearly and unequivocally denounced that the contents of the book in any way established or created any duty a physical therapist, physical therapist assistant, or student owed any patient.[32] Thus, it appears the intent of the book was not to stand for any proposition as to the standard of care owed a physical therapy patient. In fact, one disclaimer specifically states, "[t]he Guide does not contain specific treatment protocols, does not provide clinical guidelines, and does not set forth the standard of care for which a physical therapist may be legally responsible in any specific case."[33]

However, just because the *Guide to Physical Therapy Practice* has disclaimers that it does not establish duty or the standard of care for the physical therapist, physical therapist assistant, or student does not prevent expert witnesses or plaintiffs' lawyers from using it as a tool to support expert opinions that a physical therapist, physical therapist assistant, or student deviated from the prevailing standard of care in the community.

Using the hot-pack burn example may further explain. For the ailment of pain, the *Guide to Physical Therapy Practice* indicates that:

> [t]he physical therapist uses these tests and measures to determine a cause or a mechanism for the pain and to assess the intensity, quality, and temporal and physical characteristics of any pain that is important to the patient and that may result in impairments, functional limitations, or disabilities. Results of tests and measures of pain are integrated with the history and systems review findings and the results of other tests and measures. All of these data are then synthesized during the evaluation process to establish the diagnosis, the prognosis, and the plan of care, which includes the selection of interventions.[34]

The selection (decision) of which tests and measures to utilize during the evaluation of the patient depends on clinical judgment that incorporates the patient's history and systems review.[35] However, the "clinical indications for these tests and measures may include": **pathology/pathophysiology** including cardiac, endocrine, integumentary, musculoskeletal, neuromuscular or pulmonary; **impairments** of circulation, integumentary, joint integrity, muscle performance, posture or ventilation; and/or **functional limitations or disability** involving self-care, home management, work, community or leisure.[36]

As a result, the *Guide to Physical Therapy Practice*, in a plaintiff's expert's opinion, establishes that the therapist should rule out all possible causes for the pain for every back pain patient. It does not matter where the pain is located. Therefore, the physical therapist actually rules out and determines the cause of the back pain as is evidenced or substantiated in his or her documentation. Accordingly, if the physical therapist's evaluation does not document that the physical therapist ruled out all of the other possible causes for the back pain, an argument may be brought that the physical therapist had a duty to evaluate and rule out all possible causes of the pain, and because it is not documented in the evaluation that the physical therapist did the tests and measures to rule out other causes, the physical therapist breached the prevailing standard of care.

Thus, in the previous patient scenario, the physical therapist would have to mount a defense that he or she ruled out all other possible causes for the patient's back pain and determined the back pain was caused by something other than the bone metastasis to the lumbar vertebra (hypothetical). However, if the physical therapist did not document an evaluation that ruled out the other possible causes for the back pain, the plaintiff's expert can opine the physical therapist did not do all the tests and measures necessary because the tests and measures as identified in the *Guide to Physical Therapy Practice* were not documented as being completed.

Had the physical therapist conducted a comprehensive evaluation as outlined in the *Guide*, the physical therapist would have identified a problem with the patient's lungs and would have referred the patient to a pulmonologist before implementing treatment. Consequently, the physical therapist breached the duty owed the patient with regards to the evaluation of pain. Physical therapists, physical therapist assistants, and students should also realize, the younger the patient, the more sympathetic a jury will likely be when it comes time to calculate damages.

Lastly, physical therapists, physical therapist assistants, and students should recognize the low back pain example used is not uncommon and will become even more common as the profession, pursuant to Vision 2020, progresses toward physical therapists being entry-level health care practitioners. Consequently, the duty the physical therapist owes his or her patient will be raised. This should come as no surprise because the academic preparation of the doctoral physical therapist includes training in the skills of differential diagnosis. Hence, as an entry-level health care practitioner, the physical therapist may be the first health care provider to evaluate a patient presenting with new or recurrent onset of signs and symptoms.

The physical therapist will no longer have the "safety net" that a physician has already evaluated the patient and ruled out certain diagnoses such that the physician has determined the patient would benefit from physical therapy. Without the physician's prior evaluation, the responsibility to determine what is ailing the patient belongs to the physical therapist and the physical therapist must be thorough, accurate, and seek other health care providers based on evaluation results. Consequently, with the escalating responsibility comes heightened accountability for mistakes.

Thus, the *Guide to Physical Therapy Practice* is being, and will be, utilized in litigation to support experts' opinions as to what duty a physical therapist, physical therapist assistant, or student should provide in the care and treatment of patients. The utilization of this book is and will occur despite the book's disclaimer that it does not establish the standard of care owed a physical therapy patient. Accordingly, every physical therapist, physical therapist assistant, and student should not only read and understand the *Guide to Physical Therapy Practice*, but should also put into practice documentation that substantiates inclusion of available tests and measures to exclude or rule out nontreatable physical therapy pathologies.

BREACH OF DUTY

Once a duty is established, then the facts of the situation are pled to assert the duty owed and how that duty was breached. Sometimes facts are undisputed but usually facts to establish a breach of duty are disputed. One party will attempt to solicit testimony and evidence to support his or her "spin" of the facts, while the opposing party attempts to solicit testimony and evidence to support his or her theory of the case. Ultimately, jurors, "the triers of facts," listen to both sides and determine what the facts actually are. Based on the jurors' resolution of facts, one party prevails at the lawsuit.

The breach-of-duty concept is easier to digest because it is a determination of whether the previously described duties were not followed. For the legal duty, it means determining whether the physical therapist, physical therapist assistant, or student evaluated or treated the patient consistent within the established standard of care. To explain the breach of duty, the same hot-pack burn example will be used.

During the evaluation, the physical therapist either evaluated the patient's sensory system before determining that hot-pack application was appropriate for the patient's plan of care or the physical therapist did not. If the patient is subsequently burned because of a hot pack, the fact that will most assuredly be investigated is whether the physical therapist evaluated the patient's sensation prior to the application of the hot pack.

If the patient's chart demonstrates the patient's sensation was evaluated, then the plaintiff will have a tougher time arguing and trying to prove the physical therapist breached a duty; therefore, the plaintiff will have a more difficult time proving his or her case. In that case, the plaintiff will have to try and prove or argue that the physical therapist did not perform the sensation test properly, interpreted the results inaccurately or used the wrong rationale, which will be more difficult to establish.

In contrast, if the physical therapist did not assess sensation before application of the hot pack and the hot pack burns the patient, then the plaintiff's case will be that the physical therapist was under a duty to test sensation before applying a hot pack; the therapist did not test sensation, hence, the patient got burned. Had the physical therapist tested sensation, the therapist would have known the patient had impaired sensation and would have determined a hot pack was contraindicated based on the sensation test or that a modified application of a hot pack was warranted.

The remainder of this chapter will focus on medical negligence and breaches of the other duties will be discussed throughout the book. The next element a plaintiff must plead and prove in a medical malpractice or negligence cause of action against a physical therapist, physical therapist assistant, or student is causation.

CAUSATION

Although causation seems easy to understand, it is complicated because one has to prove that the breach of the duty was the legal cause of the alleged damage(s). Sometimes, although it seems some act or omission caused the harm, there may be intervening actions that ultimately are the legal cause of the damage and not the alleged breach of the duty. In order to understand causation, some additional definitions are necessary.

Causation is defined as the thing that produced "an effect or result."[37] *Actual cause* is defined as the "but-for test" or "the cause without which the event could not have occurred."[38] *Proximate cause*, also known as the *legal cause*, is defined as "a cause that directly produces an event and without which the event would not have occurred."[39] Proximate cause results in legal liability[40] and so may or may not be the actual act or omission that actually caused the harm.

For causation, there is also the requirement of foreseeability. *Foreseeability* is defined as "[t]he quality of being reasonably anticipatable. Foreseeability, along with actual causation, is an element of proximate cause in tort law."[41] Thus, for liability in the face of causation, it should have been foreseeable what harm would result for any particular breach of duty. Some lawyers will state foreseeability must be present in order for liability to lie; however, there are cases that could be argued foreseeability was not present, yet, liability was assessed.

Examples will help illustrate the differences in causation.

Using the hot-pack burn example previously discussed, this time accept that the patient had been evaluated and one of the modalities the physical therapist elected to use in the plan of care was hot packs. The physical therapist appropriately tested the patient's sensation where the hot pack was going to be applied and determined the patient's sensation was intact. The physical therapist delegated the application of the hot pack to a physical therapy aide, who had been appropriately trained and was under the direct physical supervision of the physical therapist. (The meaning of direct physical supervision as used here means the physical therapist was physically in the room where the treatment was applied and could visually see what the physical therapy aide was doing.)

The hydrocollator unit had been tested for water temperature on the day of the hot pack application and was within the appropriate range. The physical therapy aide prepared the hot pack with the appropriate layers and applied the heat to the appropriate place on the patient. All safety measures were taken with regard to the application of the hot pack. However, unbeknownst to the physical therapist, the hot pack was defective and somehow dispersed heat at a higher temperature than what was measured by the water temperature. (Remember this is a teaching example.)

Once the hot pack was applied, a greater amount of heat was delivered to the patient's skin. Despite the patient ringing the bell, moving the hot pack off their skin, and the physical therapist immediately responding, the patient still suffered a second-degree burn to the area and had to receive medical treatments. Determining causation is all this example is attempting to clarify. The placing of the defective hot pack on the patient is the actual cause of the second-degree burn. (If the therapist had not appropriately tested the sensation of the skin, another allegation could be that the actual cause of the burn was the patient's abnormal skin sensation.)

However, continuing the example with only one variable, should the product manufacturer of the defective hot pack escape liability if, in fact, the hot pack itself was made of defective material? The hot pack's defective material is a proximate cause of the second-degree burn. Hence, in order to argue a negligence claim against the hot-pack manufacturer, the plaintiff would have to assert the actual cause of the burn was the placement of the defective hot pack on the patient (plaintiff) and the proximate cause of the burn was the defective hot pack. Standing alone, the defective hot pack could not cause a burn. It was only after the defective hot pack was heated in the normal hydrocollator unit and then placed on the patient that the burn occurred.

The usual complaint that would come from this type of a scenario would be a negligence claim against the physical therapist for the application of the hot pack by the physical therapy aide, a vicarious liability claim against the physical therapist's employer, and a product liability claim against the manufacturer of the hot pack. (There are multiple other types of legal issues in the simple case, but its purpose is only to distinguish the differences between actual and proximate causation.)

Return to the same example after altering one of the facts. This time the hot pack is not defective and the physical therapist applies the hot pack; however, during application, the physical therapist forgot to provide the appropriate number of layers between the hot pack and the patient's skin. Again the patient receives a second-degree burn. This time the actual and proximate cause are one and the same: the lack of providing the appropriate layers of padding between the hot pack and the patient's skin. That is the actual and proximate cause of the second-degree burn.

This example is not all that unrealistic. In the case of *Patton v. Healthsouth of Houston, Inc.*, 2004 WL 253282 (Tex.App.–Hous. (1 Dist.) 2004), a patient sued a hospital under a theory of medical malpractice for allegedly receiving burns from an application of hot packs during a physical therapy treatment. It must be pointed out that the decision in this case illustrates another legal concept regarding the statute of limitations and conditions that must be met before filing a medical malpractice lawsuit in Texas. However, the facts of the case revolved around the single issue of whether there should be liability if the patient was burned by hot packs in the course of treatment with physical therapy.

Returning to the *Lyons* case, discussed earlier in this chapter, recall that the patient suffered a dislocated hip after undergoing a total hip replacement. During an attempted closed reduction of the dislocated hip, the patient suffered an avulsion fracture. Now, the fall in the bathroom doorway did not cause the new hip replacement to suffer an avulsion fracture, but rather the fall caused the hip to dislocate. The attempted closed reduction is what caused the avulsion fracture. The plaintiff in this case will be able to plead and likely recover damages that include those damages flowing from the dislocated hip and the subsequent avulsion fracture. Thus, using the actual causation test, the "but-for test" (but for the fall), the patient would never have undergone the attempted closed reduction to reduce the dislocated hip. Thus, the avulsion fracture directly flows from the fall and the dislocated hip. The proximate cause of the avulsion fracture in the *Lyons* case would be the failed closed reduction; however, the actual cause (but-for test) would be the fall that caused the hip dislocation.

Another case dealing with causation is *Lockett-Starks v. Weismann, Gitkin, Herkowitz.*[42] In the *Lockett-Starks* case, a physical therapy aide was employed at Weismann, Gitkin, Herkowitz, M.D., P.C. clinic.[43] The employment came at the recommendation of a vocational consultant, who was also named as a defendant in the lawsuit.[44] The plaintiff alleged the physical therapy aide sexually assaulted the plaintiff "during a physical therapy massage."[45]

The physical therapy aide had been involved in a motor vehicle accident and suffered a closed head injury prior to employment at the clinic.[46] The vocational consultant assisted the physical therapy aide in obtaining the job at the clinic.[47] After working at the clinic for approximately 9 months, the physical therapy aide was assigned to provide the plaintiff with a massage.[48] The plaintiff alleged that the physical therapy aide "touched her in a sexually inappropriate manner during the massage."[49] There had also been a patient who had been concerned with how the physical therapy aide lowered her underpants.[50]

However, the case was resolved in the defendants' favor because there was no foreseeability that the physical therapy aide could or would act in an inappropriate manner.[51] Consequently, because the defendant vocational consultant could not reasonably foresee that the physical therapy aide, despite the prior head injury, would act inappropriately, the plaintiff could not prove forseeability of the harm; therefore, the case was dismissed.[52]

The last element that a plaintiff must plead and prove by a greater weight of the evidence (also known as a preponderance of the evidence) in a medical malpractice or negligence claim is damages.

DAMAGES

Payment of monetary damages to injured parties is our society's method of compensating individuals when they are harmed because of the fault of someone else or suffered an injury to their property. Thus, the individual at fault for causing the harm is held liable and must pay money in an attempt to return the injured person as close as possible to whole. Depending on the type of cause of action (lawsuit), different damages may be available under one cause of action that are not available under a different cause of action.

As an example, suing someone for breach of contract allows the injured party to seek contract damages, whereas suing someone in negligence allows for different types of damages to be claimed. Determining an injured plaintiff's damages is always critical in every civil lawsuit because usually parties want to negotiate toward settlement in good faith and within reason. A case would not be brought unless the plaintiff was seeking remuneration for some harm the defendant allegedly caused. It is very important in medical negligence civil cases to determine what type of damages are being claimed and what is the amount of each such damage. Generally speaking, damages can be divided into economic, noneconomic, and punitive. The remainder of this chapter will discuss the different types of damages and how the physical therapist, physical therapist assistant, or student could be held liable for payment of these damages.

Economic Damages

Economic damages are generally the damages that a definite amount of money or a number can be associated with for loss of wages (past and future) or lost profits. These damages can also include past and future medical expenses. Usually a plaintiff will hire someone such as an economist to identify and project these losses. The economist will come up with a total inclusive of the predicted future losses and then, through the use of a formula, calculate an amount of money in present-value terms.

Noneconomic Damages

Noneconomic damages are those that are more subjective in nature and more difficult to assign a dollar value to. These types of damages include pain and suffering, loss of consortium, disfigurement, mental anguish, and loss of enjoyment of life, to name the most popular.

Punitive Damages

Punitive damages are used to punish the offender and send a message to others, like the defendant, that the conduct complained of will not be tolerated by society. Punitive damages are a "deterrent" to prevent and avoid future conduct like that which has led to a particular lawsuit. This type of damage is "awarded in addition to actual damages when the defendant acted with recklessness, malice, or deceit. Punitive damages, which are intended to punish and thereby deter blameworthy conduct, are generally not recoverable for breach of contract."[53]

Generally speaking, when a plaintiff files a lawsuit, there will not be a claim for punitive damages at the time the lawsuit is filed. However, as the litigation progresses and discovery is undertaken, the plaintiff may uncover certain act(s) and/or omission(s) that plaintiff's counsel believes demonstrate conduct that was reckless, wanton, and had a disregard for human safety. In those cases, the plaintiff will likely then follow the rules of procedure for the particular jurisdiction and seek to amend the complaint to add a claim for punitive damages.

In Florida, when a plaintiff files a motion to amend the complaint to add a claim for punitive damages in medical negligence cases, the plaintiff also must identify for the court the evidence it believes demonstrates the reckless, wanton, or disregard for human safety conduct. If the evidence is not already filed in the court record, then the plaintiff may "proffer" the evidence to the court for its consideration in determining whether to allow the plaintiff to amend the complaint to add the claim for punitive damages.

Whether there is a claim for punitive damages is important in negligence cases because the value of the case changes when there is the potential for the jury to decide whether the alleged act(s) and/or omission(s) rise to the level of reckless, wanton, or disregard for human safety. Generally speaking, there will be no limits to the amount of money a jury can award under the punitive damage scenario.

Case Examples

In *Pulaski*, a patient filed a lawsuit against the physical therapist and the physical therapist's employer for alleged negligence in the rehabilitation of the patient's shoulder following nonsurgical repair.[54] The case was tried before a jury that awarded the patient turned plaintiff $25,000.[55] The plaintiff, unhappy with the amount of damages awarded, filed a motion post trial for an additur or for mistrial so that there would be a new trial.[56]

An *additur* is defined as "[a] trial court's order, issued usu[ally] with the defendant's consent, that increases the damages awarded by the jury to avoid a new trial on grounds of inadequate damages,"[57] whereas a *mistrial* is defined as " [a] trial that the judge brings to an end, without a determination on the merits, because of a procedural error or serious misconduct occurring during the proceedings. A trial that ends inconclusively because the jury cannot agree on a verdict."[58] The patient had initially injured the shoulder in a fall and received a nonsurgical manipulation.[59] Thereafter, the patient was referred to physical therapy for rehabilitation.[60] The physical therapists established a plan of treatment that included flexibility exercises and manipulation of the arm.[61] On the third day of treatment, the physical therapists recommend and used the Cybex.[62]

The patient alleged that the injured shoulder was strapped to the machine such that the machine raised and lowered the arm to facilitate flexibility.[63] The plaintiff also alleged that he was left unattended while the machine was in use and that the machine malfunctioned such that the arm was jerked rapidly, causing severe pain.[64] Therefore, the plaintiff alleged that the arm was injured when the Cybex machine was used. Approximately 6 days later, the plaintiff was diagnosed with a dislocated shoulder and resultant brachial plexus injury.[65] Of significance as to damages, the plaintiff alleged there was permanent impairments to the right hand and right shoulder.[66] The lawsuit was filed under a theory of negligence against the physical therapist and the therapist's employer for treatment received in the rehabilitation of the shoulder injury.

The jury agreed with the plaintiff that the physical therapist had been negligent in the rehabilitation of the shoulder and awarded $25,000 in damages. The case was appealed by the plaintiff because the plaintiff did not believe the jury had awarded enough money in damages, thus, the plaintiff wanted the trial judge post trial to increase the amount of money awarded for damages through the additur or to grant the plaintiff a new trial so that the issue of damages could be decided again. From a defense perceptive, an award of $25,000 is not bad if the facts were as described in the appellate opinion such as leaving the patient unattended while the patient was strapped to the Cybex machine and it was operating passive range of motion to the injured shoulder.

In *Carlos v. CNA Insurance Company*, a physical therapist, the physical therapist's employer, and the insurance company were sued for allegedly exacerbating a physical therapy patient's back injury.[67] The patient initially suffered a back injury in a job-related incident.[68] Approximately 3 months later, the patient underwent a lumbar surgery.[69] After a second surgery, the physician prescribed physical therapy for the patient.[70] After 6 weeks of physical therapy, the patient was informed he was almost ready for discharge and ready to return to work.[71]

As a final progression in treatment, the physical therapist instructed the plaintiff to do leg squats with weights.[72] The physical therapist had the patient perform leg squats with 100 pounds.[73] After two attempts, the patient immediately complained of a "headache as well as pain in his back and legs."[74] The surgeon informed the patient his lifting restriction should have been 20 pounds.[75] Following this, the patient had to undergo a third surgery.[76] As a result, the patient sued the physical therapist, his employer, and the physical therapist's insurance company for alleged medical malpractice,[77] while the patient's wife sued for loss of consortium.[78]

The complaint alleged:[79]

1. [F]ailing to recognize the hazard/danger of prescribing physical therapy exercises requiring lifting weights of approximately 100 pounds;
2. [F]ailing to properly monitor and evaluate the prescribed physical therapy exercises;
3. [F]ailing to perform the proper procedures in advising and assisting with the physical therapy exercises;
4. [F]ailing to follow normal and customary lifting restrictions for a person who has endured two lumbar surgeries; and

5. [F]ailing to meet the standard of care required in the given situation.

The defendants filed a motion for summary judgment* because the plaintiff did not have any expert testimony alleging the physical therapist caused the patient's problem.[80]

The testimony the plaintiff relied on was that of the physical therapist who testified:[81]

Q: Okay. And you agree that if he was using that Smith Lift and it was 100 pounds or more, then you would agree, would you not, that there was a breach in the standard of care if that was being done pursuant to your supervision and control?

A: Again, I don't know if it was a breach in the standard of care, but it was not what I had prescribed. So it was contrary to what I prescribed for Chad for that particular lift if that answers it for you.

As usual, the plaintiff left out any evidence or testimony that did not support his case. In support of the defendants' motion for summary judgment, the defendants proffered the testimony of the patient's surgeon, who testified:[82]

A: I don't think that therapy is related to this. I think this is a natural history of this disease.

Q: What do you mean by that?

A: Well, he has two bad discs. . . . I would say 10% of the population that undergo diskectomies will end up having to have a fusion. He fell into that 10%. . . . [pp. 14–15]

Q: Did you ever tell Mr. Carlos that you thought somebody had done something wrong in the physical therapy?

A: No, I never did. . . . I don't think it is related, I don't think the therapy at all is related. . . . [pp. 15] I remember as I said I don't think the therapy at all had anything to do with it. . . . [pp. 16].

Thus, the trial court considered the evidence submitted and ruled that the plaintiff did not have any "medical evidence providing any possibility of a causal connection between the alleged incident and the alleged subsequent injury."[83] This was an excellent outcome for the physical therapist; however, the same facts in a different ju-

---

* A *motion for summary judgment* is defined as "[a] request that the court enter judgment without a trial because there is no genuine issue of material fact to be decided by a fact-finder—that is, because the evidence is legally insufficient to support a verdict in the nonmovant's favor" (Black's Law Dictionary, 1033 (Bryan A. Gardner, ed., 7th ed., West 1999).

risdiction or with different lawyers could have a different outcome because the complaints of pain were contemporaneous with the apparent exacerbation of the patient's condition and it did not appear that there had been a progressive treatment plan to lift the 100 pounds.

SUMMARY

The most probable lawsuit a physical therapist, physical therapist assistant, or student will face is a patient's claim of medical malpractice or negligence. The essential elements for a cause of action of medical malpractice or negligence are:

1. Duty
2. Breach of duty
3. Causation
4. Damages

These elements in most states will have to be proven by a greater weight of the evidence or a "tipping of the scale." If a jury finds the physical therapist, physical therapist assistant, or student is liable in a medical malpractice or negligence case, available damages will include economic, noneconomic, and possibly punitive damages.

DISCUSSION QUESTIONS

1. If you had a patient who was unsafe to drive, yet the patient continued to drive to and from your clinic for physical therapy treatments, what would you do?
2. Explain the duty a physical therapist or physical therapist assistant owes his or her physical therapy patient.
3. Identify and discuss the elements for a cause of action of medical malpractice or negligence.
4. Discuss the duties a physical therapist, physical therapist assistant, or student could owe a patient.
5. How is duty established in medical malpractice or negligence cases against a physical therapist, physical therapist assistant, or a student?
6. Discuss the use of the *Guide to Physical Therapy Practice* in litigation.
7. Discuss causation.
8. Discuss different types of damages.
9. Why would a jury award punitive damages?
10. What is a motion for summary judgment?

NOTES

[1] *Black's Law Dictionary*, 214 (Bryan A. Garner, ed., 7th ed., West Group, 1999).
[2] *Id.* at 538.
[3] *Id.* at 521.
[4] *Id.* at 522.
[5] *Id.*
[6] *Id.*
[7] *Id.*
[8] Florida Statutes, § 456.072 (2006).
[9] *Black's Law Dictionary*, 522 (Bryan A. Garner, ed., 7th ed., West Group, 1999).
[10] CNA Insurance Company, *Physical Therapy Claims Study*, CNA HealthPro, www.cna.com (December 4, 2006).
[11] *Guide to Physical Therapy Practice*, 120 (American Physical Therapy Association, 2nd ed., 2003).
[12] *Id.*
[13] *Id.*
[14] *Black's Law Dictionary*, 522 (Bryan A. Garner, ed., 7th ed., West Group, 1999).
[15] *Id.* at 1210
[16] *Id.* at 927
[17] *Id.*
[18] *Id.* at 1313
[19] *Id.* at 523
[20] *Id.*
[21] *Lyons v. Biloxi H.M.A., Inc.*, 925 So.2d 151, 155 (Ct. App. MS 2006).
[22] *Id.*
[23] *Id.* at 152.
[24] *Id.* at 152–153.
[25] *Id.* at 153.
[26] *Id.*
[27] *Id.*
[28] *Id.*
[29] *Id.* at 155.
[30] *Id.* at 155.
[31] *Guide to Physical Therapy Practice* (American Physical Therapy Association, 2nd ed., 2003).
[32] *Id.* at 17 and 27.
[33] *Id.* at 27.
[34] *Id.* at 78.
[35] *Id.*
[36] *Id.*
[37] *Black's Law Dictionary*, 86 (Bryan A. Garner, ed., 7th ed., West Group, 1999).
[38] *Id.*
[39] *Id.* at 87.
[40] *Id.*
[41] *Id.* at 660.

[42] *Lockett-Starks v. Weismann, Gitkin, Herkowitz*, 2005 WL 562683 (Mich. App. 2005).
[43] *Id.* at 1.
[44] *Id.*
[45] *Id.*
[46] *Id.*
[47] *Id.*
[48] *Id.*
[49] *Id.*
[50] *Id.* at 2.
[51] *Id.* at 4.
[52] *Id.*
[53] *Black's Law Dictionary*, 396 (Bryan A. Gardner, ed., 7th ed., West Group, 1999).
[54] *Pulaski v.Healthsouth Rehabilitation Center of Connecticut, LLC*, 2005 WL 941419 (Conn.Super. 2005).
[55] *Id.*
[56] *Id.*
[57] *Black's Law Dictionary*, 39 (Bryan A. Garner, ed., 7th ed., West Group, 1999).
[58] *Id.* at 1018.
[59] *Pulaski v. Healthsouth Rehabilitation Center of Connecticut, LLC*, 2005 WL 941419 (Conn.Super. 2005).
[60] *Id.*
[61] *Id.*
[62] *Id.*
[63] *Id.*
[64] *Id.*
[65] *Id.*
[66] *Id.*
[67] *Carlos v. CNA Insurance Company*, 900 So.2d 146 (La.App. 5th Cir. 2005).
[68] *Id.* at 147.
[69] *Id.*
[70] *Id.*
[71] *Id.*
[72] *Id.*
[73] *Id.*
[74] *Id.*
[75] *Id.*
[76] *Id.*
[77] *Id.*
[78] *Id.*
[79] *Id.*
[80] *Id.* at 148.
[81] *Id.*
[82] *Id.* at 149–150.
[83] *Id.* at 150.

CHAPTER 6

Employment Law

At any given moment, if working, every physical therapist or physical therapist assistant can be classified as either an employee or employer. The legal definition of an *employee* is "[a] person who works in the service of another person (the employer) under an expressed or implied contract of hire, under which the employer has the right to control the details of the work performance,"[1] whereas, an *employer* is defined as "[a] person who controls and directs a worker under an expressed or implied contract of hire and who pays the worker's salary or wages."[2]

A key part of the employer definition is that the employer controls or has the right to control the details of the employee's work. According to the legal concept of vicarious liability, every employer is ultimately legally liable and responsible for the act(s) and/or omission(s) of their employees. *Vicarious liability* is defined as "[l]iability that a supervisory party (such as an employer) bears for the actionable conduct of a subordinate or associate (such as an employee) because of the relationship between the two parties."[3]

This liability is also known as *respondent superior*, which in Latin means, "let the superior make answers."[4] This legal doctrine holds "an employer or principal liable for the employee's or agent's wrongful acts committed within the scope of employment or agency."[5] However, despite this legal concept, sometimes a determination must be made whether the employee's act(s) and/or omission(s) were within the employee's scope of employment to assist in defending an employer. Accordingly, as an employee, the physical therapist or physical therapist assistant needs to be cognizant of his or her duties to ensure they are performed within the scope of employment. This chapter will examine causes of action that involve vicarious liability for employers and some of the tools to assist with mitigation of liability damages.

Other causes of action and mitigation of damages tools that will be discussed in this chapter include discriminatory claims with the Equal Employment Opportunity

Commission, employment contracts, and wrongful termination. Lastly, some of the most common items involved in employment will be discussed and how these items can assist with the defense of a claim that an employee breached a prevailing standard of care to include employment applications, drug screening, reference checks, and license verification as well as having the employee work within his or her scope of employment. Policies, procedures, and orientation also will be addressed. Further, the different types of laws and the particular agency responsible for administration of those laws will be covered. Sometimes a particular law will be administrated through the state and some through the federal government.

KEY CONCEPTS

Exempt versus nonexempt employees
Fair Labor Standards Act
Equal Employment Opportunity Commission
Employment contracts
Employment at will
Progressive disciplinary action
Wrongful termination
Workers' compensation programs
Preemployment screening tools
Personnel file
Employment policy and procedures
Employee personnel files
Employee benefits
Negligent hiring, supervision, and/or retention
Federal Wage Garnishment Law
Family Medical Leave Act

EXEMPT VERSUS NONEXEMPT EMPLOYEES

Generally speaking, most employees can be classified as either exempt or nonexempt employees. The Fair Labor Standards Act defines what positions qualify for exempt status and then employers can determine which positions based on the definitions it will classify as exempt versus nonexempt.[6] Exempt employees are usually those in supervisory roles: executives, administrators or professional-level employees. Nonexempt positions are usually nonsupervisory roles and nonsalaried employees. Nonexempt employees should receive at least the minimum wage and overtime pay for hours worked in excess of 40 during a given workweek. It should be noted that no employer is required by law to provide employees breaks except in California and Maine.

FAIR LABOR STANDARDS ACT

The *Fair Labor Standards Act* is "[a] federal law, enacted in 1938, that regulates minimum wages, overtime pay and the employment of minors. 29 USCA §§ 201–219."[7] This act, administered by the Wage and Hour Division of the U.S. Department of Labor, affects almost every employer in the United States. Thus, if an employee felt his or her employer was not paying individuals at least at minimum wage, was not correctly paying for overtime, or was inappropriately employing underage children, then the correct agency to report this information to would be:

U.S. Department of Labor
Frances Perkins Building
200 Constitution Avenue, NW
Washington, DC 20210
(866) 487-2365
TTY (877) 889-5627

At the writing of this book, the minimum wage for nonexempt employees is $5.15 per hour for hours worked up to 40 hours in a workweek. A workweek can be defined by the employer and may be Monday through Sunday or Wednesday through Tuesday. There is no set rule for the definition of what constitutes a *workweek*. The minimum wage is subject to change through federal legislation. These laws also mandate that nonexempt employees be paid at least time and a half for hours worked over 40 hours in a given workweek.

EQUAL EMPLOYMENT OPPORTUNITY COMMISSION

The *Equal Employment Opportunity Commission*, also known as the EEOC, is "[a] federal agency created under the Civil Rights Act of 1964 to end discriminatory employment practices and to promote nondiscriminatory employment programs. The EEOC investigates alleged discriminatory employment practices and encourages mediation and other nonlitigious means of resolving employment disputes. A claimant is required to file a charge of discrimination with the EEOC before pursuing a claim under Title VII of the Civil Rights Act and certain other employment related statutes."[8] Thus, because this is a federal agency and the subject matter of a potential lawsuit is federal law, the appropriate court to bring a lawsuit would be the local district court within the federal court system. (Addresses have been provided in Chapter 2.)

Some discriminatory employment practices could be considered criminal; therefore, prosecution would come from the U.S. district attorney's office. Again, the local office of the U.S. district attorney would handle such a prosecution. Additionally, the same conduct (discriminatory employment practice) could lead to a civil lawsuit in the same federal court system.

Discrimination is defined as "[t]he effect of a law or established practice that confers privileges on a certain class or that denies privileges to a certain class because of race, age, sex, nationality, religion, or handicap. Federal law, including Title VII of the Civil Rights Act, prohibits employment discrimination based on any one of those characteristics. Other federal statutes, supplemented by court decisions, prohibit discrimination in voting rights, housing, credit extension, public education, and access to public facilities. State laws provide further protection against discrimination. Differential treatment; esp[ecially] a failure to treat all persons equally when no reasonable distinction can be found between those favored and those not favored."[9] Thus the different types of prohibited discrimination include age, race, and gender or sex. There is also invidious and reverse discrimination.

Age discrimination is defined as "[d]iscriminiation based on age. Federal law prohibits age discrimination in employment against people who are age 40 or older."[10] *Racial discrimination* is defined as "[d]iscrimination based on race."[11] *Gender discrimination* is synonymous with sex discrimination and is defined as "[d]iscrimination based on gender, esp[ecially] against women."[12] *Invidious discrimination* is "[d]iscrimination that is offensive or objectionable, esp[ecially] because it involves prejudice or stereotyping."[13] *Reverse discrimination* is defined as [p]referential treatment of minorities, usu[ally] through affirmative-action programs, in a way that adversely affects members of a majority group."[14]

As previously discussed, Title VII of the Civil Rights Act of 1964 prohibits employment decisions that are discriminatory based on race, color, religion, sex, or national origin.[15] Employment involves the hiring, working, promoting, and terminating of employees. Accordingly, in hiring and terminating an employee, as well as in the management of employees, an employer may not discriminate against an employee because of the individual's age, race, sex or gender, because of reverse discrimination decisions.

Enforcement of these laws is assigned to the EEOC. Such discriminatory conduct could lead to a complaint being filed with the Commission and subsequent criminal or civil litigation. There have also been additional employment acts that were legislatively passed after the Civil Rights Act of 1964 aimed at preventing and making illegal other types of discriminatory employment practices. These include Equal Pay Act of 1963; Age Discrimination in Employment Act of 1967; sections 501 and 505 of the Rehabilitation Act of 1973; Title I and V of the Americans with Disabilities Act of 1990; and the Civil Rights Act of 1991.[16]

The Equal Pay Act of 1963 was promulgated to ensure that women and men working in substantially the same job, for the same workplace, received the same pay.[17] Thus, the purpose of this federal legislation was to prevent sex-based salary differentiations.

The Age Discrimination in Employment Act of 1967 was promulgated specifically to prevent people over the age of 40 from being discriminated against in the hiring, promotion, or termination process.[18] Sections 501 and 505 of the Rehabilitation Act of 1973 were specifically promulgated to expand existing antidiscrimination laws to be effective in the employment of the federal government.[19]

Some of the previous antidiscrimination laws did not cover the employees of the federal government and additional provisions had to be enacted so that federal employees would receive the same protections. Titles I and V of the Americans with Disabilities Act of 1990 expanded the previous antidiscrimination laws to prohibit discrimination in the hiring, promoting, or termination of an employee with a disability.[20] Thus, this act prevented employment discrimination in the private sector, at the state government level, and at the local government level.[21] Lastly, the Civil Rights Act of 1991 was promulgated to allow monetary damages in cases where it could be proven there had been intentional employment discrimination.[22]

If an employee or potential employee felt he or she was being discriminated against, the first step (recommended step) would be to discuss the offensive conduct with the alleged offender. Many employment disputes could be resolved quickly, inexpensively, and fairly if the alleged victim of the discrimination simply would tell the alleged offender that the conduct was offensive. Usually alleged offenders of antidiscrimination laws, which include invidious statements, really do not perceive his or her conduct as offensive. Once he or she is made aware of the offensive conduct and the potential consequences for such conduct, he or she usually will change behavior.

However, if that does not work or if the alleged victim does not believe the alleged offender is approachable, then the next recommended step might be to report the alleged offensive conduct and the alleged offender to the alleged offender's supervisor. Again, usually the best solutions are to follow the chain of command for any organization. A chain of command is going to be successive and the alleged victim can continue up the chain until reaching the top-level executive. If satisfaction at any level is not received and the alleged victim still believes he or she has been discriminated against, then the next step (and possibly in some situations the first step) would be to file a complaint with the EEOC.

To file a complaint with the EEOC, the alleged victim can contact the local or the national office.[23] However, if the national office is contacted, that office will refer the alleged victim to the local office. It should also be noted, someone else, including an organization or other individual, may file the complaint on the alleged victim's behalf if the alleged victim is concerned about retaliation.[24] In the filed charge the alleged victim will need to provide contact information for the person filing the complaint, contact information of the employer that allegedly violated the antidiscrimination laws, and a short description of the alleged incidence of discrimination, including the date or dates.[25]

Except for the Equal Pay Act, a charge must be filed with EEOC before any lawsuit may be filed.[26] Generally speaking, the statute of limitations for an EEOC complaint (in other words the time within which the complaint must be filed) is within 180 days of the alleged discriminatory practice.[27] Thereafter, the employer is notified from the EEOC that the charge has been filed.[28] The EEOC then essentially ranks the complaint based on the alleged conduct as to how quickly it will investigate. Clearly, the more egregious the alleged conduct, the more likely there will be evidence to support there was a violation of the law and therefore the faster the EEOC will act.[29]

The investigation may involve a written request for information, interviews, on-site visits where the alleged discriminatory practice took place, or a review of documents.[30]

At any time during this process, the alleged victim and the employer may voluntarily agree to use the EEOC's mediation program or negotiate a settlement.[31] If, after the investigation, the EEOC does not find evidence to support the complaint that the alleged conduct violated the law, the complaint will be dismissed with notification to the alleged victim and the employer.[32] The alleged victim then has 90 days within which to file a lawsuit.[33]

However, if the commission finds evidence to support the complaint that the law was violated, then the EEOC will notify the alleged victim and employer in a letter of determination.[34] The commission will attempt to negotiate conciliation with the employer for a remedy for the alleged victim.[35] *Conciliation* means "[a] settlement of a dispute in an agreeable manner. A process in which a neutral person meets with the parties to a dispute (often labor) and explores how the dispute might be resolved."[36]

If the EEOC cannot negotiate a conciliation with the employer, then the Commission may decide to bring a lawsuit against the employer in federal court.[37] If the Commission does not bring a lawsuit, then the victim of the discrimination may bring a lawsuit within 90 of the EEOC's determination.[38]

Some of the damages that may be awarded in a discrimination lawsuit include back pay, being hired, being promoted, reinstatement, front pay, reasonable accommodation, payment of the victim's attorneys fees, payment of the victim's court costs, and other damages believed to be able to make the victim whole.[39]

If there is evidence the employer acted with malice or reckless indifference, then punitive damages may be available.[40] *Malice conduct* is defined as "[t]he intent, without justification or excuse, to commit a wrongful act. Reckless disregard of the law or of a person's legal rights."[41] *Reckless* is defined as "[c]haracterized by the creation of a substantial and unjustifiable risk of harm to others and by a conscious (and sometimes deliberate) disregard for or indifference to that risk; heedless, rash. Reckless conduct is much more than mere negligence: it is a gross deviation from what a reasonable person would do."[42] *Reckless disregard* is defined as "[c]onscious indifference to the consequences (of an act)."[43]

The contact information for the Equal Employment Opportunity Commission is:

Equal Employment Opportunity Commission
1801 L Street NW
Washington, DC 20507
(202) 663-4900
(TTY) (202) 663-4494
(800) 669-4000
(TTY) (800) 669-6820

EMPLOYMENT AT WILL

Employment at will governs employment relationships in most states. *At-will employment* is defined as "[e]mployment that is usu[ally] undertaken without a contract and that may be terminated at any time by either the employer or the employee, without cause."[44] Thus, if employment is without a contract, then most likely it will be an at-will employment relationship. In that type of an employment relationship, the employee essentially has no legal right to the job. Thus, the employer or employee can terminate the employment without cause at any time. In states with at-will employment, an employee can be terminated without cause but cannot be terminated based on race, gender, age, or disability because of the antidiscrimination laws.

PROGRESSIVE DISCIPLINARY ACTION

Appropriate and accurate disciplinary action can be very effective in training employees. Feedback is usually welcomed by employees and can assist in job performance and job satisfaction. However, occasionally, an employer may find that an employee has problems that must be dealt with. Most employers will have what is known as *progressive disciplinary action* policies and procedures.

In progressive disciplinary action, an employee receives discipline usually based on the severity of the rule infraction. For most employers, there will be infractions that are classified as verbal warning rule violations, with the second violation of the rule moving to a written warning and then another violation of the rule moving the employee to a final warning. If there is another infraction, then the employee would be terminated. This would be known as *termination for cause.*

Some infractions may be more severe than others and the employee may move directly to a written warning as the first step or a final warning as the first step. There are even some infractions that require immediate termination without any progressive disciplinary action. Some infractions that might require immediate termination include arriving at work under the influence of drugs or alcohol or abuse of a patient.

One of the key factors to any disciplinary action is documentation and follow-up. If the employee is being processed through progressive disciplinary action with an anticipation of termination, then whatever is listed as follow-up needs to be completed and documented in the employee's personnel file. An example of follow-up could be that the employee will complete documentation on the day the services are provided. Either the employee meets this requirement or he or she does not. Therefore, documentation should be in the employee file whether there was compliance. If the employee finds there is no follow-up, then the purpose of the disciplinary action is moot and other employees will learn the supervisor is all talk with no action. However, some caution should be used with the contents of an employee's personnel file because it may have to be produced in litigation.

WRONGFUL TERMINATION

A *wrongful termination* is defined as "[a] discharge for reasons that are illegal or that violate public policy."[45] Wrongful discharge can be for retaliation or discriminatory. Generally speaking, because there will always be particular circumstances that exempt a generality, an employee may not be terminated from his or her job out of retaliation. A *retaliatory discharge* is defined as "[a] discharge that is made in retaliation for the employee's conduct (such as reporting unlawful activity by the employer to the government) and that clearly violates public policy. Most states have statutes allowing an employee who is dismissed by retaliatory discharge to recover damages."[46]

An example of retaliatory discharge that led to a lawsuit came out of Kansas. A nurse, the director of nursing, reported to the authorities that the rehabilitation hospital she worked for was not discharging Medicaid patients at the completion of their treatments.[47] Thus, the nurse alleged to authorities the rehabilitation hospital she was working for was unlawfully billing Medicaid.[48] Thereafter, the nurse was terminated and she subsequently filed a lawsuit against the rehabilitation hospital alleging retaliatory discharge.[49]

The general elements for a cause of action that must be proven by a greater weight of the evidence ("preponderance of the evidence") for retaliatory discharge include:[50]

1. A demonstration that the employer "was involved in unlawful activity;
2. [T]he employer knew the employee reported the alleged unlawful practices; and
3. [T]he employer fired the employee in retaliation for making the report."

In this particular case, the employer alleged the director of nursing had been terminated "for an unrelated breach of patient confidentiality."[51] The case was ultimately settled without a trial.[52]

Another case, out of Nebraska known as the "whistle-blower's" doctrine, is *Wendeln v. Beatrice Manor, Inc.*, 2006 WL 903598 (Neb. April 7, 2006).[53] In the *Wendeln* case, a certified nursing assistant who was employed as the nursing home's staffing coordinator was allegedly fired after reporting to a state agency information about a resident's neglect.[54] The Nebraska Supreme Court opined the nursing home staffing coordinator had properly brought a wrongful termination case against the former employer that entitled the staffing coordinator to damages for mental suffering.[55] A jury awarded the former nursing home staffing coordinator a total of $79,000; $4,000 in actual damages and $75,000 for noneconomic damages.[56] (Remember noneconomic damages are subjective and are intended to provide remuneration for such damages as pain and suffering and mental anguish.)

Of particular interest to physical therapists, physical therapist assistants, and students, the alleged neglect involved the dropping of a wheelchair-bound resident during a transfer in which a gait belt should have been used but was not[57] and the resident suffered injury.[58] The staffing coordinator reported the incident to the state's department of health and human services (DHHS) after the staffing coordinator investigated the incident and determined the incident had been reported to the nursing home's administrator who had not reported it to the state's DHHS.[59]

After reporting the incident to the state's DHHS, the staffing coordinator was allegedly angrily reprimanded, which left the staffing coordinator feeling scared and intimidated, and thereafter terminated.[60] Ultimately, the Nebraska Supreme Court decided the former staffing coordinator had been fired after she did what the law required the staffing coordinator to do, report the incident.[61]

EMPLOYMENT CONTRACT

A *contract* is defined as "[a]n agreement between two or more parties creating obligations that are enforceable or otherwise recognizable at law. The writing that sets forth such an agreement"[62] whereas an *employment contract* is defined as "[a] contract between an employer and employee in which the terms and conditions of employment are stated."[63] Generally, an employment contract should include names of the parties to the contract and each party's address as well as each party's contact information specific for the contract. Then minimally, the employment contract should specify the wage, hours to be worked, and what type of work is to be performed.

Additional items that can be included in an employment contract include:

- the specific position being hired and by reference the employee's job description
- the duties the employee is to perform; this could be done by incorporating into the contract by reference the employee's job description
- terms of the employment contract, i.e. from when (date) to when (date)
- commencement date of employment
- whether there will be a probationary period and how long the probationary period will be
- compensation
- how often paid
- whether the employee is exempt or nonexempt for overtime pay rate purposes
- benefits
- termination of the contract to include notice required and where notice is to be given
- noncompete clause
- nonsolicitation clause
- confidentiality clause
- signatures with dates

Most of these items are self-explanatory, but some will be further defined. It is also possible to add to the employment contract that the employee will devote his or her full time to the company or in another way of saying it, the employee will devote full time, all attentions and energies to the company and will not engage in any other business activity in competition with the company. It is also possible to include in the employment contract how disputes will be resolved, which might be through binding arbitration. Binding arbitration means both parties are giving up their right to have a dispute decided by a jury.

Noncompete clauses mean "[a] contractual provision—typically found in employment, partnership, or sale-of-business agreements—in which one party agrees to refrain from conducting business similar to that of the other party. Courts generally enforce these clauses for the duration of the original business relationship, but clauses extending beyond termination must usu[ally] be reasonable in scope, time and territory."[64]

Nonsolicitation means that the employee will not attempt, during the terms of the contract and for some specified time thereafter, to recruit the employer's clients or staff. Employees should be careful when agreeing to either of these two restrictive covenants because it not only impacts the employee during employment, but for some time after the employment relationship ends.

WORKERS' COMPENSATION

Workers' compensation is defined as "[a] system of providing benefits to an employee for injuries occurring in the scope of employment. Most workers' compensation statutes both hold the employer strictly liable and bar the employee from suing in tort."[65] Thus, the statutes enacted for workers' compensation make the employer liable to the employee for coverage of injuries sustained during the scope of employment. Further, the employee cannot sue the employer for the injury.

The federal government has established an Office of Workers' Compensation Programs within the Employment Standards Administration of the U.S. Department of Labor.[66] Each state then enacts the laws and rules governing its state's workers' compensation program utilizing the federal laws. Some of the concepts generally covered in the workers' compensation programs include:

- insurance requirements for private employers
- number of employees for mandatory workers' compensation coverage
- coverage if construction type of work
- coverage if agriculture type of work
- medical benefits provided by workers' compensation statutes
- maximal and minimal compensation rates
- benefits for temporary total disability

- benefits for catastrophic temporary total disability
- benefits for temporary partial disability
- benefits for permanent partial disability
- benefits for permanent total disability
- maximal benefit payments and number of weeks for selected permanent partial disabilities
- flexible maximum benefit levels under the statutes
- disfigurement benefits
- death benefits for surviving spouse and children
- maximal burial allowance
- rehabilitation benefits available under the statutes
- state workers' compensation method of payment
- offset provisions in workers' compensation law
- attorney fees
- advisory committee
- occupational hearing loss statutes

Lastly, if you plan to be an employer, one of the things to consider is whether it will be your company's policy to drug test any employee injured on the job. The benefits of this type of policy are a drug-free work environment and, if an employee is injured and his or her drug test is positive, then the claim may not be covered under the workers' compensation insurance.

PREEMPLOYMENT SCREENING

How does an employer know what kind of an employee is being hired? It is probably one of the most difficult decisions to make and, unfortunately, as the demand for physical therapists and physical therapist assistants grows, the availability of physical therapists and physical therapist assistants is diminishing; thus, sometimes individuals are hired without being qualified. Do not be fooled into thinking a bad employee is better than no employee. A "bad" or "troubled" employee can require more administrative time than actually performing the employee's duties oneself. Also remember, under vicarious liability, employers are legally liable for the acts and/or omissions of their employees. Some of the ways to assist in hiring qualified employees and documenting the employee's file to mitigate damages will be discussed later.

The employment application is usually the first thing completed by potential employees. The employment application should include such things as:

- the person's name
- address
- phone number
- social security number
- whether he or she is eligible for employment in the United States
- if he or she is under the age of 18
- whether he or she has an employment certification
- whether he or she has been convicted or pleaded no contest to a felony* within some specified time frame
- what position the person is applying for
- the days and times the person is available to work
- the date the person is available to start work
- the person's education and any degrees with dates of confirmation
- the person's skills and qualifications
- the person's prior employment history, including the reason for leaving each prior employer
- references, which should include at least one professional reference for physical therapists and physical therapist assistants
- a signature with date certifying that all the information provided on the application is true and accurate

EMPLOYEE'S PERSONNEL FILE

In medical malpractice litigation, it is very common for the personnel file of each employee involved in a particular incident to be produced to the plaintiff's lawyer. Hence, one of the first documents looked for is the application and reference checks. If references were not checked and documented, it is likely that the lack of documentation and/or the lack of actually performing reference checks will be used to assert negligent hiring of the employee involved in the incident.

The next document a plaintiff's lawyer will look for is the orientation checklist to see what, if anything, was done to orient an employee to the job for which he or she was hired. Usually orientation involves a review of the organization's administration structure, employee benefits, and importantly the organization's policies and procedures as well as the employee's scope of employment.

---

* A *felony* is defined as "[a] serious crime usu[ally] punishable by imprisonment for more than one year or by death" (Black's Law Dictionary, 633 (Bryan A. Gardner, ed., 7th ed., West 1999).

The organization's policies and procedures likely will be used to help a plaintiff establish that a particular employee did not follow the organization's established ways of doing things. An example of how a deposition or subsequent trial testimony might go for an employee involved in an incident is:

Q: When you were hired, did you receive any type of orientation?

A: Yes.

Q: What was covered during your orientation?

A: My hours of work, who was in administration, my benefits, and what my job was.

Q: Were you shown any policies and procedures for the organization?

A: Yes.

Q: Were you told it was important to follow the organization's policies and procedures?

A: Yes.

Q: Were you told that it was optional for you to follow the policies and procedures?

A: No.

Q: OK, let's look at the policy and procedure for hot packs.

A: OK.

Q: Did you review this particular policy and procedure during your orientation?

A: I don't recall.

Q: You don't recall. Well then, tell me what policies and procedures you reviewed during you orientation.

A: I don't recall.

Q: How long did you look at the policies and procedures during your orientation?

A: It wasn't very long.

Q: Was it more or less than 5 minutes?

A: I really don't remember exactly, but it was probably more like here are the policies and procedures and that I needed to read them.

Q: Were you given time during your orientation to read all of the policies and procedures?

A: No.

Q: Now we are getting somewhere. At any time after your orientation, did you read all the policies and procedures?

A: No but I knew they were there for me to look at if I needed to.

Q: At any time after your orientation, did you specifically review the policy and procedure on hot packs?
A: I don't think so.
Q: Would you please look at paragraph four of the hot pack policy and procedure. Do you see where it says to test skin sensation every time before application of a hot pack?
A: Yes.
Q: But you never read this policy and procedure to know that the organization's policy and procedure for hot packs was to always test skin sensation before application of hot packs?
A: Correct.
Q: Thank you. I have no further questions.

Then the plaintiff's lawyer would likely also take the supervisor's deposition and it would likely go like this:

Q: When an employee is hired, does he or she receive any type of orientation?
A: Yes.
Q: What is covered during the orientation process?
A: The hours of work, the organization structure, the employee benefits, and generally the employee's job.
Q: Are the employees shown any policies and procedures for the organization?
A: Yes.
Q: Are the policies and procedures important to be followed?
A: Yes.
Q: Are the employees told they are to follow the policies and procedures?
A: Yes.
Q: Why is it important for the employees to follow the policies and procedures?
A: Because the policies and procedures tell the employee how to do things that are required of his or her job.
Q: Are the employees given time during the orientation to review all of the policies and procedures?
A: He or she is given some time and then the employee is supposed to review the policies and procedures in greater detail when he or she gets to his or her particular department.
Q: How do you ensure the policies and procedures for the physical therapy department are read and understood by new employees?
A: I don't have a specific method, but many of the policies and procedures are things the physical therapist or physical therapist assistant already knows.

Q: OK, would that include the method of applying hot packs?

A: Yes.

Q: So you are telling the jury that a physical therapist or physical therapist assistant should know through his or her educational training that the skin sensation should be tested before every application of a hot pack?

A: Yes.

Q: And then you are telling the jury that every physical therapist and physical therapist assistant should have independently reviewed the physical therapy department's policies and procedures, including the one about hot pack application?

A: Yes.

Q: OK, then do you have any explanation for why it was the physical therapist or physical therapist assistant did not test the skin sensation of my client before applying the hot pack?

A: No.

Q: Thank you. I have no further questions.

As you can see, the lawyer will establish the importance of the policies and procedures and that it is the organization's belief that the policies and procedures are to be followed at all times. Then the lawyer established that the physical therapist or physical therapist assistant did not really read the policy and procedure. The lawyer also established that the physical therapist or physical therapist assistant should have known the information from his or her educational training.

Subsequently, this will help the lawyer to plead that there was a "conscious disregard" in the application of the hot pack because the physical therapist or physical therapist assistant knew the information from his or her educational program and then the physical therapist or physical therapist assistant also had the policy and procedures that indicated what should be done. Therefore the physical therapist or physical therapist assistant consciously disregarded what he or she knew to be the right thing to do. The plaintiff's lawyer then will argue that the conscious disregard led to the burn his client received and therefore the plaintiff should be allowed to recover for punitive damages.

ACTING WITHIN SCOPE OF PRACTICE

Every physical therapist and physical therapist assistant is governed by his or her state practice act as well as the rules and regulations governing his or her state. (Recall these were discussed in Chapter 4.) If the physical therapist or physical therapist assistant works for an employer, the employer likely will have a job description for the physical therapist or physical therapist assistant. If the physical therapist or physical therapist assistant does something that is outside the scope of the duties the employer has identified the physical therapist or physical therapist assistant has been hired for, then the physical therapist or physical therapist assistant runs the risk of being accused of acting outside the scope of employment.

Additionally, if the physical therapist or physical therapist assistant does something that is outside the scope of that state's practice act or rules and regulations, the physical therapist or physical therapist assistant can be accused of practicing physical therapy outside the scope of the state's practice acts. This could also lead to a complaint being filed against the physical therapist's or physical therapist assistant's license.

NEGLIGENT HIRING, RETENTION, AND SUPERVISION

Anyone in a supervisory capacity could be named in a lawsuit or a count of a complaint alleging that the individual was negligent in the hiring, supervision, or retention of an employee. Again the elements would be the same elements as any negligent cause of action. As such, the elements would be:

1. There was a duty to hire, supervise, or retain an employee.
2. The supervisor or employer breached the duty to hire, supervise, or retain an employee.
3. The breach of the supervisor or employer was the legal cause of harm to the plaintiff.
4. There are damages associated with the breach of the duty.

This could also be the cause of action related to the supervision of students under any physical therapist's or physical therapist assistant's direction.

The reasonable employer and/or supervisor who is responsible for hiring should ensure that the policies and procedures established for any particular entity are being followed for the hiring of all potential staff. Some of the usual and business practice guidelines to follow in the hiring of employees include the completion of an application, checking references, and documenting the references that were checked. In addition, for licensed personnel, the verification of licensure in good standing should be included. Some states now require employers who work with frail elderly patients or pediatrics to complete a law enforcement background screening and a fingerprint background screening to ensure the person who is being hired has no outstanding abuse and/or neglect actions for a population identified as at risk for abuse and neglect.

It is essential to understand that supervisors can be and are held liable for negligent acts of their employees. One case example wherein the plaintiff could have added a count in the complaint for negligent supervision of a physical therapist assistant student is *Henry v. Williams*.[67] In this case, a patient fell outside while being gait trained for a step with a physical therapist assistant student.[68] This case is illustrative for many things and will be discussed for its other merits in Chapters 12 and 16. In this case, the patient had been admitted to the hospital and undergone surgery for a right knee replacement.[69] Following surgery, the surgeon prescribed physical therapy.[70]

The physical therapist delegated the therapy sessions to a physical therapist assistant trainee.[71] (The court elected to call the student a trainee.) Prior to working as a student physical therapist assistant at the hospital, the physical therapist assistant trainee had completed 1 year of an associate's degree course work and she had completed a 4-week clinical.[72] During the course of physical therapy treatment, the patient progressed to ambulating 200 feet with a rolling walker on level surfaces with stand-by assist.[73]

Prior to discharge from the hospital, the physical therapist learned that the patient would have to be able to go up and down one step in order to get in and out of the home.[74] The physical therapist directed the physical therapist assistant trainee to train the patient how to go up and down one step.[75] The physical therapist assistant trainee elected to take the patient outside to use a curb for the training instead of using a two-step piece of equipment that was available in the physical therapy department.[76]

When the physical therapist assistant trainee (student) took the patient outside and had the patient stand up, she had the patient put the walker in the left hand and the trainee walked around the back of the patient.[77] Thereafter the factual account of the circumstances differs between the patient and the physical therapist assistant trainee. Regardless, the patient took a step to go down the curb and fell.[78] The patient reinjured the knee and had to undergo additional surgery.[79]

Ultimately, the patient had a full recovery and only lacked 5 degrees extension of the operated knee.[80] The factual difference was that the patient testified the physical therapist assistant trainee stood behind her and said, "I'm trying to figure out how to tell you to do it."[81] The physical therapist assistant trainee testified she moved to the back of the patient intending to be on the right side of the patient to assist with stepping down but the patient without warning took a step down off the curb and fell.[82] Thus, there was what is called a *dispute of fact* that must be determined and resolved by a jury. Of interest, in this particular jurisdiction prior to the lawsuit being filed, a panel of three physical therapists reviewed the evidence and did not find enough evidence that either the physical therapist or the physical therapist assistant trainee breached the prevailing standard of care.[83]

Regarding negligent supervision, the student physical therapist assistant was outside with a patient teaching the patient how to go up and down one step so that the patient could be discharged home independent in this functional task. The question for this part of this chapter is whether the supervising physical therapist breached a duty for the supervision of this student and could have been named individually in this lawsuit with the count in the complaint being the negligent supervision of a student physical therapist assistant.

FEDERAL WAGE GARNISHMENT LAW

The Federal Wage Garnishment Law allows an employee's wages to be subjected to garnishment but provides for a limit.[84] The law prevents the employee from being fired because his or her wages are garnished; however, subsequent debts and garnishment may subject an employee to discharge. This law is administered through the Wage and Hour Division of the U.S. Department of Labor's Employment Standards Administration.

FAMILY MEDICAL LEAVE ACT

The Family Medical Leave Act became effective August 5, 1993. This act also is administered through the Wage and Hour Division of the U.S. Department of Labor's Employment Standards Administration. This act covers all employees of private, state, and local government. Some federal employees are covered and some are not. This act entitles employees who have been employed 12 months for at least 1250 hours who are experiencing specific family and medical problems to take up to 12 weeks of unpaid leave from work within a 12-month period of time. While on this leave, the employee's job is protected.

SUMMARY

Various employment laws and causes of actions involve employment of which physical therapists, physical therapist assistants, and students should be aware. The importance of the law or cause of action may vary depending on the job role the physical therapist or physical therapist assistant is performing. However, every physical therapist, physical therapist assistant, or student should recall ignorance of the law will never be an excuse for failure to adhere to a law.

DISCUSSION QUESTIONS

1. What is the Fair Labor Standards Act?
2. Discuss the Equal Employment Opportunity Commission.
3. Discuss progressive disciplinary action.
4. Why is progressive disciplinary action important?
5. Discuss wrongful termination.
6. Discuss employment contracts.
7. Discuss workers' compensation.
8. Discuss preemployment screening.
9. Discuss an employee's personnel file.
10. Why is an employee's personnel file important?
11. Discuss negligent hiring, supervision, or retention.
12. Discuss the Federal Wage Garnishment Law.
13. Discuss the Family Medical Leave Act.

NOTES

[1] *Black's Law Dictionary*, 543 (Bryan A. Garner, ed., 7th ed., West Group, 1999).
[2] *Id.* at 544.
[3] *Id.* at 927.
[4] *Id.* at 1313.
[5] *Id.*
[6] 29 C.F.R. Part 541, § 13(a)(1) (2004).
[7] *Id.* at 616.
[8] *Id.* at 557.
[9] *Id.* at 479.
[10] *Id.* at 480.
[11] *Id.*
[12] *Id.*
[13] *Id.*
[14] *Id.*
[15] Equal Employment Opportunity Commission, www.eeoc.gov.
[16] *Id.*
[17] *Id.*
[18] *Id.*
[19] *Id.*
[20] *Id.*
[21] *Id.*
[22] *Id.*
[23] *Id.*

[24] *Id.*
[25] *Id.*
[26] *Id.*
[27] *Id.*
[28] *Id.*
[29] *Id.*
[30] *Id.*
[31] *Id.*
[32] *Id.*
[33]*Id.*
[34] *Id.*
[35] *Id.*
[36] *Black's Law Dictionary*, 284 (Bryan A. Garner, ed., 7th ed., West Group, 1999).
[37] Equal Employment Opportunity Commission, www.eeoc.gov.
[38] *Id.*
[39] *Id.*
[40] *Id.*
[41] *Black's Law Dictionary*, 968 (Bryan A. Garner, ed., 7th ed., West Group, 1999).
[42] *Id.* at 1276.
[43] *Id.*
[44] *Id.* at 545.
[45] *Id.* at 476.
[46] *Id.* at 476.
[47] Andrews Litigation Reporter, *Nurse's Suit Survives Menon for Judgment; Retaliation Ease Ends*, page 9, April 14, 2006.
[48] *Id.*
[49] *Id.*
[50] *Id.* at 10.
[51] *Id.*
[52] *Id.*
[53] Andrews Litigation Reporter, *Nebraska High Court Upholds Whistle-blower's Award for Retaliatory Fixing*, page 7, April 28, 2006.
[54] *Id.*
[55] *Id.*
[56] *Id.*
[57] *Id.*
[58] *Id.*
[59] *Id.*
[60] *Id.*
[61] *Id.*
[62] *Id.* at 318.
[63] *Id.* at 321.
[64] *Id.* at 370.

[65] *Id.* at 1599.
[66] U.S. Department of Labor, www.dol.gov.
[67] *Henry v. Williams*, 892 So.2d 765 (La. App. 2 Cir. 2005)
[68] *Id.*
[69] *Id.* at 767.
[70] *Id.*
[71] *Id.*
[72] *Id.*
[73] *Id.*
[74] *Id.*
[75] *Id.*
[76] *Id.*
[77] *Id.*
[78] *Id.*
[79] *Id.*
[80] *Id.*
[81] *Id.*
[82] *Id.*
[83] *Id.*
[84] Title III of Consumer Credit Protection Act.

CHAPTER 7

Other Types of Lawsuits

In prior chapters, lawsuits involved negligence or medical malpractice as well as issues with employment laws. In this chapter other types of lawsuits that physical therapists and physical therapist assistants could encounter will be discussed. These include breach of fiduciary duty, breach of contract, fraud, premises liability, *res ipsa loquitur*, product liability, and assault and battery, including sexual misconduct. Each of these will be discussed in greater detail throughout this chapter.

KEY CONCEPTS

Fiduciary duty
Breach of contract
Fraud
Premises liability
Res ipsa loquitur
Product liability
Assault and battery
Pro se litigant

BREACH OF FIDUCIARY DUTY

A *fiduciary duty* is defined as "[a] duty of utmost good faith, trust, confidence, and candor owed by a fiduciary (such as a lawyer or corporate officer) to the beneficiary (such as a lawyer's client or shareholder); a duty to act with the highest degree of honesty and loyalty toward another person and in the best interests of the other person (such as the duty that one partner owes to another)."[1] A fiduciary duty is a legal relationship between two parties with one being in a fiduciary position to the other person, who is the beneficiary of the relationship. Some fiduciary relationships involve trustees, directors of companies (this will be discussed in greater detail in Chapter 14), doctors, or lawyers, and it is likely the physical therapists or physical therapist assistants could be alleged to be fiduciary. The fiduciary duty is the highest standard of care imposed on an individual. A fiduciary is expected to act with the utmost loyalty; therefore, personal interests cannot be put ahead of the beneficiary's interest in the fiduciary relationship. Thus, the physical therapist or physical therapist assistant must deal with his or her patients with the utmost loyalty, honesty, and good faith.

The elements for a cause of action alleging a breach of the fiduciary duty relative to physical therapists and physical therapist assistants would be:

1. The physical therapist or physical therapist assistant owed the patient a fiduciary duty
2. Because of the confidence placed by the patient in the physical therapist or physical therapist assistant, the patient relied on the physical therapist or physical therapist assistant
3. The physical therapist or physical therapist assistant breached the fiduciary duty
4. The breach of the fiduciary duty caused harm to the patient
5. Damages resulted to the patient

Any patient could allege he or she placed a confidence in what the physical therapist or physical therapist assistant told the patient.

Thus, the patient may make a decision based on what the physical therapist or physical therapist assistant tells the patient or the patient's family. The patient's "trust" in the physical therapist or physical therapist assistant led him or her to make certain treatment decisions. Accordingly, if the patient consents to some type of additional treatment, and these treatments are not successful, the patient may allege a breach of a fiduciary duty. This potential risk will likely grow as physical therapists become entry-level health care practitioners because the patient will be placing more confidence in the physical therapist as an entry-level health care provider and relying on information from the physical therapist for treatment decisions.

BREACH OF CONTRACT

A *contract* is defined as "[a]n agreement between two or more parties creating obligations that are enforceable or otherwise recognizable at law. A writing that sets forth such an agreement."[2] There are multiple types of contracts the physical therapists, physical therapist assistants, or students may encounter during their careers. These include an employment contract, a contract with vendors for different types of supplies or services, and a contract with patients for the payment of the physical therapy services. When one party does not perform his or her responsibilities under the contract, then a breach of the contract may be alleged to have occurred. The elements for a cause of action for breach of contract would be:

1. There was a valid enforceable contract between two parties
2. One party breached his or her duties under the enforceable contract
3. The failure of one party to perform the obligation(s) of the contract caused harm (damages) to the other party

One of the factors considered in contract law is called the statute of frauds. The *statute of frauds* is defined as "[a]n English statute enacted in 1677 declaring certain contracts judicially unenforceable (but not void) if they are not committed to writing and signed by the party to be charged."[3] The types of contracts applicable to the statute of frauds include:

1. A contract for the sale or transfer of interest in land
2. A contract that cannot be performed within 1 year
3. A contract for the sale of goods that are valued at $500 or greater
4. A contract of an executor or administrator to answer for a decedent's debt
5. A contract to guarantee the debt or duty of another
6. A contract made in consideration of marriage

The two that physical therapists, physical therapist assistants, and students should pay particular attention to are contracts for goods valued at $500 or greater and a contract that cannot be performed within 1 year.

If the physical therapist, physical therapist assistant, or student executes a contract for employment that will be for a term longer than 1 year, he or she must retain a copy of the contract that was signed by the employer. Enforcement may require an executed copy with the signature of the party the therapist wishes to hold accountable for the contract. Likewise, when dealing with vendors for supplies that are valued at $500 or greater, be sure to retain a copy of the contract executed by the vendor.

If a physical therapist or physical therapist assistant enters into any of these above types of contracts, then the party the physical therapist or physical therapist assistant enters into the contract with must sign (execute) the contract if the physical therapist or physical therapist assistant want to enforce the contract at some later time. If the other party does not sign the contract, then later breaches of the contract may not be judicially enforceable.

Another type of contract that could affect physical therapy clinic owners is the contract entered into for payment of services with health care insurance carriers. The specific language of the contract is crucial and should be completely understood by the clinic owners. A case involving this issue is *Clinton Physical Therapy Services v. John Deere Health Care, Inc.*[4]

In *Clinton*, the Clinton Physical Therapy Corporation contracted with John Deere Health Care, Inc., to provide physical therapy services as a "network provider" to John Deere Health Care, Inc., members.[5] Thereafter, Clinton Physical Therapy opened an additional office in Davenport, which was also called the Plaza office.[6] Members of John Deere Health Care, Inc., received physical therapy services at the new Davenport clinic.[7]

It took approximately 4 months from the initial contract execution for Clinton Physical Therapy to notify John Deere Health Care, Inc., of its Davenport office and that it wanted Davenport to be a covered office.[8] Initially John Deere Health Care, Inc., paid for physical therapy services at the Davenport office.[9] However, John Deere Health Care, Inc. took the position that the Davenport office was not a covered facility and notified Clinton Physical Therapy approximately 8 months later that physical therapy services provided at the Davenport facility would not be covered.[10] Prior to that time John Deere Health Care, Inc., had paid for physical therapy services.[11]

Ultimately, Clinton Physical Therapy continued to treat John Deere Health Care, Inc., members at the Clinton Physical Therapy without payment.[12] Subsequently, John Deere Health Care, Inc., refused to pay $138,750, of which $128,200 had been rendered after John Deere Health Care, Inc., notified Clinton Physical Therapy it would not pay for services.[13] The case went to trial and the jury returned a verdict for Clinton Physical Therapy in a total of $10,500.[14] However, the method the jury used to calculate the verdict appeared inconsistent and the appellate court ordered a new trial.[15]

Thus, in the end a new trial on the issue was ordered. The lesson from this case was to read any contract with third-party insurance and understand what is covered and what is not covered, including the locations and what entities are uncovered. Until there is confirmation that a particular site is a covered entity for the provision of physical therapy services, understand there may be no basis to enforce payment of the physical therapy services provided without a valid contract.

ASSAULT AND BATTERY

Assault is defined as "[t]he threat or use of force on another that causes that person to have a reasonable apprehension of imminent harmful or offensive contact; the act of putting another person in reasonable fear or apprehension of an immediate battery by means of an act amounting to an attempt or threat to commit a battery."[16] *Battery* is defined as "[t]he application of force to another, resulting in harmful or offensive contact. It is a misdemeanor under most modern statutes."[17]

There are three types of battery: aggravated battery, sexual battery, and simple battery. *Aggravated battery* is defined as "[a] criminal battery accompanied by circumstances that make it more severe, such as the use of a deadly weapon or the fact that the battery resulted in serious bodily harm."[18] *Sexual battery* is defined as "[t]he forced penetration of or contact with another's sexual organs or the sexual organs of the perpetrator."[19] *Simple battery* is defined as "[a] criminal battery not accompanied by aggravating circumstances and not resulting in serious bodily harm."[20]

Sometimes it is easier to prove a civil allegation of assault and/or battery than it is a criminal allegation because of the difference requirement in the weight of the evidence or burden of persuasion. Remember that criminal charges require proof beyond the reasonable doubt standard whereas civil allegations usually require proof at the preponderance of the evidence or greater weight of the evidence standard.

The physical therapist, physical therapist assistant, or student should be very careful in the clinical setting for potential claims of assault and battery. When a physical therapist, physical therapist assistant, or student physically touches a patient, if the physical touch is unwanted, then the patient could accuse and sue for battery. Likewise, when the physical therapist, physical therapist assistant, or student is performing an evaluation or treatment of someone that requires exposure of "private" areas, he or she may want to consider having an aide present for the comfort of the patient and as protection as a witness.

FRAUD

Fraud is defined as "[a] knowing misrepresentation of the truth or concealment of a material fact to induce another to act to his or her detriment. Fraud is usu[ally] a tort, but in some cases (esp[ecially] when the conduct is willful) it may be a crime."[21] Thus, the elements for a cause of action in fraud would be:

1. A knowing misrepresentation of the truth
2. Concealing of a material fact

3. Inducing another to act to his or her detriment

Generally speaking, the most common types of fraud the physical therapist, physical therapist assistant, or student will hear about or have the potential to commit are Medicare, Medicaid, and insurance fraud.

Medicaid is "[a] government program that provides medical aid to those who cannot afford private medical services. Medicaid is jointly funded by the federal and state governments."[22] Medicaid fraud includes billing for services not rendered or billing for services rendered but rendered by unqualified personnel. Medicaid is a state-run program that receives some federal funding. Hence, an investigation into a physical therapy practice's Medicaid billing is usually undertaken by the particular state's attorney general.

As previously discussed, authorities in New York were able to prosecute a claim for Medicaid fraud against three health care providers on Long Island.[23] Ultimately instead of the case going to trial, a settlement was reached such that the three health care providers in total agreed to pay $4,000,000. One particular health care provider billed for services rendered by unqualified personnel as well as failed to document proof that the billed treatments actually had been provided. Another health care provider submitted false cost reports that had Medicaid overpaying for services rendered, while the other health care provider submitted for Medicaid payments without being properly registered with Medicaid. Thus, the rules and regulations established by third-party reimbursement sources are created to be followed and deviation can lead to an investigation and prosecution.

RES IPSA LOQUITUR

Res ipsa loquitur is defined as "[t]he doctrine providing that, in some circumstances, the mere fact of an accident's occurrence raises an inference of negligence so as to establish a prima facie case. 'The thing speaks for itself'."[24] The physical therapist, physical therapist assistant, or student may run into this doctrine when the facts surrounding an incident seem to only have one explanation and that explanation was the negligence of the care provider.

As an example, if a patient is performing therapeutic exercises on a ball, and the physical therapist, physical therapist assistant, or student leaves that patient unattended (even for a moment!) and the patient falls off the ball, injuring himself, there would be no question the physical therapist, physical therapist assistant, or student was negligent in the supervision of that patient. The reason is that no reasonable physical therapist or physical therapist assistant would ever leave a patient alone and unsupervised when performing therapeutic exercises on a ball because of the danger of falling off and being injured. Hence, the plaintiff would assert a claim of negligence and would plead *res ipsa loquitur*.

An example of a case involving a physical therapist where the plaintiff pled *res ipsa loquitur* is *Romero v. Willis-Knighton Medical Center*.[25] In the *Romero* case, the plaintiff asserted he was undergoing physical therapy treatment for rehabilitation of his knee following surgery.[26] As part of the treatment plan, the physical therapist had the plaintiff walking on a treadmill.[27] The plaintiff asserted that the treadmill suddenly and without warning changed directions, which caused the plaintiff to fall injuring his knee and back.[28] In the complaint, the plaintiff pled *res ipsa loquitur*.[29]

Further, the plaintiff pled that the physical therapist knew or should have known that the treadmill was not functioning properly and that the physical therapist failed to warn the plaintiff (patient) of the potential harm the treadmill could cause.[30] Additionally, the claim was brought as a claim of strict liability for the defective product (treadmill) in the hospital's physical therapy clinic.[31]

Strict liability for products is defined as "[p]roducts liability arising when the buyer proves that the goods were unreasonably dangerous and that (1) the seller was in the business of selling goods, (2) the goods were defective when they were in the seller's hands, (3) the defect caused the plaintiff's injury, and (4) the product was expected to and did reach the consumer without substantial change in condition."[32]

The plaintiff's complaint asserted the following:[33]

1. Failure to use reasonable and ordinary care in order to protect patrons from a dangerous condition
2. Failure to properly inspect the premises
3. Failure to properly maintain the premises
4. Failure to warn patrons of the presence of a dangerous condition
5. Any other acts of negligence later shown

Ultimately, like many of the cases discussed in this book, this case was appealed on other grounds and the appellate court's ruling was for other issues. For this particular case, the issue on appeal was whether it had to be brought pursuant to the medical malpractice statutes or whether it could be brought as a plain negligence claim.[34] This was a critical issue to this claim because in Louisiana, medical malpractice lawsuits have to first be brought before a medical review panel.[35] Ultimately, the appellate court agreed this particular lawsuit was not really a claim for medical malpractice; therefore, it did not first need to be brought before the medical review panel.[36]

PREMISES LIABILITY

Premises liability is defined as "[a] landowner's or landholder's tort liability for conditions or activities on the premises."[37] When a physical therapist or physical therapist assistant manages a clinic, that therapist is responsible for the condition of the clinic. However, if someone gets injured because of a condition on the premises, then the owner of the clinic is ultimately responsible for the premises. If the physical therapist or physical therapist assistant also owns the clinic, then the physical therapist or physical therapist assistant also will be responsible for the damages resultant from the premises' problems.

If the landowner(s) rents or leases the property to someone else, then the landowner(s) will expect rent or lease payments at regular intervals. The time intervals for payment could be monthly, quarterly, every 6 months, or annually, but nonetheless is dictated by the terms of the contract. Thus, premises liability could also involve the landowner enforcing the terms of the contract or sometimes in the worst-case situation, evicting someone from the premises.

A case that involved eviction of a physical therapy clinic was *PTS Physical Therapy Service, Inc. v. Magnolia Rehabilitation Service, Inc.*[38] In this case, Magnolia Rehabilitation was evicted after PTS Physical Therapy Service, Inc., took eviction action.[39] Magnolia Rehabilitation argued that the contract it had with PTS Physical Therapy contained an option to buy the property, which it executed.[40] However, once Magnolia executed the option to purchase, Magnolia learned that PTS did not have clear title to the property.[41] Magnolia contacted the purported owners, Northwest Physical Medicine, L.L.C.[42]

Magnolia then asserted that Northwest guaranteed it another 1-year lease.[43] However, the trial court did not recognize the alleged new lease and essentially evicted Magnolia under the old lease (contract) with PTS Physical Therapy.[44] On appeal, the appellate court held that PTS had not established that it was the owner of the property; therefore, PTS did not have the legal right to proceed with eviction processes,[45] and the eviction was overturned.[46]

Another premises liability case involving a physical therapist is *Jenner v. the Board of Education of the North Syracuse Central School District*.[47] In this case a school physical therapist alleged she "slipped on a loose rug and fell down a set of stairs."[48] Immediate injuries were occipital lobe concussion and some bruising.[49] Later, the physical therapist began to complain of some visual problems.[50]

The physical therapist sued the school district, alleging there had been negligent maintenance of the premises.[51] The case was appealed because defendants asserted the statute of limitations had expired and therefore the claim was barred.[52] The court disagreed and allowed the claim to go forward.[53] The lesson to learn from this case is that items on the floors and/or stairs that can cause people to fall should be removed. Remember, if the physical therapist or physical therapist assistant owns the clinic, he or she will be held liable for items that cause people to fall on the premises.

PRODUCT LIABILITY

Product liability is defined as "[a] manufacturer's or seller's tort liability for any damages or injuries suffered by a buyer, user, or bystander as a result of a defective product. Product liability can be based on a theory of negligence, strict liability, or breach of warranty."[54] A physical therapist or physical therapist assistant may become involved with this type of liability when products are used in the evaluation or treatment of patients. If the patient is harmed because of something to do with a particular product, then the manufacturer or seller of the product may be brought into the lawsuit under a theory of product liability. Hence, the physical therapist, physical therapist assistant, or student should read the manufacturer warnings on all products used in a particular clinic.

PRO SE LITIGANT

A *pro se litigant* is someone who represents himself or herself throughout the litigation process and does not have a lawyer providing representation. One of the advantages to being a *pro se* litigant is that there are no attorney's fees to pay. However, the disadvantage is that the *pro se* litigant likely does not understand criminal or civil procedure nor is likely to understand the substantive law or how to research it. An example of a case involving physical therapy and a *pro se* litigant is *Faison v. Rosado*, 129 Fed.Appx. 490 (11th Cir. 2005).[55]

In the *Faison* case, a federal prisoner brought a claim against the prison's physician for failing to order physical therapy as recommended by an orthopedist.[56] The physical therapist would have allegedly instructed the prisoner in proper weight-bearing techniques to prevent the prisoner's osteoporosis from progressing.[57] Instead, the prison physician referred the prisoner to a mid-level practitioner who provided instructions to the prisoner on proper range of motion exercises and weight-bearing activities.[58] Thus, the allegation was that the physician's failure to refer the prisoner to physical therapy caused the prisoner's osteoporosis to progress. The court disagreed and found that the orthopedist's documentation for physical therapy was a recommendation and not an order.[59] The physical therapist and physical therapist assistant should understand that what he or she documents, if not clear, could be left up to a jury to interpret the meaning of the document. In this case, the failure of the prisoner to hire a lawyer who could have retained an expert to testify as to what the orthopedist documentation actually meant may have resulted in the loss of the action.

SUMMARY

In addition to medical malpractice or negligence claims, physical therapists, physical therapist assistants, or students could be involved with product liability or premises liability. Each different claim or cause of action has its own unique set of elements that give rise to the claim. The physical therapist, physical therapist assistant, and student should be aware of these types of claim to mitigate the risk exposure associated with each.

DISCUSSION QUESTIONS

1. What should a physical therapist or physical therapist assistant do when treating someone in a manner that could place the private sensitivity of the patient in question?
2. Discuss fiduciary duty.
3. Discuss breach of contract.
4. Discuss statute of frauds.
5. Discuss assault and battery.
6. Discuss fraud.
7. What is *res ipsa loquitur*?
8. How could a physical therapist, physical therapist assistant, or student become involved in litigation involving *res ipsa loquitur*?
9. What is premises liability?
10. How could a physical therapist, physical therapist assistant, or student become involved in litigation involving premises liability?
11. What is product liability?
12. How could a physical therapist, physical therapist assistant, or student become involved in litigation involving product liability?

NOTES

[1] *Black's Law Dictionary*, 523 (Bryan A. Garner, ed., 7th ed., West Group, 1999).
[2] *Id.* at 318.

[3] *Id.* at 1422.
[4] *Clinton Physical Therapy Services v. John Deere Health Care, Inc.*, 714 N.W.2d 603 (Iowa 2006).
[5] *Id.* at 606.
[6] *Id.*
[7] *Id.*
[8] *Id.*
[9] *Id.*
[10] *Id.*
[11] *Id.*
[12] *Id.*
[13] *Id.*
[14] *Id.* at 608.
[15] *Id.* at 606.
[16] *Black's Law Dictionary,* 109 (Bryan A. Garner, ed., 7th ed., West Group, 1999).
[17] *Id.* at 146.
[18] *Id.*
[19] *Id.*
[20] *Id.*
[21] *Id.* at 670.
[22] *Id.* at 996.
[23] Andrews Litigation Reporter, *N.Y. Authorities Settle Medicaid Billing Cases for Nearly $4 milion,* page 11, April 14, 2006.
[24] *Black's Law Dictionary,* 1311 (Bryan A. Garner, ed., 7th ed., West Group, 1999).
[25] *Romero v. Willis-Knighton Medical Center,* 870 So.2d 474 (La.App. 2 Cir. 2004).
[26] *Id.* at 476.
[27] *Id.*
[28] *Id.*
[29] *Id.*
[30] *Id.*
[31] *Id.* at 477.
[32] *Black's Law Dictionary,* 1226 (Bryan A. Garner, ed., 7th ed., West Group, 1999).
[33] *Romero v. Willis-Knighton Medical Center,* 870 So.2d 474, 477 (La.App. 2 Cir. 2004).
[34] *Id.*
[35] *Id.*
[36] *Id.*
[37] *Black's Law Dictionary,* 1199 (Bryan A. Garner, ed., 7th ed., West Group, 1999).
[38] *PTS Physical Therapy Service, Inc. v. Magnolia Rehabilitation Service, Inc.*, 920 So.2d 997 (La.App. 2d Cir. 2006).
[39] *Id.* at 998.
[40] *Id.*
[41] *Id.*
[42] *Id.*
[43] *Id.*

[44] *Id.* at 999.
[45] *Id.* at 1000.
[46] *Id.*
[47] *Jenner v. the Board of Education of the North Syracuse Central School District*, 803 N.Y.S.2d 18 (N.Y.Sup. Ct. 2005).
[48] *Id.*
[49] *Id.*
[50] *Id.*
[51] *Id.*
[52] *Id.*
[53] *Id.*
[54] *Black's Law Dictionary*, 1225 (Bryan A. Garner, ed., 7th ed., West Group, 1999).
[55] *Faison v. Rosado*, 129 Fed. Appx. 490 (11th Cir. 2005).
[56] *Id.* at 491.
[57] *Id.*
[58] *Id.* at 492.
[59] *Id.*

CHAPTER 8

Understanding the Role of Documentation

There is a tenet in almost every health care professional's training that says, "not documented, not done." Documentation plays an essential role in every lawsuit for medical malpractice or medical negligence. Usually the role documentation plays is one of omission; the health care provider did not document something that the plaintiff's lawyer asserts means the health care provider did not do something and that caused harm to the patient.

It is impossible for any health care provider, including physical therapists, physical therapist assistants, and students to document everything done during a physical therapy evaluation and/or treatment. Thus, physical therapists, physical therapist assistants, and students must learn to document pertinent information that includes exclusion test(s) or rationale when deviating from the accepted standards of practice, which to some degree have been reduced to writing in the *Guide to Physical Therapy Practice*.[1]

This chapter will examine some of the most critical items to include in documentation, especially informed consent, as well as provide examples wherein a lawsuit was brought to life based on a documentation entry. It should be noted that plaintiffs' lawyers often use one or two documentation entries in a medical record to provide the "spin" needed to sustain and sometimes prevail in a lawsuit.

KEY CONCEPTS

Documentation
Health Insurance Portability and Accountability Act (HIPAA)
Within normal limits (WNL) and within functional limits (WFL)

WHAT SHOULD BE INCLUDED IN DOCUMENTATION?

Essentially everything should be included in the physical therapist's, physical therapist assistant's, or student's documentation. However, because that is an unreasonable expectation, a jury usually will accept that documentation in a medical record cannot be perfect. Thus, a jury usually allows reasonable inferences for some things not to be documented and sometimes even omitted. The jury will hear that the documentation standard is "not documented, not done." Every expert is likely to agree with this tenet. Consequently, what is included in the documentation and what is omitted is often the centerpiece of medical malpractice or medical negligence causes of action.

The *physical therapy evaluation* has been defined as "[a] dynamic process in which the physical therapist makes clinical judgments based on data gathered during the examination."[2] The *examination* is defined as "[a] comprehensive screening and specific testing process leading to diagnostic classifications or, as appropriate, to a referral to another practitioner. The examination has three components: the patient/client history, the systems review, and tests and measures."[3]

According to the *Guide to Physical Therapy Practice*, the necessary component of a physical therapy evaluation is the examination.[4] Accordingly, if the physical therapy examination does not include each of those components, in the perfect world, the physical therapist should be documenting in the physical therapy evaluation why the physical therapist elected not to include all components of the "standard" evaluation. Remember, the *Guide to Physical Therapy Practice* will likely be presented to a jury as the standard under which every physical therapist should practice.

Consequently, the *Guide to Physical Therapy Practice* indicated that every evaluation should include these components of the examination. Therefore, if the physical therapist elected not to include every component, the documentation should explain why the physical therapist chose not to include some aspects. A jury then would see the physical therapist understood, comprehended, and utilized the standard of what should be included in an examination, but because of certain circumstances facing the physical therapist with that particular patient, it was not appropriate to perform the listed component(s) of evaluation documented as omitted.

This documentation of exception can help circumvent the plaintiff's lawyer from soliciting expert testimony that, because it was not documented, the physical therapist simply forgot or did not perform that component of the evaluation. Remember the elements of the cause of action for a claim of medical negligence discussed in Chapter 5; duty, breach of the duty, and causation with damages. The physical therapist is under a duty to perform an examination of the patient. If the physical therapist did not document that the physical therapist evaluated every possible component of an examination (breach of duty), and that particular omission can be causally linked (causation) to a bad outcome (damages), then the plaintiff's claim can breathe life.

Wouldn't people understand if the physical therapist didn't document a problem with all areas of an evaluation, it meant there was no problem? However, for purposes of litigation and risk management, the physical therapist, physical therapist assistant, or student must understand the tenet, not documented, not done.

In litigation, the plaintiff's lawyer will utilize the physical therapist's, physical therapist assistant's, or student's failure to document these exceptions to argue the physical therapist, physical therapist assistant, or student breached the standard of care because he or she did not document the performance of the things the therapist was obligated (duty) to evaluate, meaning the physical therapist, physical therapist assistant, or student did not evaluate them. Therefore, the plaintiff's outcome (damages) would have been different had they only performed all components of the examination.

As an example, a physical therapist has a patient who has entered the physical therapy clinic for the treatment of low back pain. One of the standards of a physical therapy evaluation—which would be established through expert testimony, use of the *Guide to Physical Therapy Practice*, and physical therapy schools' curricula—is to determine the integrity of sensation, which includes but is not limited to light touch, hot/cold discrimination, sharp/dull discrimination, and pressure, both light and deep.

The physical therapist evaluates light touch but elects not to conduct the other sensation tests. As part of the physical therapy treatment plan, the physical therapist prescribes hot packs for 20 minutes to the low back at the beginning of every treatment session. Despite utilizing the normal amount of layers between the patient and the hot pack, the patient receives a burn. The burn requires treatment and is painful to the patient. The patient retains a lawyer and sues the physical therapist (direct liability) and the physical therapist's employer (vicarious liability), if applicable. The plaintiff alleges his or her hot/cold discrimination sensation was impaired and had the physical therapist tested it during the physical therapy evaluation, he or she would have discovered this impairment and not prescribed hot packs as part of treatment or would have taken additional precautions in the application of the hot packs.

The failure to avoid hot-pack application altogether as part of the treatment plan or to take the additional precautions in the application of the hot packs was a breach in the standard of care. The patient has a burn from the hot pack (damages) as a result of this failure. The lack of documentation on the evaluation would be offered as evidence to prove the breach in the standard of care because experts, the *Guide to Physical Therapy Practice*, and physical therapy schools' curriculum all would support that hot/cold discrimination sensation should be evaluated prior to hot-pack application. Because the physical therapist did not document that he or she tested hot/cold discrimination sensation, the jury must assume the physical therapist must not have evaluated it, and the patient sustained a burn as a result.

On the other hand, consider the same example, except this time the physical therapist not only tested hot/cold discrimination sensation, but also documented that it was within normal limits. In this situation, the plaintiff still can argue through expert testimony that the physical therapist breached the standard of care because the physical therapist's rationalization and utilization of the hot packs was flawed. This is a better battleground for the defense because it forces the plaintiff to argue the merits of the decision to use hot packs versus merely showing the physical therapist's evaluation with the missing documentation. That leads to arguing the physical therapist simply did not do what the physical therapist as a professional was supposed to do.

This example also serves to further exemplify the transition the profession is undergoing in becoming entry-level health care providers. In this example, most every reader probably presumed a physician referred the patient to the physical therapist. As a result, the physician also would likely be named as a defendant in the lawsuit. However, there are times when the referring physician, called a *treater*, is supportive of the plaintiff's theory of the litigation. Hence, there are times a treater will not be named as a defendant because the treater provides supportive testimony for the plaintiff. Likewise, there are many lawsuits where all treaters are also named as defendants. In this later example, defense counsel are well-served to work together on a common defense versus pointing blame on other treaters. If all named defendants blame one another, at trial a jury would likely find liability against all of the defendants and split fault percentages amongst the group of defendants.

Under Vision 2020, with direct or consumer access and autonomous practice, the physical therapist could be performing this initial evaluation without the benefit of a physician screening the patient prior to the physical therapy evaluation. (It should be noted some states allow the physical therapist to evaluate a patient now without the requisite physician referral.) Accordingly, when a physician does not refer the patient and the physical therapist is the first health care practitioner the patient sees, the physical therapist must not only perform a thorough evaluation, but the physical therapist also is the initial determiner of what, if any, additional tests or referrals are necessary to rule out other diseases or complications.

There are many cases regarding physicians' failures to recognize signs and/or symptoms of other diseases leading to delayed diagnosis with resulting harm. Consequently, the physical therapist, in assuming the responsibility of being the initial health care practitioner, should expect the same legal risks and consequences. Thus, in the previous example, failure to perform a simple hot/cold discrimination sensation test could be used to springboard a lawsuit if the patient received a burn from the hot pack.

One case reflecting the heightened responsibility of physical therapy's autonomous and direct practice is *Bailey v. Haynes, M.D.*, 856 So.2d 1207 (LA 2003). In that case, the physical therapist actually was credited with diagnosing that a child suffered from cerebral palsy.[5] Based on the physical therapist's diagnosis, a plaintiff was afforded the information needed to file a lawsuit against the physician who delivered the child.[6] Thus, documentation has many purposes. More likely than not, the physical therapist in the *Bailey* case had no intention of her documentation being used to support a claim for physician medical malpractice, but it did.

Additionally and equally as important is the information communicated to a patient and/or the patient's family. In *Bailey*, the court made its ruling based on the physical therapist's date of diagnosing the cerebral palsy.[7] Obviously there could be instances where the evidence relied on would be the date or content of information provided by the physical therapist, physical therapist assistant, or student. Consequently, every physical therapist, physical therapy assistant, and student should recognize his or her documentation, or lack thereof, as well as information communicated verbally to the patient or patient's family, could see the inside of a courtroom one day.

Likewise, the inclusion of information observed or discussed during an evaluation and/or treatment can prove invaluable in the defense of a lawsuit. Just like one note can breath life into a lawsuit, the right note can sometimes slam the door shut on a lawsuit. The dilemma is what to include in the documentation and what is essentially frivolous writing. The recommended rule is to include everything actually performed during an evaluation and explain any deviation from what is considered a normal evaluation. If the physical therapist, physical therapist assistant, or student is uncertain what to include in the documentation, review the *Guide to Physical Therapy Practice*; call the American Physical Therapy Association; call mentors or experts in the field; speak with local practitioners and ask what they include in their evaluations of similar patients; ask physicians what they consider important; and obtain clinical competence through continuing education.

Another case wherein documentation played a key role to exonerate the defendants was *Biggs v. Clyburn, et. al.*, 2003 WL 21197151 (Tex. App. Hous. 1st Dist. 2003). In *Biggs*, a patient who had undergone a shoulder replacement sued the hospital and surgeon alleging the surgery was a failure as the patient's shoulder continued to dislocate.[8] However, the surgeon documented "the patient himself was moving the shoulder in directions and in positions that were causing the shoulder to dislocate."[9] Further, the physical therapist documented warnings and instructions to the patient to "stop moving his shoulder in certain positions."[10] Both the surgeon's and the physical therapist's documentation supported and was evidence that the patient himself was moving his arm into directions that were causing the shoulder to dislocate. Thus, there was no breach of duty on behalf of the surgeon to the patient with regards to the surgery. Accordingly, the plaintiff lost the lawsuit.[11]

From these examples, it should be clear that documentation is critical evidence during any litigation or trial. With regard to medical malpractice lawsuits, it is often one of the key pieces of evidence—or lack of evidence—to support the factual assertions of one party or the other. It must be recognized that all too often, the lack of documentation or omission of documentation is the crux of the issue during litigation or trial.

PROGRESS NOTES

The *progress note* is what details and contemporaneously documents what occurred during each physical therapy treatment. Most physical therapists, physical therapist assistants, and students document progress notes in the SOAP format. This format stands for:

S—**Subjective** part of the note that includes the patient's or patient's family comments that are relevant to the condition being treated,

O—**Objective** part of the note that indicates specifically what was done with the patient including the treatment, examinations, and patient's response to the treatment,

A—**Assessment** part of the note should specifically document how the patient is progressing toward the goals and what changes are needed to the plan of treatment,

P—**Plan** part of the note should reflect what is going to be done at the next visit and what is going to be done to progress the patient toward discharge.

However, all too often in a retrospective review of documentation, it is found that the progress notes all look very similar and really do not uniquely document what occurred during each treatment. Instead what is found is repetitive documentation that essentially states the same thing occurred over and over for each treatment There is essentially nothing unique about any particular note, which not only questions the level of skill involved in the treatment but also gives the appearance that contemporaneous documentation is not being completed.

Progress notes should include information about how the patient responded to the last treatment in detail, what the patient has refrained from doing that could irritate or exacerbate the patient's symptoms, what treatment was delivered with specific parameters, what tests were utilized prior to the application of the treatment to ensure that patient was still appropriate for the treatment, what instructions the patient was given, and what is planned for the next visit and over the course of the plan of care. These notes should be specific and unique to the patient and to the particular treatment.

Obviously not everything can be included in the progress note, but remember if this particular patient's chart goes into litigation, whatever is not documented could be argued as an omission in the care because of the tenet. Therefore, as an example, the following are examples from various physical therapy progress notes with identifying information redacted:

1. **Outpatient Clinic**
   S: No complaints
   O: Continued with plan of treatment to include HP × 20 minutes, stretching exercises × 15 repetitions, bike × 15 minutes, Cybex at 120 degrees × 3 sets of 10 repetitions, cool-down stretches × 15 repetitions
   A: Doing well, ROM increased 5 degrees
   P: Continue current plan of treatment

2. **Nursing Home**
   S: Blank
   O: Continued with skilled physical therapy for ambulation, therapeutic exercises, transfers, and balance training
   A: Doing well
   P: Continue

3. **Home Health**
   S: No complaints

O: Transferred from bed to wheelchair; able to perform therapeutic exercises × 10 repetitions × 2 sets; worked on wheelchair mobility within the house and then worked on transfers to/from wheelchair and toilet

A: Tolerated well but still requires skilled physical therapy as strength is still poor

P: Continue plan of treatment 3 times per week

You will note from these examples that essentially the patients all seem to have no complaints and nothing needs to be changed or upgraded in the treatment plan. However, example one is an outpatient note, example number two is a progress note from a nursing home patient, and example number three is a progress note from a home health chart. Some of the specific questions that these notes raise collectively are:

1. Regarding the Subjective part of the note:
   a. How did the previous treatment impact the patient? Did the patient regress, stay the same, or demonstrate any improvement?
   b. What happened functionally to the patient as a result of the last treatment?
   c. As a result of the last treatment has the patient—if complaining of pain—experienced an increase, decrease, or or no change in pain level?
   d. Did the patient perform or not perform any exercises or treatments prescribed for a home program?
   e. What is the patient's understanding of the plan of treatment?
2. Regarding the Objective part of the note:
   a. The area receiving treatment: What is its status upon entering physical therapy and what is its status upon physical therapy being completed this treatment?
   b. What exactly was done during the treatment session? (No, there were no worksheets or check-off sheets indicating specifics of the treatment program.)
   c. What of the treatment required the skill and knowledge of the physical therapists or physical therapist assistants?
   d. Was there any part of the session that increased or decreased from the last physical therapy treatment session?
   e. What assistance did the patient need to perform or participate in the physical therapy treatment session? Was the patient total assistance or did the patient required minimal physical assistance but required complete verbal instructions whereas last treatment only required infrequent reminders or

cues? (Then in the assessment part of the note the physical therapists or physical therapist assistants would assess whether this impacted treatment and whether this was a significant change that might need a referral to other services.)

3. Regarding the Assessment part of the note:
   a. Was the performance at this physical therapy session an improvement, regression, or status quo from the last treatment session?
   b. Had any area of treatment improved, regressed, or stayed the same?
   c. Based on the objective measurements, how far is the patient from reaching the goals?
   d. Is the treatment effective and reasonable?
   e. What is it about the treatment that is requiring the skill and knowledge of the physical therapist or physical therapist assistant?
4. Regarding the Plan part of the note:
   a. What is going to be changed for the next treatment session?
   b. What additional physical therapy is needed and why?
   c. Who else needs to be involved in this patient's treatment or care?
   d. Is the patient on target to meet the goals of physical therapy in the time frame originally expected? If not, why not and what is the physical therapist or physical therapist assistant going to do to change the course of action or request additional physical therapy time?
   e. What education and what equipment may the patient need?

Thus, these progress notes highlight how unoriginal these examples are. Consequently, these example progress notes are not helpful for reimbursement or for the defense of a lawsuit. In fact these progress notes could actually assist the plaintiff's theory of the case.

The reason these progress notes can assist a plaintiff's theory of cases is because the progress notes demonstrate how the treatments are either not in line with the plan of care or appear to not have been performed by skilled professionals. Also a trend beginning is that some plaintiffs' lawyers are asserting fraudulent billing because these progress notes do not demonstrate skilled physical therapy was delivered; still, physical therapy services were billed as if given by a physical therapist or physical therapist assistant. Thus, each progress note should be individually written for the patient for the particular treatment session.

REEVALUATION

Reevaluation is synonymous with reexamination. *Reexamination* is defined as "[t]he process of performing selected tests and measures after the initial examination to evaluate progress and to modify or redirect interventions."[12] There is no specific time during the treatment of a patient that a reexamination needs to be done; however, it needs to be done when the plan of treatment needs to be modified or different interventions need to be attempted.

DISCHARGE SUMMARY

A *discharge* is defined as "[t]he process of ending physical therapy services that have been provided during a single episode of care, when the anticipated goals and expected outcomes have been achieved. Discharge does not occur with a transfer (that is, when the patient is moved from one site to another site within the same setting or across setting during a single episode of care)."[13] Thus, a discharge summary is the documentation that summarizes all the care the patient received during the episode of care. This discharge summary should include the patient's initial status and the patient's discharge status as well as the treatments received and the outcome from the treatment received.

To emphasize how important documentation is, including the discharge summary, consider the case of *Polidoro v. Chubb Corporation*, 386 F.Supp.2d 334 (S.D.N.Y 2005). In this case, the plaintiff essentially alleged the physician terminated her physical therapy services prematurely after a workers' compensation injury, which subsequently led to further injuries.[14] However, upon review of all the documentation, the court disagreed.

In June 1998 the plaintiff was injured at work and suffered a left wrist and right knee injury.[15] Plaintiff's injuries were covered under workers' compensation for medical treatments and disability.[16] Eleven months later, the plaintiff's previously injured right knee gave way and the plaintiff suffered a fracture to her right foot.[17] After another 11 months, the employer terminated the physical therapy benefits based on a physician's report that the left wrist and right knee had recovered.[18] Four months later, a workers' compensation hearing was held and there was apparently an agreement between the employer and the plaintiff that the plaintiff's weekly compensation payment would be reduced in return for an authorization for continued physical therapy.[19]

The plaintiff alleged in the complaint that because the physical therapy services were terminated after 11 months of treatment, the failure to receive ongoing physical therapy services caused the joints that were injured in the first fall to weaken.[20] The weakened joints led to the plaintiff sustaining a fractured left hip and torn right knee meniscus 2 and one half years after the initial injury.[21] Thereafter, the plaintiff was going to require a left hip replacement and a right knee replacement.[22]

The plaintiff demanded $16 million in compensatory damages (economic and noneconomic damages combined), $15 million in punitive damages, and two times the amount of expenses that had been covered by Medicare.[22] Ultimately the plaintiff's nine-count complaint was partially dismissed after the appellate court's ruling.[23] What is instructional with this case is that the physician's report documenting that the plaintiff had recovered from the original injuries led to the physical therapy services being discontinued. As a result, the physician also was named as a defendant in the lawsuit. Physical therapists, physical therapist assistants, and students should realize the discharge summary will be utilized to justify continuance or discontinuance of services and some plaintiffs may allege improper discharges from physical therapy.

MISSING DOCUMENTATION

The idea that documentation could be missing from a patient's chart seems ludicrous, however, it is a recurrent theme in many medical malpractice cases. In fact, many hours are spent in storage rooms looking through boxes and boxes of records in hope that missing documentation can be found. The important legal concept that needs to be understood regarding missing documentation is that if a plaintiff believes there is missing documentation from his or her medical record, he or she also can add a cause of action to the lawsuit for spoliation of evidence.

Spoliation of evidence is defined as "[t]he intentional destruction, mutilation, alteration, or concealment of evidence, usu[ally] a document. If proved, spoliation may be used to establish that the evidence was unfavorable to the party responsible."[24] Thus, a party also can assert that the missing documentation is actually missing because it was harmful evidence to the party whose responsibility it was to secure the documentation. If this were a case in Florida, the party seeking the missing documentation at trial might request the judge to give the jury a *Valcin* jury instruction.[25]

The *Valcin* jury instruction generally means the jury is to presume that the missing documentation would be favorable to the party requesting the documentation. The party that is unable to produce the documentation has the opportunity to prove to the jury, by a greater weight of the evidence, that "the 'records are not missing due to an intentional or deliberate act or omission' of the hospital or its employees."[26]

In the *Valcin* case, a patient suffered a ruptured tubal pregnancy 1 and one half years after the hospital staff performed a tubal ligation.[27] The court noted that generally the law in Florida is that a plaintiff has the burden to establish medical malpractice (*citing Atkins v. Humes*, 110 So.2d 663 [Fla. 1959]).[28] However, in the *Valcin* case, the "operation report" of the tubal ligation was missing.[29] Hence, experts could not determine if the standard of care had been followed before, during, and after the tubal ligation surgery despite the standard being that there was to be an operative report.[30]

Further, the court found that the hospital had a statutory duty to maintain such records as the operative report and that "where evidence peculiarly within the knowledge of the adversary is, as here, not made available to the party who has the burden of proof, other rules must be fashioned."[31] Hence, the court established a rule that, because the records were missing, the hospital had the burden to establish the record was not missing because of an intentional or deliberate act.[32]

It is clear courts are not forgiving of individuals or entities that have a duty to maintain records and the records are not maintained. Of course there are exceptions to record destruction such as natural acts of God, like a hurricane. However, short of a natural disaster, if there is a duty to maintain the records, then the records need to be maintained. Sometimes those records will not be good for the defense, but that does not obviate the duty to maintain the records. Therefore, the loss of records, whether accidental or intentional, could lead to a claim for damages under a spoliation of evidence theory and the request for a special jury instruction that the party deliberately destroyed the records because the records would establish the adversary's case.

LATE-ENTRY DOCUMENTATION

Sometimes a physical therapist, physical therapist assistant, and student might forget to write a note or might forget to include information in a note. It is normal that this can happen on an occasion; however, this should not become the normal way of practicing. Documentation should be completed contemporaneously at the time of the evaluation or treatment. However, when documentation has been forgotten, it is legally acceptable to do what is called a late-entry note. When a late-entry note is written, the physical therapist, physical therapist assistant, and student should label the entry as "late entry" and include the date of the late entry. Write the information and then sign the note.

If the physical therapist, physical therapist assistant, and student is making a corrective note, then one line needs to be marked through the incorrect documentation and labeled as "incorrect entry" or "error." There is debate over which label is better than the other, but from a defense lawyer's perspective, it really makes no difference. The incorrect entry or error also needs to be dated and the physical therapist or physical therapist assistant needs to sign the entry.

As an example:

S: No complaints

O: Doing well, continued with therapeutic exercises of quad sets, ham sets, SLR [straight leg raise], TKE [terminal knee extension], hip abduction and adduction, and ankle pumps of dorsiflexion and plantarflexion all performed with 3 pounds for 15 repetitions by 2 sets; rode Fitron by 15 minutes at 45 rpm

A: Good muscle strength increase such that able to do leg exercises with 3 pounds over 2 pounds last session; however, not able to descend steps without using handrail; therefore, eccentric strength still needs strengthening exercises

P: Continue with current home program with instruction to increase weight to 3 pounds and will add wall slides to next sessions

Error or incorrect entry: 10/31/06—Sheila K. Nicholson, PT

A single line is drawn through the documentation with the label of "incorrect entry" or "error" with the date and signature. This way someone can still read the note and understand the signatory is stating this was a mistake in documentation and is not accurate. Do not scratch through or in some way try to obliterate the writing.

PRIVILEGED DOCUMENTATION

Sometimes there are documents that lawyers will privilege and not produce to an opposing party. Some of these documents include incident reports and personnel evaluations. There is a rule in evidence that documents created in anticipation of litigation are usually not required to be produced to the other party in litigation.[33] However, in order for this privilege to be maintained, the party creating the document must not waive the privilege by producing it or discussing the contents of it with third parties. The documents this rule will likely apply to most are incident reports.

Incident reports are generally created to document something that occurred that was out of the ordinary or not expected. The unusual event may or may not be related to a negative outcome. The incident report usually provides a place to document the circumstances surrounding the event and an opportunity for the investigation of what happened, how it happened, and what can be done to prevent it from happening again. At the time the incident occurs, there may or may not be the threat of litigation; however, if the document is created "in anticipation of litigation," then the document is usually protected from subsequent production under the attorney work product, quality assurance, and/or attorney-client communication privileges.

One method to help ensure the appropriate documents are privileged is to print on the document "prepared in anticipation of litigation" and have counsel review the documents and offer legal advice about the occurrence. Another way to protect the privileges is to have the incident report prepared and maintained in the custody of the risk-management department. If the practice is too small to have a risk-management office then designate someone in the clinic, most likely the owner of the clinic, as the risk manager. Then the risk manager is charged with the duty of investigating the incident and maintenance of the incident report.

It should be noted, however, that even when these steps are taken, there are times when a judge may order production of the document. Usually the side that wants the document believes there will be information contained in the document that cannot be obtained from any other source. The opposing side usually has the burden to establish there is no other way to obtain the information such that it is unfairly prejudicial to the client not to have the information.

One example of where the court might require production of an incident report is when objective measurements associated with the patient were taken at the time of the incident but not recorded (documented) anywhere except on the incident report. When the person involved in the incident is questioned during a deposition whether he or she, for example, took the patient's vital signs immediately after the incident to determine what, if any, medical treatment needed to be summoned and the deponent testifies yes, but the notes associated with the event do not document vital signs, then the judge might order the production of the incident report.

From a legal defensive perspective, it might be beneficial to produce such an incident report; however, if the defense ever waived the privilege in the one lawsuit, there would be the argument that the party has waived its privilege to the document in subsequent lawsuits. Hence, there could be a dilemma whether to produce a defensively beneficial incident report and run the risk of waiving the privilege in subsequent litigation. Obviously, if this is an issue in any lawsuit the physical therapist, physical therapist assistant, and student will want to discuss all options, strengths, and weaknesses of the privilege.

Personnel evaluations are necessary tools for the training of staff members. However, sometimes the personnel evaluations contain criticisms that plaintiff lawyers like to use in litigation. Therefore, defense lawyers will attempt to privilege these documents to prevent discovery so that these tools can continue to document employees' weaknesses and strengths without the fear that this information could be used in litigation.

HIPAA

HIPAA stands for Health Insurance Portability and Accountability Act of 1996. This legislation is federal and is administered through the U.S. Department of Health and Human Services. This act was essentially the first time there had been legislation regarding the privacy rule related to individuals' medical information. This act regulates, as a privacy rule, the use and disclosure of individuals' health information.[34]

The average health care provider under these laws must:

1. Notify a patient about his or her privacy right and how his or her information can be used,
2. Adopt and implement privacy procedures for its practice,
3. Train employees in privacy procedures,
4. Designate someone responsible for privacy procedures and enforcement,
5. Secure patients records.

The laws do allow for the disclosure of protected health information to another health care provider for treatment purposes.[35] There are also provisions for disclosure when a patient puts his or her health care at issue in a lawsuit. Complaints for violation of the HIPAA laws should be forwarded to the Office for Civil Rights, www.hhs.gov. Complaints must be filed within 180 days of the violation.

CASES INVOLVING DOCUMENTATION

The case of *Roberts v. State Farm Mutual Automobile Insurance Company*, 802 N.E.2d. 157 (Ohio 2d DCA 2003) demonstrates how physical therapists and physical therapist assistants sometimes document their own negligence to support liability. In the *Roberts'* case, a patient was referred to physical therapy for treatment of a foot injury sustained on the job.[36] The case was ultimately appealed on the issue of whether the trial court erred when it did not instruct the jury on the consequences of subsequent medical malpractice.[37] Thus, the defendant in the trial case wanted the jury to be instructed that the defendant could not be held liable for the medical malpractice of the subsequent physical therapy.

The patient sustained a foot injury when a piece of steel fell on the patient's foot[38] and the patient was referred to physical therapy.[39] During physical therapy, the patient complained of back pain when using the leg press.[40] The physical therapist discontinued using the leg press, however, the patient continued to complain of back pain.[41] The patient also complained of rib pain after using the sled with weights.[42] Subsequently, a physician expert testified that the patient was further injured during her rehabilitation for the foot injury. The physical therapy documentation indicated "client tends to hyperextend the back to increase momentum for heavier overhead lifts."[43] In other words, the physical therapist documented that the treatment being delivered was resulting in problems for the patient and that the treatment was actually what had injured the patient. It should be evident that if a patient is hyperextending his or her back to increase momentum to lift heavier objects, then the patient had not developed the strength to do the lift.

WNL AND WFL

Often physical therapists, physical therapist assistants, and students document WNL (within normal limits) or WFL (within functional limits) in the objective section of notes for assessment of range of motion or strength. Somehow these terms have gotten confused with actual objective goniometric measurements or muscle strength testing. WNL and WFL are assessments and are NOT objective measurements. Accordingly, physical therapists, physical therapist assistants, and students should not use these assessments tools as objective measurements.

SUMMARY

Documentation is a vital piece of evidence in medical malpractice or medical negligence cases. The recurring theme used in litigation related to documentation is "not documented, not done." Therefore, physical therapists, physical therapist assistants, and students should contemporaneously document pertinent findings of a patient's evaluations, treatments, and progress toward goals as well as any information obtained or communicated to the patient and/or the patient's family.

DISCUSSION QUESTIONS

1. What are the basic pieces of physical therapy documentation?
2. What should be included in a physical therapy evaluation?
3. Is there only one way to document a physical therapy progress note? If yes, what is the one way? If no, what are the different ways?
4. When should documentation be completed?
5. Who should complete the documentation and why?
6. When should a reevaluation be completed?
7. What is spoliation of evidence?
8. How should a late-entry or inaccurate documentation be corrected?
9. What is privileged documentation?
10. What is HIPAA?
11. Why is documentation important?
12. What should be included in a physical therapy progress note?
13. Discuss reevaluation.
14. What is a discharge summary?
15. Why is a discharge summary important?
16. How can a document become privileged?
17. Discuss HIPAA.
18. When and how should WFL and WNL be used?

NOTES

[1] *Guide to Physical Therapy Practice,* 679 (American Physical Therapy Association, 2nd ed., 2003).
[2] *Id.*
[3] *Id.*
[4] *Id.*
[5] *Bailey v. Haynes,* 856 So.2d 1207, 1211 (LA 2003).
[6] *Id.*
[7] *Id.*
[8] *Biggs v. Clyburn, et. al.,* 2003 WL 21197151 (Tex. App. Hous. 1st Dist.).
[9] *Id.* at 6.
[10] *Id.*
[11] *Id.* at 7.
[12] *Guide to Physical Therapy Practice,* 682 (American Physical Therapy Association, 2nd ed., 2003).
[13] *Id.* at 678.
[14] *Polidoro v. Chubb Corp.,* 386 F.Supp.2d 334, 335 (S.D.N.Y. 2005).
[15] *Id.*

[16] *Id.*
[17] *Id.*
[18] *Id.* at 335–336.
[19] *Id.* at 335.
[20] *Id.* at 336.
[21] *Id.*
[22] *Id.*
[23] *Id.*
[24] *Id.* at 342.
[25] *Black's Law Dictionary*, 1409 (Bryan A. Garner, ed., 7th ed., West Group, 1999).
[26] *Public Health Trust of Dade County v. Valcin*, 507 So.2d 596 (Fla. 1987).
[27] *Id.* at 598.
[28] *Id.* at 597.
[29] *Id.*
[30] *Id.*
[31] *Id.* at 597–598.
[32] *Id.* at 598.
[33] *Id.*
[34] Fed. R. Evid. 502 (2001).
[35] 45 C.F.R. §§ 160, 162 and 164 (2006).
[36] *Id.*
[37] *Roberts v. State Farm Mutual Automobile Insurance Company*, 802 N.E.2d. 157, 160 (Ohio 2d DCA 2003).
[38] *Id.* at 159.
[39] *Id.* at 160.
[40] *Id.*
[41] *Id.* at 162.
[42] *Id.*
[43] *Id.*
[44] *Id.* at 163.

CHAPTER 9

Liability with Various Practice Settings

This chapter will discuss liability issues associated with different types of practice settings. Every physical therapy clinical setting will have the risk of medical malpractice; however, there are some clinical settings that present unique liability risks.

Different types of practice settings include and involve various clinical settings and various associated business entities. Clinical settings include hospitals, outpatient clinics, nursing homes, rehabilitation hospitals, home health settings, and school systems/pediatric clinics. Further, the personal liability risk associated with a clinical setting is sometimes predicated on the clinical setting's organizational structure.

Organizational structure is different than the type of business entity; however, both are important issues in litigation. The organizational structure becomes critically important in litigation because a plaintiff's lawyer wants to determine the person or group of persons or entity or entities that directed, controlled, and determined day-to-day operations that ultimately affected what happened to the plaintiff. Usually, the plaintiff's lawyer believes that the higher in the organizational structure it can be alleged that there was control, direction, and decisions that affected the negative outcome for the plaintiff, the more money that will be available to pay for plaintiff's damages. Hence, this chapter will examine the organizational structure of several clinical settings and explain how the clinical setting's organizational structure affects liability risks. The various business entities and their impact on liability will be discussed in Chapter 14.

KEY CONCEPTS

Organizational structures
Liability risk associated with various clinical settings
Liability risk associated with organizational structure

HOSPITALS

Generally speaking, hospitals will be privately, publicly, or corporately owned. When privately owned, an individual or group of individuals or an entity will own the hospital. There will be fewer layers of management to go through for approvals of equipment, supplies, or policy and procedures. When the hospital is publicly owned, there will usually be a board of directors that is either appointed or elected and will have the ultimate authority over the hospital's operations.

The board of directors will not have the day-to-day oversight of operations for the hospital, because that is usually delegated to the chief executive officer (CEO). Lastly, corporate-owned hospitals will likely have local and distant management structures. These concepts are important, because in a lawsuit, it is not uncommon for plaintiffs' lawyers to want to sue any and all parties or entities that may have had some authority over the day-to-day decisions that occur at the hospital level.

The organizational structure for a privately owned hospital might look similar to **Figure 9-1**.

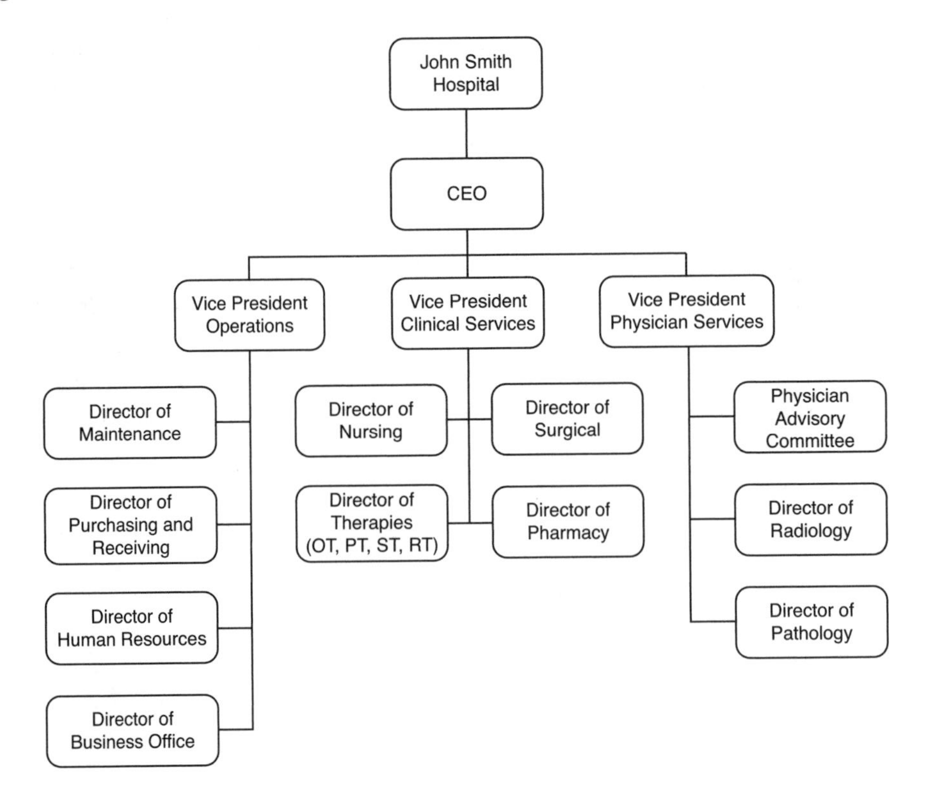

Figure 9-1 Privately Owned Hospital

Thus, in this organizational structure, if a lawsuit resulted from treatment in the physical therapy department, then the vice president of clinical services, the CEO and the private owner of John Smith Hospital could also be named as defendants in the lawsuit alleging each controlled and directed what happened in the physical therapy department.

The organizational structure for a publicly-owned hospital might look like **Figure 9-2**.

Thus, as can be seen, there are multiple levels that could be sued if the plaintiff wants to attempt to reach the highest level of authority. In fact, for a lawsuit based on a happening in physical therapy, additional defendants could be the vice president of clinical services, the CEO, every member of the board of directors, the county of Smith and the state of Smith. The purpose of naming more defendants is an attempt to find more money to pay for damages to the plaintiff as well as possibly establishing conduct that would sustain a claim for punitive damages.

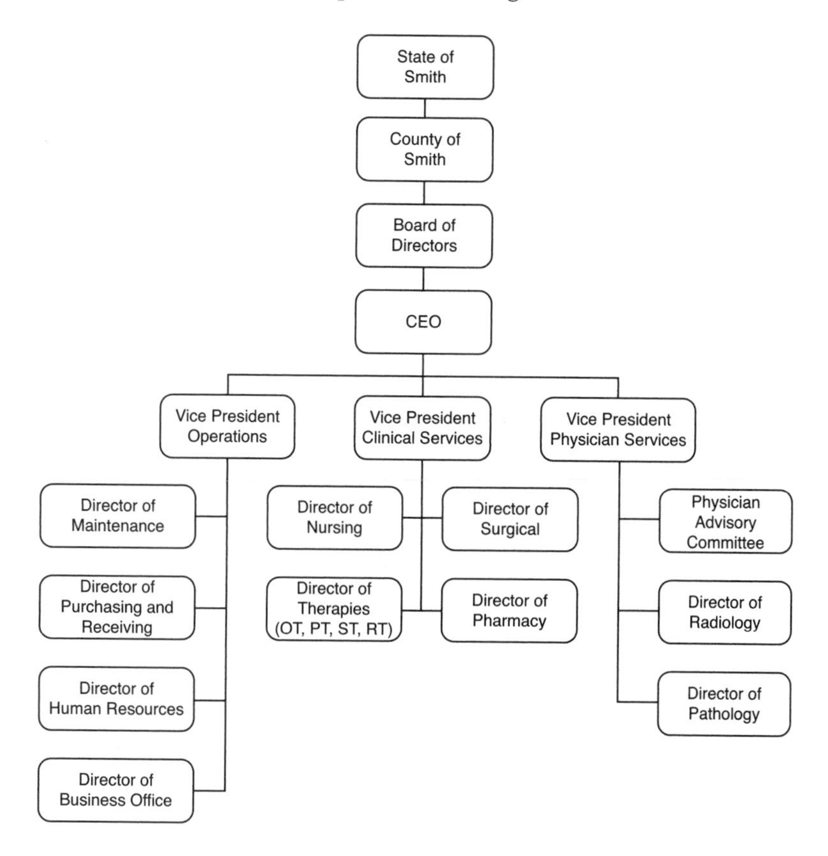

Figure 9-2 Publicly-Owned Hospital

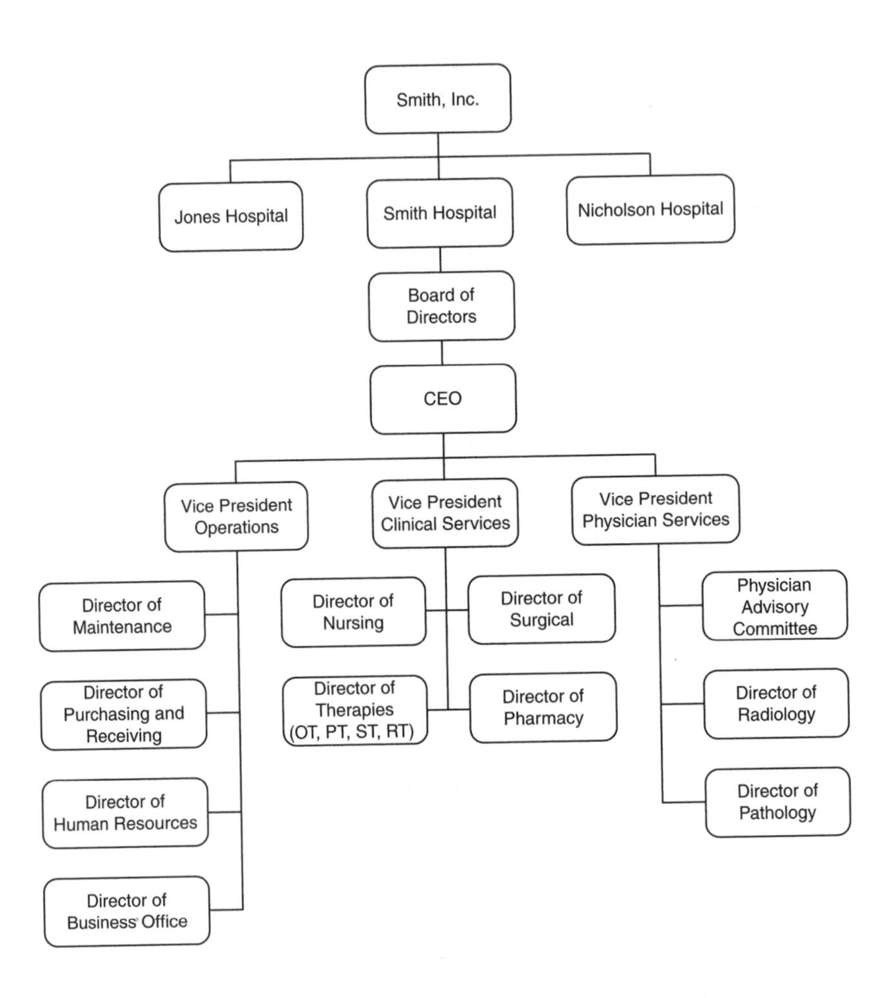

Figure 9-3 Corporate-Owned Hospital

Figure 9-3 represents what the organizational chart might look like for a hospital that is corporately owned. This diagram shows that the parent company owns several hospitals. However, at the local level, the organization is the same as if this were a privately owned hospital. Again, as in the private and publicly owned hospital examples, there are more potential defendants, which in plaintiff terms means more potential money to pay for damages.

The structure of the actual corporate entity, whether incorporated or a limited liability company, will dictate how a plaintiff's lawyer might be able to pierce the corporate veil. (Corporate entities and piercing the corporate veil will be discussed in Chapter 14.) Thus, when a lawsuit arises based on the act(s) and/or omission(s) in the physical therapy department, everyone involved up the chain of command may be named in the lawsuit, depending on the facts surrounding the lawsuit. Some of the high risks facing the physical therapy departments in hospitals are related to the acuity of the patients.

When patients are hospitalized, it is generally related to an acute illness, trauma, or the need for surgery. These patients will be weaker, under the influence of medications, and, more likely than not, in some degree of pain. These factors make it critical for the physical therapist, physical therapist assistant, or student to always know, understand, and appreciate the complications associated with the condition of the patient he or she is treating.

Likewise, the physical therapist, assistant, or student and especially the director of the department, should ensure supportive staff are well trained in their particular job duties and the potential complications associated with each patient they may be assisting. Some of these complications include cardiopulmonary resuscitation (CPR), choking, and first aid. If a supportive staff member fails in his or her duties, the supervising physical therapist or physical therapist assistant and director of the department also should expect to be named in a lawsuit.

An example is *Budner v. Allegheny General Hospital*.[1] In the *Budner* case, the plaintiff sued the hospital for the alleged negligence of a physical therapist.[2] The plaintiff was receiving physical therapy whirlpool treatments to her feet.[3] In order to receive the treatment, the plaintiff had to sit in a chair that could swivel around so the plaintiff could put her feet in the whirlpool.[4] On the date of the incident, the plaintiff alleged she got up in the swivel chair, which was tall, and received her treatment.[5]

At the conclusion of the treatment, the chair was swiveled 90 degrees so the physical therapist could dry the plaintiff's feet.[6] However, instead of waiting for the chair to be completely turned before getting down, the plaintiff attempted to stand up without the chair being in the proper position.[7] When the plaintiff attempted to stand, she fell and alleged injuries to her neck, back, ribs, coccyx, and right shoulder.[8]

The issue for the appellate court was whether this was medical malpractice or premises liability.[9] If the claim was for medical malpractice, then there were certain statutory requirements the plaintiff had not met, which meant the case should be dismissed.[10] However, if the case was grounded in premises liability, then the statutory requirements of certification of merit were not required.[11]

Ultimately, the court decided the facts asserted were for a claim of professional negligence; therefore, it was a claim for medical malpractice and not premises liability.[12] Thus, a hospital can sometimes be sued for problems that occur in the physical therapy clinic under different theories of liability other than professional malpractice.

OUTPATIENT CLINICS

An outpatient clinic may be privately or corporately owned and most likely the organizational chart is less complicated than that of a hospital. Usually there will be a clinic director who is responsible for the clinic's day-to-day operations. This director may also be the owner of the clinic or employed by the owner(s) of the clinic or employed by the corporate owner. **Figure 9-4** demonstrates the variations.

Unlike hospitals, outpatient clinics usually do not treat acutely ill patients. Instead the general population of outpatient clinics is chronic disease with acute exacerbations, various pain problems, and rehabilitation from surgical procedures. Accordingly, the high-liability risks are associated with premises liability or inappropriate rehabilitation following surgical repairs.

Premises liability is "[a] landowner's or landholder's tort liability for conditions or activities on the premises."[13] The owner of the clinic will be responsible for ensuring the premises are safe. As an example, the restroom used by patients will most likely have a handrail of some variation to assist patients getting on and off the toilet. If the handrail loosens and a patient uses the loosened handrail and falls, sustaining an injury, then the patient may file a lawsuit for negligent maintenance of the premises. The owner of the clinic is the person or entity who could be held liable.

Variation in the liability could occur if the space was being rented or leased or if there was a group with whom the clinic contracted to maintain the premises. All of these variations would be explored by the attorneys for both parties. Ultimately the party responsible for the maintenance of the premises will most likely be the party that carries insurance for the property.

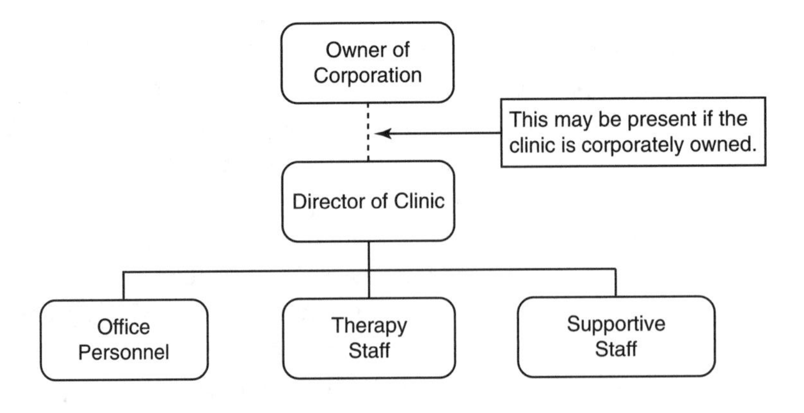

Figure 9-4 Outpatient Clinic

The outpatient clinic also will likely face lawsuits wherein negligent hiring, supervision, and retention are alleged. The other possible cause of actions an outpatient clinic may face is false advertising. *False advertising* is defined as "[t]he tortuous and sometimes criminal act of distributing an advertisement that is untrue, deceptive, or misleading."[14] Thus, the elements for a cause of action of false advertising are (1) distributing an advertisement (2) that is untrue, deceptive, or misleading.

If the outpatient clinic advertises in some type of media that it provides a certain service, and the patient is somehow injured because of that service, then the clinic may face a lawsuit under this cause of action.

NURSING HOMES

The physical therapy provided in nursing homes has advanced significantly in the last 20 years. It is not unusual or uncommon for nursing home physical therapy departments to treat subacute ill patients and postsurgical patients. The critical factor for nursing home physical therapy departments is that the patients are usually elderly and usually have multiple comorbidities that must be considered in the physical therapy plan of treatment.

Additionally, an unfortunate factor is that nursing homes have experienced a plethora of litigation claims against them. As such, nursing home physical therapists, physical therapist assistants, and students should expect to be involved either directly or indirectly with lawsuits many times in their careers. The management or organizational chart for a nursing home also is important because, generally speaking, the ultimate decision maker in a nursing home will be the administrator. An example of the organizational chart for a nursing home is found in **Figure 9-5**.

This example represents a privately owned nursing home. When the nursing home is owned by a corporation, the organizational chart would add the corporate owner at the top. It is very common now for a nursing home to be a limited liability company, which then is owned by another limited liability company or a corporation. This method of ownership limits the liability for a nursing home to the nursing home and not its parent owner(s). This tactic forces plaintiffs' lawyers to pierce the corporate veil (to be discussed in Chapter 19) to get liability adjudicated against the parent corporation.

The highest risks for physical therapists, physical therapist assistants, and students in nursing home practices are identifying functional problems and doing nothing to address the problem under the auspices of reimbursement constraints. Other high-risk areas include a failure to account for the nursing home resident's other comorbidities and attempting to progress the patient too rapidly, leading to possible falls during physical therapy sessions.

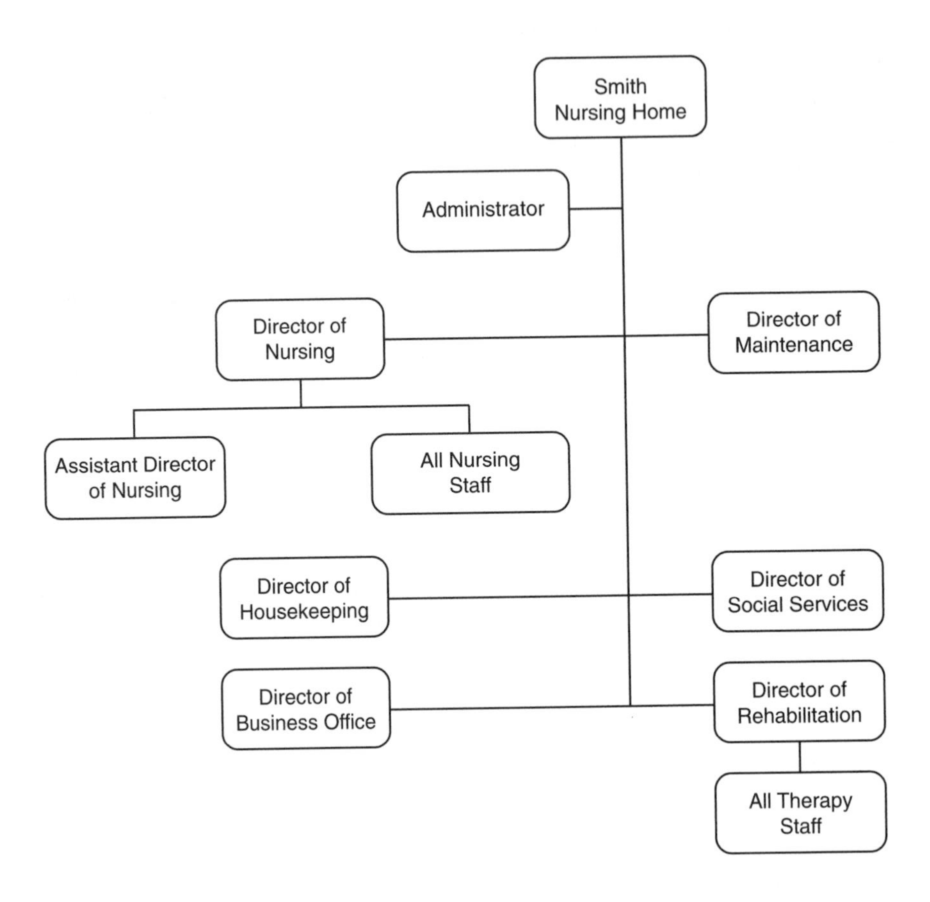

Figure 9-5 Example of Nursing Home Organizational Chart

The other interesting challenge facing nursing home physical therapists, physical therapist assistants, and students is managed-care Medicare patients. These types of patients usually will have a case manager who aggressively oversees the care and treatment the patient receives at the nursing home. It is not uncommon for managed-care Medicare patients to be admitted to and discharged from the nursing home within 20 days. This means the physical therapist, physical therapist assistant, or student might not agree that the patient is ready for discharge from the nursing home to a lesser level of care such as an assisted-living facility or home. However, if they disagree with the patient's case manager, the case manager no longer may refer patients to that nursing home. In these situations, the physical therapist or physical therapist assistant needs to do everything possible to make the discharge as safe as possible and document the nursing home resident's status at the time of discharge in the discharge summary.

From the initial evaluation, it should be evident what discharge status of the patient is necessary to meet the conditions of the discharge location. When the physical therapist, physical therapist assistant, or student documents the discharge status, he or she is documenting whether the patient met the status requirement for the discharge location. Additionally, if the patient did not meet the necessary functional status for the discharge location, then the therapist or assistant also is documenting the interventions or recommendations that have been made to the patient and/or the patient's family to overcome the discharge deficits.

This is a professional way to deal with potential disagreements with dictated discharges. If the patient goes home and has a negative outcome, the physical therapist, physical therapist assistant, or student may still be named in a subsequent lawsuit, but ultimately he or she would not be the one who made the discharge decision or documented that the patient met the necessary level for discharge to the location. Thus, liability for the discharge generally should not be with the physical therapist, physical therapist assistant, or student.

If the physical therapist, physical therapist assistant, or student feels adamant, he or she should document disagreement with the discharge; it is recommended that he or she seek advice from his or her supervisor before entering that type of documentation. Remember: the patient's medical record should document the care and treatment the patient received, not departmental or business disagreements about the patient's care and treatment.

The following example is a case not specifically identified as having occurred in the physical therapy clinic but has characteristics of circumstances giving rise to possible lawsuits that could occur in nursing home physical therapy clinics. In *Taryley v. Kindred Healthcare*, a nursing home resident's daughter sued the nursing home because of alleged injuries she sustained when a mechanical standing lift that was being utilized with her father (the nursing home resident) fell over and hit her.[15] The complaint alleged the employee using the mechanical lift operated it negligently and improperly.[16]

Overall, the actual reason this case was published was related to an issue of diversity of jurisdiction.[17] However, the case has implications for physical therapists, physical therapist assistants, and students because a mechanical lift device is a common piece of equipment used in nursing homes. Therefore, failure to operate the device correctly can lead to lawsuits if the patient or an innocent bystander gets injured as a result of the operation of the lift. Further, it should be recognized that if it was the physical therapist assistant or student operating the device when the injury occurred, the physical therapist and department manager could be sued under a theory of negligent supervision as discussed in Chapter 6.

REHABILITATION HOSPITALS

Rehabilitation hospitals generally treat subacute patients who have been deemed able to tolerate at least 3 hours of therapy combination, including occupational therapy, physical therapy, and speech therapy. These patients stay at the rehabilitation hospital and are there for the sole purpose of being rehabilitated. Thus, the highest risks facing physical therapists, physical therapist assistants, and students working in rehabilitation hospitals probably is discharging the patient to a lesser level of care before the patient is ready for discharge. Again, based on the initial evaluation, there should be an understanding between the physical therapist, physical therapist assistant, or student and the patient what level the patient needs to reach functionally before the patient will be ready for discharge to that location.

Then, throughout physical therapy, there is a measure of what still needs to be accomplished in order for that patient to reach the necessary discharge functional level. The other type of lawsuit the physical therapist, physical therapist assistant, or student may face in a rehabilitation hospital is related to falls.

HOME HEALTH

Home health lawsuits are on the rise. The usual circumstances revolve around whether the patient received all the physical therapy that was ordered or whether the physical therapy was discontinued before the patient had reached maximum benefit. Generally, the physical therapy will be ordered by a discharging physician; however, the insurance carrier paying for the physical therapy may not cover what the physician ordered. Thus, the physical therapist, when conducting the evaluation, may be telling the patient that, despite what the physician ordered, the patient's insurance company is only going to cover one half of the visits. It is imperative the physical therapist give the patient the opportunity to pay for more services privately if the patient wants to do so or provide the patient the information necessary to undertake an appeal.

Further, it is not uncommon for the physical therapist, physical therapist assistant, or student doing home health services to be very specific in treatment and not look at the patient as a whole. When this happens, there could be problems the patient is experiencing that the physical therapist, physical therapist assistant, or student overlooks. Be thorough and complete.

SCHOOL SYSTEM/PEDIATRIC CLINICS

School systems present unique opportunities and sometimes unique liabilities to the physical therapist and physical therapist assistant. In the school system, the physical therapist or physical therapist assistant is treating children and reporting to the parent(s). Hence reports should be complete and thorough, and when there needs to be follow-through with home programs, the physical therapist or physical therapist assistant should document whether there is compliance with home programs. The usual complaint involving school systems is that the parent(s) were unaware of problems the children were experiencing or that the parent(s) needed to do anything at home.

SUMMARY

There are a multitude of clinical settings where physical therapists, physical therapist assistants, and students practice. Each practice setting can face the various lawsuits discussed in previous chapters, but each setting tends to have unique litigation opportunities associated with it. Understanding the various clinical settings will assist the physical therapist, physical therapist assistant, or student in mitigating risk exposure with his or her physical therapy practice.

DISCUSSION QUESTIONS

1. Why is organizational structure important in litigation?
2. Explain the different types of litigation unique to three clinical settings.
3. What clinical setting faces increased risk from early discharges?
4. What are the unique liability risks facing school system physical therapists?
5. Which practice setting is currently experiencing a rise in lawsuits? Discuss what could be causing this.
6. How should clinicians protect themselves when early discharge is forced by payor restrictions?
7. What liability is unique to a therapist practicing in the hospital?
8. What is premises liability?

NOTES

[1] *Budner v. Allegheny General Hospital*, 2005 WL 3843620 (Comm. Pleas. PA 2005).

[2] *Id.*

[3] *Id.*

[4] *Id.*
[5] *Id.*
[6] *Id.*
[7] *Id.*
[8] *Id.*
[9] *Id.*
[10] *Id.*
[11] *Id.*
[12] *Id.*
[13] *Black's Law Dictionary,* 1199 (Bryan A. Gardner, ed., 7th ed., West Group 1999).
[14] *Id.* at 618.
[15] Andrews Litigation Reporter, *Mechanical-Lift Suit Removed to Ga. Federal Court, Tarpley v. Kindred Healthcare,* page 10, September 30, 2005.
[16] *Id.*
[17] *Id.*

CHAPTER 10

Private Malpractice Insurance

Whether to carry personal malpractice insurance can be a very difficult decision. This chapter will discuss types of malpractice insurance and the benefits and risks of carrying malpractice insurance. This chapter also will discuss different types of insurance coverage and what constitutes an issue that requires putting your insurance carrier on notice of a potential claim.

KEY CONCEPTS

Malpractice insurance
Insured's rights
Declaratory actions
Types of insurance
Bad faith
Subrogation
Reservation of rights

INSURANCE

Insurance is defined as "[a]n agreement by which one party (the insurer) commits to do something of value for another party (the insured) upon the occurrence of some specified contingency; esp[ecially] an agreement by which one party assumes a risk faced by another party in return for a premium payment."[1] There are many different types of insurance, including homeowner's, automobile, life, health, dental, disability, and malpractice. *Malpractice insurance* is defined as "[a]n agreement to indemnify a professional person, such as a doctor or lawyer, against negligence claims."[2]

Whether a physical therapist, physical therapist assistant, or student should carry malpractice insurance is one of the most common questions presented to medical malpractice defense lawyers. Generally, the decision to carry medical malpractice insurance is personal. Some of the factors to consider when deciding include the type of practice in which the physical therapist, physical therapist assistant, or student works and what the high risks in that type of practice are. Additionally, the physical therapist, physical therapist assistant, or student should determine what, if any, malpractice insurance the employer is carrying for act(s) and/or omission(s) that occur within the clinic where the physical therapist, physical therapist assistant, or student is working.

Also, the physical therapist, physical therapist assistant, or student should consider, based on the population they are treating, what the potential damages that the population could assert in a lawsuit are. As an example, if the physical therapist, physical therapist assistant, or student is working in a nursing home, the likelihood that lost wages could be asserted as damage is slim. However, if the physical therapist, physical therapist assistant, or student is working in an outpatient clinic and treating individuals during their working years, then lost wages are potential damages if the alleged negligent act prevents the individual from returning to work.

The concern that physical therapists, physical therapist assistants, or students should have about not carrying malpractice insurance is what personal assets they have that could be liquidated to pay damages awarded in a lawsuit. Obviously, the more personal assets, the greater the need for insurance to protect these assets.

MALPRACTICE INSURANCE

The American Physical Therapy Association (APTA) endorses the insurance plan offered through Health Providers Service Organization (HPSO) that is underwritten by American Casualty Company of Reading, Pennsylvania, which is a CNA company. Generally, malpractice policies through HPSO are for $1 million per occurrence with a $3 million aggregate per policy year. HPSO also offers an insurance product line that provides for license protection coverage. As of December 4, 2006, CNA indicated that in 2005 the average physical therapist policy cost was $348.00 per year.[3] This premium varied depending on the type of employment and whether the physical therapist was full time or part time.[4]

EXCESSIVE INSURANCE

Excessive insurance is defined as "[a]n agreement to indemnify against any loss that exceeds the amount of coverage under another policy."[5] Essentially, if the physical therapist or physical therapist assistant had the HPSO coverage of $1 million per occurrence and a damage award exceeded the $1 million, then excessive insurance would begin to pay the excess damage award over the $1 million up to the limits of the excess insurance policy. It should be understood that most of these polices including paying the costs of defense; therefore, as previously discussed, the policies are known as defense-cost depleting. Hence, although the physical therapist or physical therapist assistant might have a policy of $1 million per occurrence, the $1 million would be depleted as payments were made to the defense lawyer for attorneys' fees and costs associated with defense.

WORKERS' COMPENSATION INSURANCE

Physical therapists or physical therapist assistants who own their own practice must carry workers' compensation insurance for employees. The physical therapist or physical therapist assistant who is a member of APTA can contact APTA for referrals to insurance companies that write these types of insurance policies.

DECLARATORY ACTIONS

Sometimes a party might want to know how the law might be interpreted with a given set of facts. Thus, there are actions brought forth called declaratory actions that seek declaratory judgments. A *declaratory judgment* is "[a] binding adjudication that establishes the rights and other legal relations of the parties without providing for or ordering enforcement."[6] Noteworthy is that "[d]eclaratory judgments are often sought, for example, by insurance companies in determining whether a policy covers a given insured or peril."[7]

Accordingly, a declaratory action could be brought by an insurance carrier to determine whether the law would rule that the insurance carrier legally had to cover a claim. Likewise, a physical therapist, physical therapist assistant, or student could bring a declaratory action against his or her insurance carrier if the insurance carrier denied there was coverage under the therapist's insurance policy. Thus, a physical therapist might decide to file a declaratory action against his or her insurance carrier to determine his or her legal rights under the insurance policy.

INSURED'S RIGHTS

When a physical therapist, physical therapist assistant, or student pays for malpractice insurance coverage, he or she should be familiar with the insurance and understand exactly what the insurance policy covers and how the insurance carrier will defend the insured. The insured is the person who pays for the insurance and is effectively insured; the insurer is generally known as the insurance company or insurance carrier.

It is common for an insurance company to have a law firm it prefers to work with and therefore refers cases to that law firm for defense of a claim. Thus, if a physical therapist, physical therapist assistant, or student pays for malpractice insurance and has to report a claim at any time, the insurance carrier likely will select and retain the counsel. However, the physical therapist, physical therapist assistant, or student should understand that as the insured, he or she has certain rights under the law and should not be intimidated or shy about making sure his or her needs are met in the defense of the claim. Note, however, that not every claim will lead to a lawsuit.

Therefore, you should be very familiar with what your insurance carrier defines as a claim and when you are required to report it. This is known as putting your insurance carrier on notice of a potential claim.

The insured's rights generally are sent to the insured as a statement of insured's rights. The letter usually will have an introduction, such as the insurance company has selected a lawyer to defend the lawsuit or claim against you. This statement of insured's rights is being given to you to assure that you are aware of your rights regarding your legal representation. This disclosure statement highlights many, but not all, of your rights when your legal representation is being provided by the insurance company.

1. **Your Lawyer:** If you have questions concerning the selection of the lawyer by the insurance company, you should discuss the matter with the insurance company and the lawyer. As a client, you have the right to know about the lawyer's education, training, and experience. If you ask, the lawyer should tell you specifically about his or her actual experience dealing with cases similar to yours and should give you this information in writing, if you request it. Your lawyer is responsible for keeping you reasonably informed regarding the case and promptly complying with your reasonable requests for information. You are entitled to be informed of the final disposition of your case within a reasonable time.
2. **Fees and Costs:** Usually the insurance company pays all of the fees and costs of defending the claim. If you are responsible for directly paying the lawyer for any fees or costs, your lawyer must promptly inform you of that.
3. **Directing the Lawyer:** If your policy, like most insurance policies, provides for the insurance company to control the defense of the lawsuit, the lawyer will be taking instructions from the insurance company. Under such policies, the lawyer cannot act solely on your instructions, and at the same time, cannot act contrary to your interests. Your preferences should be communicated to the lawyer.

4. **Litigation Guidelines:** Many insurance companies establish guidelines governing how lawyers are to proceed in defending a claim. Sometimes those guidelines affect the range of actions the lawyer can take and may require authorization of the insurance company before certain actions are undertaken. You are entitled to know the guidelines affecting the extent and level of legal services being provided to you. Upon request, the lawyer or the insurance company should either explain the guidelines to you or provide you with a copy. If the lawyer is denied authorization to provide a service or undertake an action the lawyer believes necessary to your defense, you are entitled to be informed that the insurance company has declined authorization for the service or action.
5. **Confidentiality:** Lawyers have a general duty to keep secret the confidential information a client provides, subject to limited exceptions. However, the lawyer chosen to represent you also may have a duty to share with the insurance company information relating to the defense or settlement of the claim. If the lawyer learns of information indicating that the insurance company is not obligated under the policy to cover the claim or provide a defense, the lawyer's duty is to maintain that information in confidence. If the lawyer cannot do so, the lawyer may be required to withdraw from the representation without disclosing to the insurance company the nature of the conflict of interest that has arisen. Whenever a waiver of the lawyer-client confidentiality privilege is needed, your lawyer has a duty to consult with you and obtain your informed consent. Some insurance companies retain auditing companies to review the billings and files of the lawyers they hire to represent policy holders. If the lawyer believes a bill review or other action releases information in a manner that is contrary to your interests, the lawyer should advise you regarding the matter.
6. **Conflicts of Interest:** Most insurance policies state that the insurance company will provide a lawyer to represent your interests as well as those of the insurance company. The lawyer is responsible for identifying conflicts of interest and advising you of them. If at any time you believe the lawyer provided by the insurance company cannot fairly represent you because of conflicts of interest between you and the company (such as whether there is insurance coverage for the claim against you), you should discuss this with the lawyer and explain why you believe there is a conflict. If an actual conflict of interest arises that cannot be resolved, the insurance company may be required to provide you with another lawyer.
7. **Settlement:** Many policies state that the insurance company alone may make a final decision regarding settlement of a claim, but under some policies your agreement is required. If you want to object to or encourage a settlement within

policy limits, you should discuss your concerns with your lawyer to learn your rights and possible consequences. No settlement of the case requiring you to pay money in excess of your policy limits can be reached without your agreement, following full disclosure.

8. **Your Risk:** If you lose the case, there might be a judgment entered against you for more than the amount of your insurance, and you might have to pay it. Your lawyer has a duty to advise you about this risk and other reasonably foreseeable adverse results.
9. **Own Lawyer:** The lawyer provided by the insurance company is representing you only to defend the lawsuit. If you desire to pursue a claim against the other side, or desire legal services not directly related to the defense of the lawsuit against you, you will need to make your own arrangements with this or another lawyer. You also may hire another lawyer, at your own expense, to monitor the defense being provided by the insurance company. If there is a reasonable risk that the claim made against you exceeds the amount of coverage under your policy, you should consider consulting another lawyer.
10. **Reporting Violations:** If at any time you believe that your lawyer has acted in violation of your rights, you have the right to report the matter to the bar of that state, which is the agency that oversees the practice and behavior of all lawyers in that state.

Lastly, the letter should provide the physical therapist, physical therapist assistant, or student the information on how to contact the bar for the particular state.

One of the disputes that can occur between the insured and the insurance carrier is the insured's belief that the insurance carrier is not dealing or negotiating for resolution of the claim in good faith. Once a physical therapist, physical therapist assistant, or student is sued, it is likely he or she will want the issue resolved as quickly as possible and to ensure it is resolved within the insurance policy's limits. Thus, many insureds would rather the insurance carrier pay more money for a claim so that it resolves quickly versus aggressively defending the claim, which can make it last for years.

The problem that arises when claims are resolved quickly, usually for more money than the claim is worth, is that when other claims are brought that are also of little value, the plaintiffs' lawyers know a particular defendant will pay more money than a claim is worth just to resolve it quickly. Thus, paying more for frivolous claims tends to lead to more frivolous claims. Consequently, the goal for claim resolution between insured and insurer should be to resolve those claims that have some legitimate basis as quickly as possible for as little as possible and aggressively contest the claims that have little or no merit.

In insurance defense, there are claims called bad-faith claims. *Bad faith,* with regards to insurance, is defined as "[a]n insurance company's unreasonable and unfounded (though not necessarily fraudulent) refusal to provide coverage in violation of the duties of good faith and fair dealing owed to an insured."[8] Bad faith often involves an insurer's failure to pay the insured's claim or claim brought by a third party. The insured usually feels the insurer (insurance company) failed to act in the insured's best interests. Therefore, an insured's claim against an insurance company for an unreasonable and unfounded refusal to provide coverage is known as a bad-faith claim.[9]

When the insured believes a claim should be paid at policy limits and an opposing party would accept policy limits as settlement for the claim, some insureds believe they may have a bad-faith claim against the insurance carrier for not tendering policy limits for settlement. However, what must be recognized and understood by the insured is that most plaintiffs' attorneys will overvalue claims in an attempt to force a wedge between the insured and the insurer by demanding policy limits for the case to resolve and aggressively intimidating the insured.

What the physical therapist, physical therapist assistant, or student must realize, as the insured, is that generally the lawyers working with the insurance carrier will work diligently to resolve the matter for a reasonable value; doing so is in the physical therapist's, physical therapist assistant's, or student's best interest. Generally speaking, it is doubtful many claims, if any, would be valued at or above policy limits.

To determine the value of a case, the lawyer must consider the cause of action being pled and the damages being asserted. Based on that information and factoring in the skill level of the plaintiff's attorney, the defense lawyer will attempt to calculate the total sum of damages that are likely attributable to the insured's act or omission. This, of course, is assuming that after the defense lawyer's investigation, the defense lawyer believes denial of liability is unlikely; hence, there is some liability exposure based on the insured's act(s) and/or omission(s).

If, after the defense lawyer investigates the claim, the defense lawyer is of the opinion the insured acted within the standard of care and has no liability, then the decision has to be whether to defend the matter through trial so that a potential defense verdict is possible. Trials intimidate many people because of the risks associated with an unknown jury and the potential a jury could render a verdict in excess of the insured's policy limits.

However, what must be explained is that defense lawyers are well-trained to work with insurance carriers and insureds to provide estimates and likelihoods of victory at trial. Not every prediction is correct, but most defense lawyers can explain the risks involved, the typical jury pool for that given region, and the strengths and weaknesses of the case, so informed decisions can be made. Sometimes the goal at trial is not necessarily to win a defense verdict but rather to mitigate damages so that the jury renders a reasonable verdict because the plaintiff or plaintiff's lawyer was being unreasonable.

Using the hot-pack burn scenario, assume the insurance carrier and defense lawyer might value the case for $50,000 to $75,000 and the plaintiff will only agree to settle the matter for $150,000. The insurance carrier refuses to pay $150,000; thus, the matter is taken to trial. If the verdict is for the defense or an award for the plaintiff is less than $150,000, then the insured physical therapist, physical therapist assistant, or student would likely feel the insurance carrier made the right decision.

However, if the jury came back with a plaintiff's verdict and awarded $500,000 for compensatory damages (medical bills and lost wages), $500,000 in noneconomic damages (pain and suffering, disfigurement, and mental anguish), and $1,000,000 for punitive damages (punish conduct), then the insured might feel the insurance carrier did not act in good faith by negotiating and offering the $150,000 to resolve the matter prior to trial. In that case, the insured physical therapist, physical therapist assistant, or student might be able to bring a bad-faith claim against the insurance carrier.

A real example of a bad-faith claim is *Jurinko v. Medical Protective Co.* This particular case may be the largest bad-faith claim awarded in Pennsylvania history—$7,900,000.[10] In the case, a plaintiff successfully sued an insurance carrier for failure to tender the physician's medical malpractice policy limits, which led to a $2,500,000 verdict against the physician.[11] The physician repeatedly requested the insurance carrier tender his policy limits of $200,000 but the insurance carrier would only offer $50,000.[12] Of note, two justices (judges) had valued the case at $1,500,000.[13]

Once a jury returned a verdict against the physician of $2,500,000, which clearly exceeded his policy limits, the plaintiff and physician agreed that the plaintiff would accept an assignment of the physician's bad-faith claim against the insurance carrier.[14] Recall the physician would be liable for any verdict awarded in excess of his policy limits because he did not have any excess professional malpractice insurance. In the second lawsuit (the physician's bad-faith claim against the insurance carrier), the jury awarded $1,600,000 in compensatory damages and $6,250,000 in punitive damages.[15] (Remember punitive damages are society's way to punish conduct and deter the conduct from occurring again, not just by this particular party but also as a message to other potential offenders.)

Thus, this example should help establish how important it is for the insured to stay very involved in the litigation process.

SUBROGATION

Sometimes the physical therapist, physical therapist assistant, or student may come in contact with an insurance carrier wanting to subrogate a claim against him or her. *Subrogation* is defined as "[t]he substitution of one party for another whose debt the party pays, entitling the paying party to rights, remedies, or securities that would otherwise belong to the debtor. The principle under which an insurer that has paid a loss under an insurance policy is entitled to all the rights and remedies belonging to the insured against a third party with respect to any loss covered by the policy."[16] Thus, the insurance carrier wants to stand in the shoes of the physical therapist, physical therapist assistant, or student to attempt recovery of monies paid under the policy.

RESERVATION OF RIGHTS

Lastly, sometimes the physical therapist, physical therapist assistant, or student might receive a letter from the insurance carrier stating that it is going to defend and pay the claim under a reservation of rights. A *reservation of rights* means "[a] contract (supplementing a liability-insurance policy) in which the insured acknowledges that the insurer's investigation or defense of a claim against the insured does not waive the insurer's right to contest coverage later."[17] Thus, if there is something that turns up during the investigation of the claim that eliminates the insurance carrier's obligation under the policy to pay and defend, the physical therapist, physical therapist assistant, or student will be left to pay and defend the claim without insurance money.

SUMMARY

There are many nuances to insurance defense of a medical malpractice or medical negligence claim. When the physical therapist, physical therapist assistant, or student is involved in such a defense, he or she should remain in contact with the defense lawyer and insurance carrier. There will be times when a physical therapist, physical therapist assistant, or student may want an insurance carrier to pay more for a claim just to have the claim resolved. However, an insurance carrier's duty is to negotiate in good faith for resolution, not to overpay claims so claims can be resolved quickly.

DISCUSSION QUESTIONS

1. Discuss the different types of insurance.
2. What is a declaratory action?
3. What is the difference between an insured and an insurer?
4. What is putting an insurance carrier "on notice" of a potential claim?
5. Discuss an insured's rights.
6. Discuss bad faith.
7. Discuss subrogation.
8. What is a reservation of rights?
9. What duty does the insurance carrier owe the insured?

NOTES

[1] *Black's Law Dictionary,* 802 (Bryan A. Gardner, ed., 7th ed., West Group 1999).
[2] *Id.* at 806.
[3] CNA Insurance Web page, www.cna.com, *CNA Study Analyzes Professional Liability Claims, Offers Risk Management Solutions for Physical Therapists,* 14 (December 4, 2006).
[4] *Id.*
[5] *Black's Law Dictionary,* 804 (Bryan A. Gardner, ed., 7th ed., West Group 1999).
[6] *Id.* at 846.
[7] *Id.*
[8] www.dictionary.com.
[9] *Black's Law Dictionary,* 846 (Bryan A. Gardner, ed., 7th ed., West Group 1999).
[10] *Jurinko v. Medical Protective Co.,* 2006 WL 785234 (E.D. PA March 24, 2006); and Andrews Litigation Reporter, page 13, April 14, 2006.
[11] *Id.*
[12] *Id.*
[13] *Id.*
[14] *Id.*
[15] *Id.*
[16] *Black's Law Dictionary,* 1440 (Bryan A. Gardner, ed., 7th ed., West Group 1999).
[17] *Id.* at 1082.

CHAPTER 11

Trends in Current Case Law

This chapter will cover some previously discussed cases as well as some new cases. However, it should be noted that, even as this book is being written, the precedents some of these cases set could have changed before the publication of the book. In law, cases are decided every day, leading to new interpretations of prior case decisions. These new interpretations can change what laws actually mean and can overturn prior decisions. Hence, any time someone researches to determine the latest interpretation for a particular issue, that person also must be mindful that interpretation could be changed and ongoing research is necessary. Thus, a review of how some cases could affect trends in the future of the physical therapy profession will be discussed.

KEY CONCEPTS

Acting within the scope of practice
Negligent instruction in use of equipment

POTENTIAL PROBLEMS

There are many cases wherein a physical therapist, physical therapist assistant, or student is mentioned in the facts of the case but the issue resolved through the case does not affect him or her. Many lessons can be learned through a review of these cases because eventually the physical therapist, physical therapist assistant, or student likely will become the center of attention and the facts discussed will involve whether the therapist had any liability. A review of some examples will help establish this point.

In *Mitter v. Touro Infirmary*, a patient was hospitalized following knee surgery. (The specific type of knee surgery was not identified.) During the patient's rehabilitation program, a physical therapist assistant was accused of pushing too hard on the patient's knee wherein a "pop" was heard.[1] The allegedly excessive force caused further damage that required the patient to undergo a second surgery related to a rupturing of the medial collateral ligament.[2] Besides the physical therapist assistant's alleged malpractice action, there was also an allegation that a nurse negligently dropped the leg of a wheelchair on the surgically repaired leg.[3] Thus, the two acts combined allegedly caused the medial collateral ligament to rupture, necessitating another knee surgery.[4] After the second knee surgery, it was alleged that a nurse "improperly set" a continuous passive motion machine.[5]

The case revolved around whether the infirmary was liable for the alleged negligent or malpractice acts of its nonphysician employees: the nurses and the physical therapist assistant. In reviewing the elements of a cause of action for negligence or malpractice, the elements a plaintiff must prove are: (1) duty; (2) breach of the duty; (3) causation; and (4) damages. Likewise, because this was a civil matter, the burden of proof and/or persuasion was by a preponderance of the evidence or a greater weight of the evidence. Hence, the issue in the case was whether the employees of the infirmary breached the prevailing standard of care, resulting in the patient suffering another injury to her knee that required surgery.

Ultimately, the patient was awarded $1500 for pain and suffering as well as the costs of the litigation and some legal fees and legal interests for the prosecution of the claim. It should be noted that the legal fees likely were significantly higher than the damage award. Accordingly, the total damages the infirmary was ordered to pay included the $1500 pain and suffering of the plaintiff, $1000 of the plaintiff's expert's fee of $2012, and the plaintiff's attorney fees and costs of litigation as well as interest. Needless to say, the attorney fees and costs of the matter likely added up to several thousand dollars. Therefore, realistic valueing of cases up front helps eliminate situations wherein the actual damages awarded are less than the attorney fees to litigate the case.

As a learning tool, it should be noted that had the physical therapist assistant had private malpractice insurance, the plaintiff may have elected to individually name that person in the lawsuit. Additionally, the physical therapist responsible for that patient who delegated the treatment to the physical therapist assistant could have been named individually under a theory of negligent supervision. One question to ponder about this particular case is whether the physical therapist assistant acted within his scope of practice. (Remember the state practice act would delineate the scope of practice, and consideration should be given to the Louisiana Physical Therapy Association's and

APTA's guidelines, including the *Guide to Physical Therapy Practice.*) Other questions include whether the physical therapist inappropriately delegated to the physical therapist assistant. Did the physical therapist assistant report to the physical therapist what occurred when it occurred? Did the physical therapist evaluate the patient after the alleged "pop"? Lastly, did the physical therapist assistant and physical therapist document their findings? These would be some of the questions both the plaintiff and defense lawyers would ask.

The previous case and subsequent cases demonstrate that, although the primary issue on appeal has nothing to do with the liability of the physical therapist, physical therapist assistant, or student, the underlying case does involve a physical therapist, physical therapist assistant, or student. Remember, when a case goes through an appeal, it is usually based on a narrow issue or issues that the appellate court is being asked to resolve, not whether the defendant—in this case the physical therapist, physical therapist assistant, or student—is liable for the act(s) or omission(s) litigated in the underlying case.

In the case of *Woodger v. Christ Hospital*, the hospital and physical therapist were sued for medical malpractice. Again, the primary issue on appeal had nothing to do with the liability of the physical therapist regarding his act(s) and/or omission(s), but rather whether the plaintiff's contribution payment to the disability fund of Social Security should be a set off to the collateral source deduction for disability payments she received related to the injury. However, the underlying facts involving the physical therapist are instructive.

The jury in the trial case awarded $100,000 for past lost income, $96,000 for anticipated future lost income, and $100,000 for subjective pain and suffering.[6] In the underlying case, the plaintiff alleged she was diagnosed with a patellofemoral disease resulting from a malalignment of the patella that resulted in degenerative and arthritic conditions in one knee.[7] Subsequently she was diagnosed with the same condition of the other knee.[8] For these conditions she was prescribed a treatment plan with physical therapy, which she undertook at the hospital involved in the lawsuit.[9]

After 19 sessions of physical therapy, including the use of a Kinetron machine, "she underwent an arthroscopic repair of a torn lateral meniscus in the right knee."[10] Thereafter, she again went through rehabilitation involving physical therapy and again was placed on the Kinetron machine.[11] The plaintiff alleged in the lawsuit that she injured and/or reinjured her right knee because the physical therapist negligently instructed her on the use of the Kinetron machine.[12]

Thus, because of the physical therapist's negligence and/or medical malpractice, she injured the knee resulting in "significant" loss of mobility and required the permanent use of a cane for assistance with ambulation.[13] Of significance, the plaintiff was a registered nurse.[14] Hence, although the case was taken to appeal on different issues, the underlying facts of the case support that a jury found the physical therapist negligent in the instruction and/or use of the Kinetron machine that was part of the plan of treatment for this patient following knee surgery.

EMPLOYER-REQUIRED TEST

An interesting case wherein a physical therapist followed a physician's order but documented the patient had not yet achieved the necessary skills to undergo a particular test is the case of *Williams v. Tri-State Physical Therapy, Inc.* In *Williams*, a truck driver injured his lower back while performing his job duties.[15] One of his treating physicians referred him to a physical therapy clinic for conservative treatment.[16] One of the key facts in the case was that "the relationship between [the doctor] and [the physical therapy clinic] was such that [the physician] would order certain physical therapy routines and tests for [the patient], and [the physical therapy clinic] in turn would report to [the physician] regarding [the patient's] therapy performance and tests results."[17] The physical therapy clinic "made no decisions relative to [the patient's] therapy regimen and relied solely on the therapy procedure directives of [the physician]."[18] Interestingly, during the course of therapy, the employer required the patient to undergo a functional capacity evaluation (FCE) at the physical therapy clinic.[19] The physician in turn ordered the physical therapy clinic "to ascertain [the patient's] medical standing for returning to work."[20]

Approximately 6 months after his injury, the patient was lifting 25 pounds successfully.[21] This was a requirement in order for the patient to return to work.[22] Within a week, the physician reported to the physical therapy clinic that, although the patient had achieved his lifting potential of 48 pounds, he (the physician) "was concerned that the FCE requirement of lifting 100 pounds would expose [the patient] to an undue risk of re-injuring his back."[23] Despite this warning or concern, the physical therapist conducted the functional capacity evaluation a few weeks later.[24] During the 100-pound lift, the patient "experienced severe pain in his lower back."[25] The physician's subsequent notes indicated the 100-pound lift was of concern but the employer required the patient to successfully lift 100 pounds during the functional capacity evaluation.[26]

Thereafter, the patient continued treatment with the physician and the physical therapy clinic for approximately 4 more months.[27] The patient continued to complain of pain.[28] Subsequently, the physician informed the patient "that his injury sustained during the functional capacity evaluation on February 13, 1998 had 'aggravated his situation and set him back significantly'."[29] Thereafter, the physician discontinued physical therapy and treated the patient with medication only.[30]

The physician then ordered a repeat MRI, which demonstrated the "degenerative and bulging disk at L_5–S_1 was 'worse' than reflected on the previous [ ] MRI."[31] Therefore, the physician determined conservative treatment had failed and ordered surgery.[32] The physical therapist and the physical therapy clinic were sued for medical malpractice.

EXCESSIVE FORCE

In *Butler v. Martins*, the plaintiff alleged a hand physical therapist used excessive force that caused a fracture to the plaintiff's ulna.[33] The physical therapist was a certified hand therapist,[34] but during a treatment, the plaintiff alleged that the physical therapist pushed down too hard on the left arm and "a loud crack was heard."[35] Thereafter, X-rays confirmed there was a fracture to the left ulna.[36]

The plaintiff underwent surgery for an open reduction internal fixation to the ulna fracture 2 days later.[37] It was undisputed that the ulna fracture was indeed a new fracture.[38] The plaintiff sued for personal injuries that allegedly resulted from the negligence of the therapist.[39] During the litigation came the battle of the experts.

The plaintiff's expert physician opined the physical therapist breached the standard of care utilizing a theory of *res ipsa loquitor*.[40] Recall that *res ipsa loquitor* means, "[t]he doctrine providing that, in some circumstances, the mere fact of an accident's occurrence raises an inference of negligence so as to establish a prima facie case. 'The thing speaks for itself'."[41] The plaintiff's expert opined "this type of fracture would not have occurred without excessive force being applied."[42] The physical therapist's (defendant) expert, however, opined "there was no departure from the accepted physical therapy practice in any of the care and treatment rendered" by the physical therapist.[43]

Ultimately the case was resolved on whether a motion for summary judgment in favor of the defendants should be granted.[44] The court denied the defendants' motion for summary judgment because there was a genuine issue of fact, which was whether the physical therapist had used excessive force.[45] The case proceeded for a jury to resolve whether the physical therapist used excessive force with the plaintiff's expert basically opining this type of fracture does not occur in the absence of negligence.[46]

A case appealed on different grounds was brought against a hospital because a patient was allegedly injured during a physical therapy session when the patient fell off a large therapeutic ball.[47] The alleged breach of duty was associated with an alleged failure to assist and supervise the patient during the physical therapy session.[48] The case was appealed on different grounds; however, this case does provide another example of activities performed during the physical therapy session that can lead to claims. Thus, therapeutic balls now account for at least one lawsuit.

The plaintiff specifically alleged the physical therapist failed to supervise and assist the plaintiff during the physical therapy session.[49] Ultimately, the case was appealed on an issue of whether the statutory conditions had been met prior to the filing of the lawsuit.[50] Still, the case provides a lesson on providing the proper supervision and assistance when a patient is using a therapeutic ball in the physical therapy clinic. A therapeutic ball likely will be viewed as a piece of equipment in the physical therapy clinic.

There was also a civil suit as a result of the *Teston* case out of Arkansas.[51] The patient filed a medical malpractice case against the physical therapist and physical therapist's employer.[52] The patient alleged she received negligent treatment from the physical therapist and that the employer, through *respondeat superior*, was responsible for the physical therapist's actions.[53]

Part of the appeal was to exclude the findings of the Arkansas Board of Chiropractors as evidence in this civil case, in which the Board fined the physical therapist for practicing chiropractic medicine, which was outside the scope of the Physical Therapy Practice Act.[54] Further, in the civil action, the plaintiff wanted to use a chiropractor as the plaintiff's expert witness to testify that the physical therapist had breached the physical therapy standard of care.[55] Ultimately, the court held a chiropractor could testify as to the standard of care required by a physical therapist but that the board of chiropractic examiner's findings could not be used in the civil action.[56]

SUMMARY

Although the cases that have reached the appellate courts regarding direct liability for physical therapists, physical therapist assistants, or students are few, other cases in which the treatments rendered by physical therapists, physical therapist assistants, and students have led to liability for others are instructional. Hence, physical therapists, physical therapist assistants, and the students should not be lulled into complacency merely because there are not a plethora of cases directly on point wherein physical therapists, physical therapist assistants, or students were found liable of medical malpractice for medical negligence.

DISCUSSION QUESTIONS

1. Discuss negligent instruction on the use of equipment.
2. Discuss failure to adhere to a physician's warning regarding a patient's treatment.

NOTES

[1] *Mitter v. Touro Infirmary*, 874 So.2d 265, 267–268 (La. App. 4 Cir. 2004).
[2] *Id.*
[3] *Id.*
[4] *Id.*
[5] *Id.* at 268.
[6] *Woodger v. Christ Hospital*, 834 A.2d 1047 (N.J. Super. Ct. 2003).
[7] *Id.*
[8] *Id.*
[9] *Id.*
[10] *Id.*
[11] *Id.* at 1048.
[12] *Id.*
[13] *Id.*
[14] *Id.*
[15] *Williams v. Tri-State Physical Therapy, Inc.*, 850 So.2d 991, 993 (La. App. 2 Cir. 2003).
[16] *Id.*
[17] *Id.*
[18] *Id.*
[19] *Id.*
[20] *Id.*
[21] Id.
[22] *Id.*
[23] *Id.*
[24] *Id.*
[25] *Id.*
[26] *Id.*
[27] *Id.*
[28] *Id.*
[29] *Id.*
[30] *Id.* at 994.
[31] *Id.*
[32] *Id.*
[33] *Butler v. Martins*, 2005 WL 3501583 (N.Y. Sup. 2005).
[34] *Id.*
[35] *Id.*

[36] *Id.*
[37] *Id.*
[38] *Id.*
[39] *Id.*
[40] Id.
[41] *Black's Law Dictionary,* 1311 (Bryan A. Gardner, ed., 7th ed., West Group 1999).
[42] *Butler v. Martins,* 2005 WL 3501583 (N.Y. Sup. 2005).
[43] *Id.*
[44] *Id.* at 2.
[45] *Id.*
[46] *Id.* at 2.
[47] *Barnum v. Lawrence & Memorial Hospital,* 2004 WL 870679, 1 (Conn. Super. 2004).
[48] *Id.*
[49] *Id.* at 1.
[50] *Id.*
[51] *Fryar v. Touchstone Physical Therapy, Inc.,* 2006 WL 348334 (Ark. 2006).
[52] *Id.* at 1.
[53] *Id.*
[54] *Id.*
[55] *Id.*
[56] *Id.*

CHAPTER 12

Surviving a Lawsuit

This chapter discusses what the physical therapist, physical therapist assistant, or student can expect and should do when served with a complaint or notice that someone intends to sue him or her. It should be noted that in some states the process of a lawsuit may begin with a statutorily mandated presuit prior to the filing of any lawsuit. Consequently, the first indication of an impending lawsuit may be the receipt of a presuit notice. Additionally, even if a presuit is not required, some states—like Louisiana—require the claim be reviewed by a medical review panel as provided under the Medical Malpractice Act.[1] Lastly, the first indication of an impending lawsuit might be the receipt of a records request from the person or representative of a potential plaintiff. The remainder of this chapter will discuss the life and tribulations of a lawsuit.

KEY CONCEPTS

Selecting an attorney
Records request
Presuit
Complaint
Answering a complaint
Discovery
Depositions
Hearing
Trial
Arbitration
Mediation
Appeals
Settlement

CHOOSING AN ATTORNEY

One of the difficult aspects of being insured is that the insurance carrier often chooses defense counsel. Some physical therapists, physical therapist assistants, or students might find it difficult to accept that they will not be in control of the selection of counsel. Generally, insurance carriers have determined what defense counsel they will retain in different venues throughout the country. The insured physical therapist, physical therapist assistant, or student usually will not be consulted prior to or with regard to the selection and retention of defense counsel. However, the insured should be kept apprised of what defense counsel has been retained and then defense counsel should keep the insured therapist informed throughout the litigation. (Please refer back to the insured's rights discussed in Chapter 10.)

Generally speaking, the claims adjuster for the insurance carrier will make the decision about what, if any, settlement offer will be made at any time during litigation. However, an insured physical therapist, physical therapist assistant, or student retains the right to hire independent defense counsel at his or her own expense at any time during litigation. When this occurs, the privately hired lawyer usually monitors the insurance carrier's retained defense counsel and privately reports to the insured physical therapist, physical therapist assistant, or student who retained the lawyer.

This is a typical occurrence when the insured professional (physical therapist, physical therapist assistant, or student) believes a claim may exceed his or her insurance policy limits and some of the insured physical therapist's, physical therapist assistant's, or student's private assets might be exposed should a verdict award exceed insurance policy limits. Thus, the insured professional may decide it is beneficial to have a lawyer looking out for his or her interests only and not the dual interests of the insured and the insurance carrier.

There are also occasions when the insurance carrier denies coverage and thereby denies retention of defense counsel. Other times, the physical therapist, physical therapist assistant, or student might not have insurance; thus, a physical therapist, physical therapist assistant, or student will find the need to hire his or her own defense counsel. Some of the things that should be considered when hiring a lawyer are:

1. What is the lawyer's experience with physical therapy or medical malpractice?
2. How many cases has the lawyer handled with the issue that the physical therapist, physical therapist assistant, or student has?
3. Has anyone recommended the lawyer to the physical therapist, physical therapist assistant, or student?

4. Does the lawyer have any disciplinary actions pending or prosecuted against him or her by the state's bar?
5. How much does the lawyer charge and how are the charges based? (It is common practice for lawyers to bill in 6-minute increments.)
6. How often will you receive a bill?
7. How quickly must the lawyer's bill be paid?
8. Who else will work on your case with the lawyer?

There are times when the insurance carrier may deny coverage for a claim, and it is later determined that the insurance carrier is responsible for coverage. In that case the insured physical therapist, physical therapist assistant, or student may have already retained private counsel and subsequently the insurance carrier becomes financially responsible for the payment of that defense counsel. An example of a case where the insurance carrier denied coverage and the insured privately retained counsel is *Bellsouth Telecommunications, Inc. v. Church Tower of Florida, Inc.*

In the case of *Bellsouth*, Liberty Mutual Fire Insurance Company insured Bellsouth Telecommunications.[2] The insurer initially denied coverage in a personal injury lawsuit.[3] Once the insured received notification that the insurer was denying coverage, the insured retained its own defense counsel.[4] As the litigation progressed, the insurer changed its position and agreed to assume the responsibility for a defense.[5] However, the insured objected to changing defense counsel.[6]

The court cited what was a well-established law in Florida: "[i]t is well-settled law that, when an insurer agrees to defend under a reservation of rights or refuses to defend, the insurer transfers to the insured the power to conduct its own defense, and if it is later determined that the insured was entitled to coverage, the insured will be entitled to full reimbursement of the insured's litigation costs. Additionally, if the insurer offers to defend under a reservation of rights, the insured has the right to reject the defense and hire its own attorneys and control the defense" (citing *Aguero v. First Am. Ins. Co.*).[7] Thus, physical therapists, physical therapist assistants, and students should be prepared to retain defense counsel when necessary.

REQUEST FOR RECORDS

For many lawsuits, the initiating process is the receipt of a records request. In the records request, someone, usually a plaintiff's lawyer, will request a copy of a physical therapist's or physical therapist assistant's entire records for a particular patient, including medical records, billing records, photographs, incident reports, and internal documentation and/or communication. In the records request, the requesting party should indicate who is requesting the records and what legal authority he or she has to obtain a copy of the records.

There are many opinions as to whether the physical therapist, physical therapist assistant, or student should retain a defense lawyer at this stage of the process. The benefit of having a lawyer at this stage is that the attorney should advise the defendant regarding which documents are privileged. Physical therapists, physical therapist assistants, and students must understand that once information is produced, any privilege that would or could be associated with that document is considered waived.

As an example, in many states, incident reports still are considered a privileged document and are not required to be produced in litigation. The privileges asserted for incident reports are attorney/client privileged communication, attorney work product, and/or quality assurance privilege. The *attorney/client privileged communication* is defined as "[t]he client's right to refuse to disclose and to prevent any other person from disclosing confidential communications between the client and the attorney."[8]

The *attorney work product* is defined as "[t]angible material or its intangible equivalent—in unwritten or oral form—that was either prepared by or for a lawyer or prepared for litigation, either planned or in progress. Work product is generally exempt from discovery or other compelled disclosure. The term is also used to describe the products of a party's investigation or communications concerning the subject matter of a lawsuit if made (1) to assist in the prosecution or defense of a pending suit, or (2) in reasonable anticipation of litigation."[9] Lastly, the *quality-assurance privilege*, also known as *peer-review privilege*, is defined as "[a] privilege that protects from disclosure the proceedings and reports of a medical facility's peer-review committee, which reviews and oversees the patient care and medical services provided by the staff."[10]

The key to sustaining these privileges is whether the document in question was created in response to an internal investigation of an incident; that is, prepared in anticipation of litigation, or prepared at the request of the physical therapist's, physical therapist assistant's, or student's counsel to contemporaneously document an occurrence. Accordingly, the physical therapist, physical therapist assistant, or student does not want to produce these documents in a records request even though the requesting party may ask for them. It is very common for plaintiff lawyers to request these documents even though it is known the document might be privileged. As such, an unknowing person could produce for lack of knowledge and once produced, a court would likely deem the privilege waived. Accordingly, one of the advantages to hiring a lawyer when a records request is received is that the lawyer will review all documents before production to ensure no privileged documents are produced.

The other thing the physical therapist, physical therapist assistant, or student will need to do when a records request is received is notify the physical therapist's, physical therapist assistant's, or student's insurance carrier, if applicable, of the potential claim. In other words, if the physical therapist, physical therapist assistant, or student has professional malpractice insurance, he or she will need to notify the carrier of the request for records. This is known as putting the insurance carrier on notice. The insurance carrier might hire a lawyer to represent the physical therapist's, physical therapist assistant's, or student's and insurance carrier's interest during the records request phase of litigation. (Please refer back to Chapter 10 on personal malpractice insurance for the discussion of some of the physical therapist's, physical therapist assistant's, or student's rights as an insured.)

At no time should the physical therapist, physical therapist assistant, or student alter the records. This may seem the simplest of statements, but some individuals may get scared at the thought of their records being requested for review by a plaintiff's attorney. In the emotion of it all, people sometimes go back and review the records only to identify omissions in the documentation or descriptions they wish had been documented in more detail.

In that fear, the physical therapist, physical therapist assistant, or student may subsequently add documentation or change documentation without clearly indicating the date the documentation is being added and/or changed. Do not succumb to that temptation. **NEVER** alter a medical record after the fact. If the physical therapist, physical therapist assistant, or student chooses to add or change any documentation, do it correctly and put the date the change or addition is being made along with the appropriate signature. (Please refer to Chapter 8 on documentation for more of a discussion on this issue.)

Lastly, always keep a copy of whatever is sent to a party or a party's lawyer. The physical therapist, physical therapist assistant, or student always will want to be able to review the same documents that a plaintiff's lawyer has to review.

Verify the Legal Authority to Obtain the Records

Before producing records to anyone, the physical therapist, physical therapist assistant, or student must verify the requesting party has the legal authority to obtain the records. Under Health Insurance Portability and Accountability Act (HIPAA), every patient is guaranteed under federal law the right to privacy of his or her medical records.[11] Lastly, know the state's timeline for the production of records. Many states statutorily specify the length of time a health care provider has to produce a copy of a patient's medical records.

PRESUIT

Some states have implemented presuit statutes wherein the parties (plaintiff and defendant) must complete a presuit investigation of any claim relative to medical malpractice. Of note, during presuit, the plaintiff is usually called a *claimant,* and the defendant is usually called the *respondent.* The time frame of the presuit varies. In Florida, the medical malpractice act is defined in Chapter 766. Chapter 766, Florida Statutes, has a 90-day presuit period for claims alleging medical malpractice of health care providers.[12]

However, it should be noted that occupational therapists and speech language pathologists, as well as nursing homes (as of the writing of this book), are not considered health care providers in Florida under Chapter 766; thus, these individuals do not receive the protections of the Florida Medical Malpractice Act. Likewise, under Louisiana law, it was questionable whether physical therapists were covered health care practitioners as "physical therapists [were] not listed among those health care providers covered under the special periods for prescription (statute of limitations) set forth in La. R.S. 9:5628, regulating actions for medical malpractice."[13] However, in Louisiana, the *Williams* case ultimately held that physical therapists were subject to the provisions of the Louisiana Medical Malpractice Act.[14] Consequently, each state's statutes and case law will determine what, if any, protections in liability cases are afforded physical therapists, physical therapists assistants, and/or students.

During presuit, both sides can usually take unsworn statements of key witnesses and conduct limited discovery. An *unsworn statement* is a statement taken of a witness without the witness being placed under oath to tell the truth. The interesting thing about the presuit is that usually the discovery that is obtained during presuit is not discoverable or cannot subsequently be used in the actual lawsuit. Now, the parties can reask for the same discovery in the lawsuit and it is usually provided. Thus, the caveat that the discovery during presuit is not useable in the actual lawsuit actually has very little benefit except that information obtained from an unsworn statement cannot be used for impeachment (discrediting) of a witness later. The concept of presuit is for the parties to effectively evaluate each party's position and attempt to negotiate and resolve the matter before undertaking extensive and costly litigation.

During presuit, some cases resolve without a complaint ever being filed. In this author's experience, it is rare for a case to resolve in presuit, but it does happen occasionally.

LAWSUIT FILED

Whether the state has mandatory presuit or not, the beginning of a lawsuit occurs with the filing of a complaint with the clerk of the court in the jurisdiction where the lawsuit is being brought. In determining which jurisdiction to file the complaint, the plaintiff must consider how much money will be alleged as damages, because most jurisdictions determine subject matter jurisdiction based on the amount of the alleged damages.

Recall from Chapter 2 the multitude of various courts that are available for the filing of a lawsuit. In order to get the case into civil court, the plaintiff usually has to allege a certain amount of money in damages; otherwise, the case will be assigned to county court. As an example, in Florida, the plaintiff must allege the amount of damages are more than $15,000 in order for the case to be assigned to circuit court. Anything less than $15,000 will be assigned to county court.

One of the key issues that should be scrutinized first is whether the case has been filed within the statute of limitations. *Statute of limitations* is defined as "[a] statute establishing a time limit for suing in a civil case, based on the date when the claim accrued (as when the injury occurred or was discovered). The purpose of such a statute is to require diligent prosecution of known claims, thereby providing finality and predictability in legal affairs and ensuring that claims will be resolved while evidence is reasonably available and fresh."[15]

If the matter is not filed within the statute of limitations, then usually the case can be dismissed on a motion to dismiss asserting the statute of limitations has expired, unless the plaintiff is able to plead that a particular exception should be applied to the statute of limitations. Examples of types of exceptions that can be pled may be the injury was a latent injury that was not discovered until something happened or that the defendant did something to hide the information needed to discover the injury.

A case involving a physical therapist that was dismissed on the grounds that the statute of limitations expired is *Levinson v. Health South Manhattan*.[16] In the *Levinson* case, the plaintiff alleged negligence against the physical therapist in the use of electrical stimulation.[17] The complaint alleged the physical therapist incorrectly used the electrical stimulation and that the incorrect usage led to an injury of the plaintiff.[18] The court ordered the dismissal of the complaint because the statute of limitations had expired. Once the statute of limitations expires, the plaintiff must be able to plead and prove that one of the exceptions to the statute of limitations applies in order for the claim to not be dismissed.

Once the complaint is filed, the complaint must be served on the defendant. The person allowed by law to serve the complaint will be specified in the jurisdiction's laws. There is usually a specified time frame during which the complaint must be served and then there will be a specified time in which the defendant must file a response in order to avoid a default judgment.

RESPONDING TO THE COMPLAINT

Once the defendant is served with the complaint, the next step for the defendant is to respond to the complaint. There are generally two alternatives for this response: the defendant may file a motion to dismiss the complaint or the defendant may answer the complaint. There are certain defenses, depending on the jurisdiction, that must be pled in the first responsive pleading or the defenses are forever waived.

If the defendant files a motion to dismiss, it must be based on a good-faith belief of the attorney that grounds exists for the dismissal of the complaint. A motion to dismiss is defined as "[a] request that the court dismiss the case because of settlement, voluntary withdrawal, or a procedural defect."[19] Usually, the parties' attorneys will discuss the merits of the motion to dismiss and may or may not agree on the grounds. Sometimes, the parties' attorneys can reach an agreement such that the plaintiff's lawyer files an amended complaint to address the grounds raised in the motion to dismiss. At this point in the litigation, if all of the grounds raised in the motion to dismiss have been addressed effectively, then the next response may be to answer the complaint.

However, sometimes the parties' attorneys cannot agree on the grounds raised in the motion to dismiss and the attorneys schedule a hearing before the judge assigned to the case so that the judge can decide the merits of the motion to dismiss. Usually, unless there is some dispositive issue raised in the motion to dismiss, the motion may be granted but the plaintiff will be allowed to amend the complaint to address the issues raised. It is rare for a case to be dismissed at this stage in the litigation without the plaintiff having further recourse for the alleged wrong. The standard that is usually applied to a motion to dismiss is that the facts alleged as construed as true in favor of the nonmoving party. Once there is a valid complaint filed with the court, the next step is for the defendant to answer the complaint.

ANSWERING THE COMPLAINT

Once it is time to answer the complaint, each paragraph in the complaint must be answered with either admit, deny, or without knowledge; therefore, denied. Sometimes there may be the need to admit part of an allegation contained in a paragraph and then deny the remainder of the allegation with an explanation as to why the paragraph cannot be completely admitted or denied. Once each of the paragraphs of the complaint is answered, then the defense may put forth affirmative defenses.

Affirmative defenses are defined as "[a] defendant's assertion raising new facts and arguments that, if true, will defeat the plaintiff's or prosecutor's claim, even if all allegations in the complaint are true."[20] Some of the affirmative defenses that may be applicable to cases involving physical therapists, physical therapist assistants, or students are that the statute of limitations has expired, failure of the plaintiff to perform all conditions precedent to bringing the action, collateral estoppel, and/or issue preclusion. Some other types of defenses that are usually pled include collateral payments, a third party is at fault, or the plaintiff was contributorily negligent or failed to mitigate the damages.

The important thing to remember when pleading affirmative defenses is to include all potentially available defenses that, in good faith, have the potential to be proven. Although the defendant might be able to seek court permission to amend the answer and affirmative defenses later, if sought after a certain time frame, it will usually take a court order and the plaintiff will likely argue against the amendment because it will prejudice the plaintiff. Thus, the lawyer defending the physical therapist, physical therapist assistant, or student wants to be as thorough as possible from the beginning. However, it is understood that as discovery is undertaken, new facts may be discovered that necessitate an amendment. Generally speaking, the standard that must be met for an amendment is one of reason and courts are usually fairly liberal in the granting of orders to amend answers and complaints.

The case of *Henry v. Williams* is an illustration of how affirmative defenses are important. The jury found that the patient was 25 percent at fault for a fall that occurred while undergoing gait training with a physical therapist assistant trainee. The patient had been admitted to the hospital and undergone surgery for a right knee replacement.[20] Following surgery, the surgeon prescribed physical therapy.[21] The physical therapist delegated the physical therapy sessions to a physical therapist assistant trainee (student).[22] Prior to working as a student physical therapist assistant at the hospital, the physical therapist assistant trainee had completed 1 year of an associate's degree course work and she had completed a 4-week clinical.[23]

During the course of physical therapy treatment, the patient progressed to ambulating 200 feet with a rolling walker on level surfaces with stand-by assist.[24] Prior to discharge from the hospital, the physical therapist learned that the patient would have to be able to go up and down one step in order to get in and out of the home.[25] The physical therapist directed the physical therapist assistant trainee to train the patient on how to go up and down one step.[26] The physical therapist assistant trainee elected to take the patient outside to use a curb for the training instead of using a two-step piece of equipment that was available in the physical therapy department.[27]

When the physical therapist assistant trainee had the patient stand up, she had the patient put the walker in the left hand and the trainee walked around the back of the patient.[28] Thereafter the factual account of the circumstances differed between the patient and the physical therapist assistant trainee. Regardless, the patient took a step to go down the curb and fell.[29] The patient re-injured the knee and had to undergo additional surgery.[30] Ultimately, the patient had a full recovery and only lacked 5 degrees of extension.[31]

The factual difference was that the patient testified the physical therapist assistant trainee stood behind her and said, "I'm trying to figure out how to tell you to do it."[32] Whereas the physical therapist assistant trainee testified she moved to the back of the patient intending to be on the right side of the patient to assist with stepping down but the patient without warning took a step down off the curb and fell.[33] Thus, there was what is called a dispute of fact that must be determined by a jury. Prior to the lawsuit being filed, a panel of three physical therapists reviewed the evidence and did not find enough evidence that either the physical therapist or the physical therapist assistant trainee breached the prevailing standard of care.[34]

The lesson from this case relative to affirmative defenses is that the defense counsel pled the patient also was comparatively negligent and that a jury should assign some fault to the patient. In this case, the jury assigned some fault to the patient in the amount of 25 percent. This case was also discussed in Chapter 6, as another cause of action to the complaint could have been for negligent supervision of the delegating physical therapist. Additionally, this case will be discussed in Chapter 16 as an ethical issue relative to supervision of the student physical therapist assistant.

DISCOVERY

Different types of discovery can be undertaken during litigation. *Discovery* is defined as "[t]he act or process of finding or learning something that was previously unknown."[35] Some of the most common types of discovery are interrogatories, request for production, request for admissions, and depositions. There is no specific order or method that one party has to undertake in the discovery process.

Interrogatories are questions that the other party must answer within a specified period of time. The lawyer who propounds the question must artfully craft the question to narrow the information sought. It is not uncommon for the party receiving the interrogatory to object to answering.

Most jurisdictions limit the number of interrogatories one party can propound on the other and specify how long the party answering has to answer. Some types of interrogatories might be to determine what damages the party is claiming, or what other sources have paid some medical bills, or who knows anything about the facts of the case. Usually interrogatories must be answered under oath; therefore, the party answering the questions usually executes a notarized jurat page.

Requests for production generally are not limited, but must be relevant to the cause of action. Usually in medical malpractice cases, the defense wants to obtain as many medical records as possible from other health care providers in order to have a complete understanding of the plaintiff's medical conditions. Other items requested in this type of discovery include policies and procedures, personnel files, time cards, payroll records, tax returns, employee rosters, death certificates, and autopsy reports. All of this information can be useful to one side or the other to prove or disprove issues within a lawsuit. Again, there is usually a time limit within which the information has to be provided to the other side. Sometimes, there are documents or other items that are considered privileged and that are not produced and instead, appropriate privilege logs are produced.

Requests for admissions are a discovery tool wherein one party requests the other party to admit to certain facts. The purpose of this type of discovery is to narrow the facts in dispute. Remember, once the case goes to trial, the facts in dispute will be resolved by the jury. As an example, in a medical malpractice case, one thing that may be in a request for admission is that the plaintiff received an explanation of the risks and benefits of a certain procedure. Once the matter is at trial, if the plaintiff admits that the risks and benefits of the treatment were explained, then the defense does not need to prove that fact. Instead, the defendant can use that fact in opening statement and in closing without having to prove it. The use of request for admissions usually occurs later in the litigation process once facts and issues of the case have been narrowed.

Request for entry on the land for inspection is another discovery tool that is sometimes used in medical malpractice cases. This is especially true when medical equipment is involved in litigation. The plaintiff, if injured by a piece of equipment, may want to have his or her expert evaluate the piece of equipment. Thus, when a piece of equipment is involved in an incident, it may be necessary to take the equipment out of usage and store it until after litigation is over.

Sometimes a party may object to answering or producing items that are requested. When a party objects to answering or the production of items, then the party objecting must state the grounds for the objection. The party receiving the objection then determines whether the objection is well taken or if that party disagrees and believes the question should be answered or the information produced. At that point the party requesting the information can file a motion to compel the other party to answer or produce the information. If the attorneys cannot resolve the issue, then the motion to compel is scheduled for a hearing before the judge who has been assigned the case. At the hearing, the parties' attorneys will appear and make oral arguments to the judge (court) for the court to resolve the issue. In federal court, it is rare that the attorneys will be granted a hearing before the judge; instead the judge will make a ruling based upon the pleadings (papers filed with the court).

DEPOSITIONS

Depositions are an expensive way of doing discovery. The party who schedules the deposition is customarily responsible for the costs associated with the expense of the court reporter and the original transcript of the deposition. Other than parties, one party cannot compel a nonparty to appear for a deposition outside of the county in which the deponent lives. The deponent is the person being scheduled for the deposition. Hence, travel expenses to and from the deposition location can also get quite expensive. Some methods often utilized to reduce the expense associated with out-of-state depositions include video conferencing or telephonic depositions. The disadvantage to these types of depositions is the lawyer's inability to assess how a jury might respond to the deponent.

The purpose of a deposition is to ask questions of a party who might appear as a witness at trial to try and determine what knowledge of the facts in dispute this person has. It is a way to discover information about a case and to assess the credibility of a witness. It is not uncommon for depositions to be videotaped. Sometimes, if it is doubtful whether a deponent who is expected to testify at trial will be able to be present at trial, the party might decide to videotape the witness so the party can show the video to the jury versus just having to read a transcript to the jury, which is considered to be one of the most boring portions of a trial.

Lastly, the lawyer scheduling the deposition can make the witness bring documents to the deposition for inspection. This is called a *deposition duces tecum.* When this occurs, the witness who has been subpoenaed or agreed to appear must come to the deposition bringing with him or her whatever has been identified on the subpoena for production at the time of the deposition. Usually lawyers on both sides attempt to work together to schedule these depositions at a convenient time and place for the parties as well as nonparties. However, sometimes it cannot be accomplished and a motion to compel depositions must be filed.

Once the parties complete discovery, then one party can file a pleading to the court that the matter is ready to be set for trial. However, usually the plaintiff's lawyer will file the notice that the matter is ready to be set for trial long before the defense lawyer believes the matter is ready to be set for trial. When that happens, the defense lawyer will likely file an objection that the matter is not ready for trial and then it is left to the discretion of the judge when to set the matter for trial.

HEARINGS

Throughout the litigation process there are a variety of motions that can be filed and the lawyers for the parties might have to appear before the judge for a determination of a particular issue. The physical therapist, physical therapist assistant, or student should be kept informed of what motions have been filed and whenever the lawyer for the physical therapist, physical therapist assistant, or student is going to appear before the judge on behalf of the physical therapist, physical therapist assistant, or student. Some of the motions that might lead to the lawyers appearing before the judge include motions to dismiss, motions to compel, motions for protective orders, motions for summary judgments, or motions for partial summary judgments.

PRETRIAL MATTERS

Once the matter is set for trial, the judge will issue a trial order. In the trial order there will be certain deadlines for the parties to meet as the trial date approaches. Usually the different deadlines are relative to the trial date and a pretrial conference. Such things as discovery, witness disclosure, and dispositive motions will have deadlines relative to the trial date. Usually the plaintiffs will disclose the experts they intend to call at trial and identify the subject matter about which the expert will testify. Usually some time later, the defense will have to disclose their experts. Once the experts are disclosed, then the depositions of the experts are scheduled and taken; usually the plaintiff's experts are deposed before the defense's experts. This way the deposition transcripts from the plaintiff's experts can be sent to the defense's experts so that the issues of the matter are narrowed.

Other pretrial matters include motions *in limine* and sometimes motions that will narrow issues for the trial. *Motions in limine* are one party's attempt to restrict or eliminate the use of certain evidence at trial. As an example, a motion *in limine* from the plaintiff on a case involving a pressure ulcer might be that defense counsel cannot discuss with the jury or use the example of Christopher Reeve's development and ultimate death from a pressure ulcer. As many will recall, Christopher Reeve received some of the best health care available and still developed pressure ulcers as a complication of his quadriplegia. The pressure ulcer ultimately became infected and led to sepsis and death. Thus, plaintiffs do not want jurors to understand that even with the best of health care, sometimes bad things happen.

TRIAL

Once the trial date arrives, the trial is ready to begin. It is not unusual for multiple trials to be set on the same date at the same time because many cases will be settled on the courthouse doorsteps. The case that is first on the docket will be the case that starts its trial on the trial date if it does not settle. Consequently, it also is possible the case that is number nine on the docket may be the case that goes to trial if cases numbered one through eight settle before the trial date. As a result, there is really no way to know whether a particular case is really going to go to trial on the date set unless that case is number one on the docket and it does not settle prior. Once the trial starts, the first thing that usually occurs is for any last-minute preliminary matters to be decided by the judge. Then the potential jurors are brought in for the jury-selection process to begin.

Jury Selection

Jury selection is called *voir dire. Voir dire* is defined as "[a] preliminary examination of a prospective juror by a judge or lawyer to decide whether the prospect is qualified and suitable to serve on a jury."[36] During this process, the judge usually will ask the preliminary questions to eliminate jurors for various reasons, including determining that they are not qualified to sit on a jury panel or cannot reasonably sit through the length of the trial. However, the juror will not know he or she essentially has been eliminated until the final jury selection takes place. Then the plaintiff's counsel is allowed to ask questions of the prospective jurors. Once the plaintiff's lawyer is finished, the defense's lawyer is allowed to ask questions of the jurors. After the questioning is completed, then the lawyers decide which jurors will sit on the trial jury panel. There are two ways for the lawyers to eliminate a juror. One way is for cause and the other way is a preemptive challenge.

For cause means there is a reason that the juror should be eliminated from the jury panel because there is some type of bias one party believes the juror cannot overcome. Usually what happens is that one party wants the juror on the panel because of the bias and the other party wants the juror removed because of the bias. Thus, the party wanting to remove the juror will argue to the judge why the juror should be removed from the panel for cause.

As an example, a potential juror on a medical malpractice case may state during *voir dire* that he or she agrees with tort reform. This information would tell the plaintiff's lawyer that this potential juror might not be sympathetic to the plaintiff's cause or be willing to award big money and the plaintiff's attorney would likely want to remove this potential juror from the jury panel. Thus, the plaintiff's lawyer would likely argue to the judge that this potential juror is biased and cannot overcome the bias to render an impartial verdict in the matter. The defense lawyer during questioning would likely attempt to rehabilitate the juror so that in order for the plaintiff's lawyer to eliminate the juror from the panel, the plaintiff's lawyer will have to expend a preemptive challenge. Usually there is no limit to the number of jurors that one side can eliminate for cause.

A *preemptive challenge* is the ability of a lawyer to remove a potential juror from the jury panel without having to give a reason. Usually each side in a civil trial will have three preemptive challenges. The lawyers want to use these sparingly in an attempt to seat a jury panel the lawyer believes will best serve his or her client's interest. Sometimes the parties can stipulate to additional preemptive challenges; however, it is the judge's responsibility to maintain fairness amongst the parties. One of the restrictions to using a preemptive challenge is that the use of the preemptive challenge must be race neutral. In other words, a lawyer may not attempt to remove a potential juror because of the juror's race.

Once the lawyers and judge agree on the jury panel, then the panel is sworn in to hear the issues in the case. The remainder of the potential jurors then are dismissed. Usually, for a civil trial, there are one or two alternate jurors sat to hear the matter in case one of the other jurors becomes unable to complete the trial. The alternate jurors do not know they are the alternate jurors until the jury is ready to deliberate. Usually the judge will dismiss the alternate juror(s) at the time the jury gets the case to deliberate. Once the jury is seated and impanelled, then both parties' lawyers make an opening statement to the jury.

Opening Statement

An opening statement is the party's first opportunity to present an overview of the case to the jury. An *opening statement* is defined as "[a]t the outset of a trial, an advocate's statement giving the fact-finder a preview of the case and of the evidence to be presented, but not containing argument."[37] The information presented in opening statement is not evidence and should not be considered evidence. Additionally, the opening statement is not allowed to be what is called argumentative. The opening statement should lay out for the jury what the party expects to prove at trial and who will present the different pieces of the evidence. The plaintiff will go first and the defense follows. Prior to trial, the lawyers for each party usually agree on the amount of time each side will have to present the party's opening statement.

Plaintiff's Case-in-Chief

Once the opening statements are completed, the plaintiff will present the plaintiff's case. This is known as the plaintiff's *case-in-chief.* During this phase of the trial, the plaintiff will call its witnesses and through the witnesses' testimony admit for the jury's consideration various pieces of evidence. There are rules that the lawyers are trained in regarding what is admissible and what is not admissible as evidence. During the presentation of a witness, one lawyer may object to various questions asked by the other party's lawyer or may object to the introduction of evidence. The judge makes rulings throughout the trial based on the objections. It is this process of preserving the record that courts use later when a party takes the case up on appeal. The party taking the appeal usually will argue to the appellate court that the trial judge erred in his or her ruling(s).

The plaintiff's lawyer will conduct what is known as direct examination of the witnesses called. During direct examination, the lawyer is not allowed to lead a witness in the questioning. Thus, the questions will usually revolve around who, what, where, when, how, and explain. Once the plaintiff's lawyer completes the direct examination, the defense lawyer is allowed to cross-examine the witness. On cross-examination, the lawyer may ask leading questions. Again there are various rules of procedure and evidentiary rules that lawyers are required to follow that guide how the examinations are conducted.

Once the plaintiff has called all of its witnesses and admitted into evidence all its evidence, then the plaintiff rests. At the time the plaintiff rests, the defense usually will make a motion outside the presence of the jury called a motion for directed verdict. The motion is to ask the judge to direct the verdict in favor of the defense because the plaintiff failed to present evidence to support its claim such that a jury could find for the plaintiff. These motions rarely are granted. If not granted, the defense then puts on its case-in-chief.

Defendant's Case-in-Chief

Just like the plaintiff's case-in-chief, the defense will call witnesses and present evidence to support the defense's interpretation of the case. At this stage of the trial, the defense team will call witnesses and do what is called direct examination. Just like during the plaintiff's case-in-chief, the questions of direct examination are usually who, what, where, when, how, why, and explain. Following the direct examination of a witness, the plaintiff's counsel may conduct cross-examination. Once the plaintiff's lawyer completes cross-examination of the witness, the defense lawyer may then conduct a redirect examination to rehabilitate anything necessary based on the cross-examination.

Once the defense team completes their case-in-chief, then the defense will rest. At that time, the defense likely will renew its motion for a directed verdict. Again this motion and oral argument will be made outside the presence of the jury. This motion rarely will be granted, but is necessary to preserve some appellate issues. If this motion is denied, the next phase of the trial will be closing arguments.

Closing Argument

Closing argument is the final opportunity for the parties to address the jury. *Closing argument* is defined as "a lawyer's final statement to the judge or jury before deliberations begins, in which the lawyer requests the judge or jury to consider the evidence and to apply the law in his or her client's favor. Usu[ally] in a jury trial, the judge afterwards instructs the jury on the law that governs the case."[38] The plaintiff will be allowed to go first and may reserve a portion of the allocated time for a rebuttal argument. Once the plaintiff completes the closing argument, the defense will present its closing argument. Thereafter, the plaintiff may present a rebuttal argument for whatever the remainder of the allocated time the plaintiff has reserved. After closing argument, the judge will give the jury its jury instructions.

Jury Instructions

The jury instructions will have been submitted by the parties and the judge will make final determination of which instructions will be given to the jury. *Jury instructions* are defined as "[a] jury direction or guideline that a judge gives a jury concerning the law of the case."[39] Generally speaking, most jury instructions are now standardized in an attempt to remove some of the potential appellate issues based on judges' drafting individual case jury instructions. The jury instructions tell the jury the law and issues that are before it to resolve. Lastly, the judge will explain the verdict form; however, more likely than not, both parties have explained the verdict form to the jury during each party's closing argument. Once the judge has completed giving the jury its instructions and verdict form, the jury will then retire for deliberations. Prior to adjournment to the jury room, any alternate jurors who had been seated usually will be dismissed and not participate in the deliberations.

Jury Deliberations

There is no time limit for how long a jury may deliberate on a matter. *Jury deliberations* are defined as "[t]he act of carefully considering issues and options before making a decision or taking some action; esp[ecially], the process by which a jury reaches a verdict, as by analyzing, discussing, and weighing the evidence." [40] Once the jury retires to the jury deliberation room, the first thing the jury is charged with doing is electing a foreperson to speak for the jury. Thereafter, how the jury conducts its deliberations is unique to each panel. Any evidence admitted into evidence throughout the trial will be taken into the jury deliberation room for the jury members to examine and discuss. Once the jury reaches a verdict, which in most jurisdictions and most cases has to be unanimous, the foreperson will notify the judge's clerk of the court that a verdict has been reached.

The clerk then will begin contacting the attorneys for all parties so that the lawyers and parties can return to the courtroom. Once all of the parties and lawyers have returned to the courtroom, the judge will bring the jury back in. There is a formal process wherein the judge will ask if the jury has reached a verdict. The jury foreperson, responding in the affirmative, will lead to the clerk obtaining the verdict form from the foreperson and giving it to the judge. Once the judge checks the verdict form for completeness and correctness, the judge will ask the clerk to post the verdict. At that time, the clerk reads the verdict form.

After the verdict is read, whichever party the verdict went against, may ask the judge for a JNOV verdict. JNOV stands for judgment notwithstanding the verdict. A *JNOV* is defined as "[a] judgment entered for one party even though a jury verdict has been rendered for the opposing party."[41] Again, these are rarely granted, but sometimes the jury simply gets it wrong. When that happens, this is the party's last resort to have the judge correct the mistake of the jury without the necessity of an appeal.

Posttrial Motions and Final Judgment

Just because the trial is over does not mean that the lawsuit is finished. After the trial, whether with a judge or jury, the winning party will file a motion to enter judgment against the other party. The losing party may file a motion for a new trial or offsets to the verdict based on other entities' payment of some damages. The latter motion is commonly used in medical malpractice cases. In medical malpractice cases, generally an insurance company or Medicare has already paid the plaintiff's medical bills. Medical bills that have already been paid on plaintiff's behalf should not then be paid again to the plaintiff as a damage award. If that occurred, the plaintiff would receive double payments. Thus, if the defendant lost, he or she would want the damages the jury or judge awarded reduced by the amount that insurance or Medicare has already paid for the medical expenses.

On the other hand, if the insurance carrier or Medicare placed a lien against the trial awards, then the plaintiff will attempt to prevent reduction of the damage award because the plaintiff will have to pay off the liens. A *lien* is defined as "[a] legal right or interest that a creditor has in another's property, lasting usu[ually] until a debt or duty that it secures is satisfied."[42]

Once the trial judge rules on the posttrial motions, a final judgment can be entered. However, if one party has filed a motion for a new trial and the trial judge denies the motion, then the party may file an appeal. If an appeal is filed, then the conclusion of the matter is delayed.

ALTERNATIVE DISPUTE RESOLUTION

There are two other ways to resolve disputes without the necessity of a trial. These two means are arbitration and mediation. Usually before any civil case actually goes to trial, the presiding judge over the case with require the parties to go to at least one mediation. *Arbitration* is defined as "[a] method of dispute resolution involving one ore more neutral third parties who are usu[ally] agreed to by the disputing parties and whose decision is binding."[43] *Mediation* is defined as "[a] method of nonbinding dispute resolution involving a neutral third party who tries to help the disputing parties reach a mutually agreeable solution."[44]

APPEALS

In many of the cases to which this book refers, the appellate judges' rulings created what is known as case law. An appeal can occur during the litigation of a matter based on the trial judge's ruling affecting the case. There are various rules and reasons why some matters during litigation are not available for appeal while other matters can be appealed. It is sufficient for this book to know that after the trial, the losing party may file an appeal if something occurred during litigation or the trial that the party believes affected the outcome and the judge was wrong. Appeals are time consuming and costly; however, errors in the litigation can result in the wrong or erroneous results that can only be corrected on appeal.

Where the matter is appealed will depend on which court had jurisdiction over the case from the beginning. If the case was in a state court, then the appeal will go to the next higher state court. If the case was litigated in federal court, then the appeal will go to the circuit court for that particular jurisdiction. Whether the appellate court's decision can be appealed depends on multiple factors. For this book, suffice to know that sometimes the appellate court's decision can be appealed to the highest court in the state or the U.S. Supreme Court. Once the highest court makes it decision, usually the appellate options are over. Once the matter is finally over, the losing side is obligated to abide by the results.

SETTLEMENT

Settlement is defined as "[a]n agreement ending a dispute or lawsuit."[45] A settlement may be reached between the opposing parties at any time during the litigation process. There are even times that the parties can reach an agreement of settlement long before the litigation process begins. The key to settlement is requiring the plaintiff to execute (sign) a settlement agreement that bars the plaintiff from pursuing any further action against the defendant. The settlement agreement usually also contains a confidentiality agreement, which means no party can discuss the settlement, or that the defendant was sued, and especially cannot discuss the terms of the settlement agreement. However, sometimes when other parties are still in the litigation process, the judge may require the amount of the settlement to be known or the settlement agreement to be produced. When that occurs, the party having to do the production should take appropriate steps to try and ensure that the agreement remains confidential and that a court order is required for the document to be viewed. This is called sealing the document in the court file.

SUMMARY

The litigation process is complicated, long, and fraught with details. Medical malpractice cases are usually lengthy and take several years to resolve unless one party decides to end the litigation by either a settlement or withdrawal of the claim. This seldom happens early in the litigation. If the defendant has insurance coverage for the claim, then usually the insurance carrier will select defense counsel and the insured's policy limits are depleted based on defense attorney's fees and costs. Some of the costs associated with litigation include travel expenses, copies of records, depositions, and hearings.

DISCUSSION QUESTIONS

1. In a physical therapy malpractice case, what are some of the interrogatory questions a plaintiff's lawyer might ask?
2. In a physical therapy malpractice case, what are some of the documents a plaintiff's lawyer would request be produced?
3. In a physical therapy malpractice case, what are some of the questions a plaintiff's lawyer might ask during a deposition?
4. What should be considered when selecting an attorney?
5. Discuss a records request.
6. Define and discuss presuit.
7. What is the statute of limitations?
8. Discuss the different stages of litigation.
9. Discuss the different types of discovery.
10. What is jury selection?
11. Discuss the various phases of a trial.

NOTES

[1] La. R.S. 40:1299.47
[2] *Bellsouth Telecommunications, Inc. v. Church Tower of Florida, Inc.*, 2006 WL 626071 (Fla. 3d DCA 2006).
[3] *Id.*
[4] *Id.*
[5] *Id.*
[6] *Id.*
[7] *Id.* at 2.
[8] *Black's Law Dictionary*, 1215 (Bryan A. Gardner, ed., 7th ed., West Group 1999).
[9] *Id.* at 1600–1601.
[10] *Id.* at 1216.
[11] HIPAA, www.hhs.gov/policies/#hippa.
[12] Fla. Stats. Chapter 766.
[13] *Williams v. Tri-State Physical Therapy, Inc.*, 850 So.2d 991, 994 (La. App. 2 Cir. 2003).
[14] *Id.*
[15] *Black's Law Dictionary*, 1422 (Bryan A. Gardner, ed., 7th ed., West Group 1999).
[16] *Levinson v. Health South Manhattan*, 793 N.Y.S.2d. 401 (N.Y. Supr. 2005).
[17] *Id.* at 501.
[18] *Id.*
[19] *Black's Law Dictionary*, 1034 (Bryan A. Gardner, ed., 7th ed., West Group 1999).
[20] *Id.* at 431
[21] *Henry v. Williams*, 892 So.2d 765, 767 (LA 2d Cir. 2005).
[22] *Id.*

[23] *Id.*
[24] *Id.*
[25] *Id.*
[26] *Id.*
[27] *Id.*
[28] *Id.*
[29] *Id.*
[30] *Id.*
[31] *Id.*
[32] *Id.*
[33] *Id.*
[34] *Id.*
[35] *Id.*
[36] *Black's Law Dictionary,* 478 (Bryan A. Gardner, ed., 7th ed., West Group 1999).
[37] *Id.* at 1569.
[38] *Id.* at 1118.
[39] *Id.* at 248.
[40] *Id.* at 861.
[41] *Id.* at 438–439.
[42] *Id.* at 847.
[43] *Id.* at 933.
[44] *Id.* at 100.
[45] *Id.* at 996.
[46] *Id.* at 1377.

CHAPTER 13

Managing Risk

One of the first steps to protecting the physical therapist, physical therapist assistant, or student from lawsuits is to understand what practice behaviors increase liability risks. For physical therapists, physical therapist assistants, and students, the liability risks will increase as the profession transitions toward that of an entry-level health care professional. In fact, in a 2006 report from CNA insurance company about physical therapy liability claims, the company that insures physical therapists, physical therapist assistants, and students stated, "[t]his expanding and changing role means increasing potential liability."[1]

The reason for this progression will be that a physician will not be overseeing and diagnostically ruling out diseases that could be causing the patient's complaints. The physical therapist, as an entry-level health care practitioner, will have to rule out diseases and complications that are not treatable through physical therapy and refer the patient elsewhere. Failure to refer could lead to devastating malpractice claims.

In a report released by CNA insurance in December 2006, liability claims against physical therapists, physical therapist assistants, and students were examined from 1993 through March 31, 2006.[2] During that time, CNA narrowed the claims for analysis down to 1464.[3] Of the 1464 claims, 1117 were closed and 347 remained open.[4] Of those closed claims, CNA insurance, through HPSO (Healthcare Providers Service Organization), paid $43,367,287 in indemnity and expenses.[5]

Indemnity is defined as "[a] duty to make good any loss, damage, or liability incurred by another."[6] An additional $13,326,657 had been reserved for the 347 claims that remained open and $3,000,000 had been paid in associated expenses.[7] Thus, this chapter will examine some of the allegations and claims against physical therapists, physical therapist assistants, and students as well as some risk management techniques that clinicians may utilize in order to reduce their risk.

KEY CONCEPTS

Risk management
Primary allegations against physical therapists, physical therapist assistants, and students
Quality improvement

RISK MANAGEMENT

Risk management is the process of identifying the liability risks and determining ways to reduce them. One of the first things that must be done is to identify what the physical therapist, physical therapist assistant, or student does that may put his or her practice at a liability risk. After the risks are identified, various tools can be used to put processes in place to help reduce the exposure. Some of the specific items that will be further explored in this chapter are what risks physical therapists, physical therapist assistants, or students are facing and the different tools used to help reduce the exposure to these risks.

For the physical therapist, physical therapist assistant, or student who has never done any type of risk-management analysis, a recommended starting point is to review the primary allegations and primary injuries that are listed later in this chapter. Then determine which allegation or allegations could be applicable to the physical therapist's, physical therapist assistant's, or student's practice. Next, the physical therapist, physical therapist assistant, or student should identify honestly what different situations occur in his or her daily practice that could lead to the identified allegation being brought against him or her. Identify improvements in the practice that could reduce the risks of that allegation based on an honest assessment of what the practice needs.

INHERENT RISK

One of the most difficult tasks to undertake is identification of what constitutes a potential risk in a physical therapy clinic. It does not matter whether the clinic is a hospital, outpatient setting, home health, industrial clinic, school, or nursing home. With the 2006 insurance report on physical therapy claims, the states, practice settings, and types of claims presenting liability risks to physical therapists, physical therapist assistants, and students have been identified.

First, the states that have the most or the most severe physical therapy liability claims are California, New York, Florida, Texas, Pennsylvania, Louisiana, Illinois, and New Jersey.[8] The states with the fewest claims were Wyoming, Maine, Puerto Rico, Nebraska, South Dakota, Hawaii, and New Mexico.[9] However, it should be noted that a physical therapist, physical therapist assistant, or student had at least one claim reported in every state during the time period of 1996 through March 31, 2006.[10]

Second, the overall practice setting with the most claims were physical therapy clinics outside of hospital settings, which accounted for 77 percent of the claims.[11] Practice settings outside of the hospital included home health, nursing homes, outpatient clinics, schools, and industrial rehabilitation clinics.[12] The percentage allocation of claims by practice setting was as follows[13]:

Physical therapy clinic outside hospital	77%
Patient's home (assuming home health)	7%
Nursing home	6%
Hospital physical therapy clinic	2%
School	2%
Physician's office	<1%
Industrial rehabilitation clinic	<1%

Although nursing homes only accounted for 6 percent of the claims, these claims were the most severe, with the average claim indemnity being $76,215.[14] The next most severe claims occurred in the industrial rehabilitation clinic, with an average cost of $75,000.[15]

The most common claims alleged damages for fractures and burns.[16] The next most common allegation that resulted in indemnity was a delay in recovery.[17] The most severe claims involved a patient's allegation that the physical therapist, physical therapist assistant, or student failed to report the patient's condition to a physician or other licensed health care practitioner who was responsible for the patient's overall medical care.[18] The most common primary allegations in order of severity were[19]:

Failure to report patient's condition
Failure to complete proper patient assessment
Failure to follow established policy
Retained foreign body
Improper positioning
Failure to refer/seek consultation
Injury during active resistance/assistive range of motion exercises
Injury during gait or elevation training
Provider functioning outside accepted scope of practice
Injury during training for assistive devices or equipment (such as canes, crutches, walker, wheelchair, etc.)
Improper technique

Improper management of course of treatment
Improper use of equipment
Injury during manipulation
Inappropriate behavior by clinician (including physical, sexual, or emotional abuse and/or misconduct)
Delay in treatment
Injury during resistance exercise or stretching
Patient injured while carrying out self-care treatment plan
Failure to supervise treatment/procedure
Injury during passive range of motion
Failure to properly test equipment
Injury during heat therapy or hot packs
Premature discharge or abandonment
Equipment malfunction or failure
Allegation unknown
Failure to monitor patient
Failure to respond to patient
Improper performance of test
Injury from cold packs/ice massage
Injury during traction
Injury during electrotherapy
Lack of informed consent
Injury during connective tissue manipulation or massage
Iontophoresis related
Injury during endurance activities (including weights, treadmills, ergonomics, etc.)

Other allegations included improper management of course of treatment; injury during electrotherapy; equipment malfunction or failure; failure to maintain proper infection control; unnecessary treatment; failure to diagnose; injury during aquatic exercise; improper management of a surgical patient; wrong medication administered; failure to treat; delay in treatment; breach of confidentiality or privacy; inadequate record keeping/documentation; hydrotherapy related; injury during training for assistive devices or equipment; and improper/inadequate pain management.[20]

The specific allocations of damages or injuries were[21]:

Trauma including fractures	27%
Burns	18%
Delay in recovery	11%
Additional procedure required	9%

Injury not specified	6%
Loss of limb or use of limb	6%
Abrasion/irritation/laceration	6%
Emotional distress (as primary injury)	5%
Unknown	3%
Bruise or contusion	2%
Sprain/strain	2%
Neurological related	2%

The injuries accounting for 1 percent were "cracked/broken teeth; death from disease; infection; and brain injury and/or paralysis."[22] The injuries accounting for less than 1 percent were "death from trauma; no injury; personal injury—e.g., slip and fall, hit by object, etc.; death not otherwise classified; loss of organ or organ function; suicide; addiction; and cardiopulmonary arrest."[23]

As the physical therapist, physical therapist assistant, or student can see, there are a multitude of claims that can be made in the delivery of physical therapy. Once the physical therapist, physical therapist assistant, or student identifies which of these types of services are delivered in his or her clinic, then the next step is to identify risk management behaviors to undertake.

PERSONNEL MANAGEMENT

Essentially, every lawsuit involving physical therapy will begin and revolve around some staff member. As discussed in Chapter 6, various issues associated with personnel can lead to litigation or additional allegations in a lawsuit. Some of the risk-management areas to consider in personnel management include the application process, ongoing training, and adherence to policy and procedures.

The application process is critical to the selection of staff members to work in the physical therapy clinic. There should be a completed application for every staff member, regardless of the position applied for, as well as references checked for every staff member. Anyone who is working in the physical therapy department that requires licensure should have his or her license verified as being active and in good standing.

If there is any work history gap for the individual applying for a position in the physical therapy clinic, the work history gap should be explored and documentation of why the person had any gaps in employment should be provided. Other background checks that could be undertaken include federal criminal background screenings, state criminal background screenings, and a review of the national or state sex offenders list. However, it should be pointed out that once the process of doing additional background screenings occurs, it should not be stopped because the standard of practice for the clinic has been established. Thus, once started, do not stop. Remember, the goal of the initial hiring process is to attempt to verify the person is qualified for the position for which he or she applied and that there are no reasons to exclude the person from employment.

Thereafter, initial and ongoing training to ensure competency is essential. Every employee, regardless of the position, should go through some type of initial orientation. Failure to orient an employee to his or her position will appear of itself to be negligent. After the initial orientation, all staff members should receive ongoing training and education. Whatever the continuing educational requirements for a particular state, the physical therapist, physical therapist assistant, and student must track and document completion of the minimal hours. It is recommended to keep track of all continuing education, because the physical therapist, physical therapist assistant, or student may some day need to provide a certification of attendance at some particular continuing education seminar as proof of competency.

Additionally, the new employee should receive a copy of his or her job description and be provided access to the department's policies and procedures. As discussed in Chapter 6, the new employee should be allocated time during the initial orientation process to read and understand the department's policies and procedures.

Next, physical therapists and physical therapist assistants should receive, at minimum, annual performance evaluations. These evaluations should include checks to document that the clinician remains competent to perform his or her job duties. If the physical therapist or physical therapist assistant is not competent in any particular area of practice, then he or she should not receive patients on caseload that require that particular type of practice. A plan should be put in place so that the physical therapist or physical therapist assistant can obtain proficiency in that area of practice.

Lastly, when the physical therapy clinic is working with independent contractors, the clinic supervisor should always ensure there is a copy of the independent contractor's liability insurance on file in case of litigation. If the physical therapy clinic is using independent contractors, then the contractor should carry professional malpractice insurance. If a lawsuit ensues that involves the independent contractor, the defense attorney for the physical therapy clinic will attempt to posture the litigation so that the independent contractor's insurance is the first source of liability coverage and the physical therapy clinic's insurance is second in line for coverage of any incident involving the independent contractor.

One recommendation many employers may not favor, but should implement, is that physical therapists and physical therapist assistants should belong to the American Physical Therapy Association. If a physical therapist or physical therapist assistant is sued, one of the questions that undoubtedly will be asked is whether he or she belongs to the organization that represents the physical therapy profession. If the answer is no, then the physical therapist or physical therapist assistant will have to explain how he or she maintain competency in the delivery of physical therapy.

It should also be understood that the plaintiff's lawyer will likely calculate the physical therapist's or physical therapist assistant's salary in relation to the cost of membership in the organization, which will likely be less than 1 percent, and use that evidence to argue the physical therapist or physical therapist assistant is less than professional. In other words, the physical therapist, physical therapist assistant, or student could not be competent because he or she would not expend the small amount of money necessary to belong to the organization charged with providing the latest and most important information on the profession of physical therapy.

QUALITY IMPROVEMENT

Quality improvement is an approach, usually formal, that analyzes performance and then formulates ways to improve performance. This process can help reduce liability risks because structure, processes, and/or outcomes can be improved through quality improvement. Years ago, quality improvement was called quality assurance, but now quality improvement offers more than quality assurance. There are numerous models available for use and what model best fits the physical therapy clinic will depend on the individuals involved in the program. Some of the most common models are FADE, PDSA, six sigma (DMAIC), CQI and TQM.

Models Available for Quality Improvement

FADE is an acronym for focus, analyze, develop, execute, and evaluate. It is a process-improvement-driven model. The focus (F) of the process is for the team to identify the processes that will be improved. Once the processes are identified, then the team has to analyze (A) information that is collected to establish baselines, identify root causes, and identify possible solutions. Root-cause analysis is really just identifying the true cause of a problem and possible solutions. Once the process to improve has been identified and the process analyzed, then the team develops (D) action plans to improve the process. One of the keys to an action plan is a way to measure and monitor the action taken to determine whether it actually improved the process. Once the action plan(s) has been developed, then the action plan(s) is put into action or executed (E). Thereafter, the measures and monitors are evaluated to determine whether the process that was being tested should be installed.

An example of a process that could undergo the FADE model might be the process of obtaining insurance verification for treatment in a physical therapy clinic. Recall that one of the primary allegations from the CNA insurance company study was a delay in treatment. Accordingly, if the delay in treatment is related to having to wait for insurance verification, then this might be a process the physical therapist or physical therapist assistant wants to improve. Thus, the focus of the quality-improvement process would be the way in which the clinic handles insurance verification. Data would be collected on the current process, especially how much time it takes and how much follow-up is being performed. The root-cause analysis might identify it is the person doing the verification who is not completing the forms, it might be the insurance carrier is not responding, or it might be a whole host of other problems. The action plan that is developed might be a meeting with each insurance carrier to determine how best to process insurance verifications or it might be to do additional training with the person doing the verification. Once the improvement is identified and implemented, then remonitor and assess to determine if the time it is taking to get insurance verification processed has improved or gotten worse. The process continues on an ongoing basis.

The PDSA model stands for plan, do, study, and act. This process does not necessarily require the identification of a process that needs to be improved, it just requires the team to decide to plan to change or test a particular process. Once the process is identified to change or test, then the plan is carried out and the process is studied. Once the process is studied, the team decides what, if any, action(s) should be undertaken to improve the process. This process is continued until some goal is achieved.

The six sigma model is a measurement-based quality-improvement method. There are two models called DMAIC and DMADV. DMAIC stands for define, measure, analyze, improve, and control. DMADV stands for define, measure, analyze, design, and verify. Like the FADE and PDSA models, the six sigma models are designed to improve a department with the focus on customers. Thus, determine a process to study for improvement and then measure whether the improved process worked. As an example, in a physical therapy clinic, determine a patient's wait time. The goal might be that no patient will wait more than 10 minutes for a scheduled appointment. Data is collected to ascertain what the wait time actually is. If the data demonstrates the wait time is greater than 10 minutes, then a program or process is developed or designed to improve the clinic's performance to decrease the wait time below 10 minutes. After the program/process is implemented, then data is again collected to determine if the process was successful. Thereafter, additional programs/processes can be reviewed. It should be noted that sometimes a process will be studied and after the data is reviewed the decision could be that no improvement is necessary.

CQI stands for continuous quality improvement. CQI builds on some of the traditional quality assurance methods with emphasis on the organization and the organization's systems. Like PDSA, CQI focuses on processes and process improvement. CQI, like the other models, collects data and from the data decisions are made in an attempt to improve practices so that quality is improved.

TQM is total quality management. This last method seeks to involve the entire organization's management to integrate all departments' functions to meet the needs of the customers. TQM is a management style that is demonstrated by top-level managers. The principles of TQM include commitment of management; the empowering of the organization's employees; decision making based on facts; continuous improvement; and a focus on the customer.

It does not matter what type of quality improvement the physical therapist or physical therapist assistant undertakes; however, it is essential some type of program is in place on a continuing basis to assist in liability risk reduction. Ultimately, the goal for any administration will be to improve efficiency in the workplace, while, for physical therapy services, the ultimate goal will be the delivery of quality effective services with reduced errors.

OTHER METHODS TO REDUCE LIABILITY RISKS

Some of the other methods to assess for improvement that can reduce liability risks include developing relationships with other providers, infection control, insurance at the appropriate level, and having a definite process whereby informed consent for treatment is obtained and documented. Developing relationships with other health care providers is essential to reduce liability risks, especially as physical therapists transition to entry-level health care practitioners.

If the physical therapists, physical therapist assistants, or students alienate themselves from other health care practitioners, when a claim arises, it is likely the other health care practitioners will be less than supportive. Likewise, when there is a lawsuit and there are multiple defendants, the physical therapist or physical therapist assistant might find that the other defendants are blaming the physical therapist or physical therapist assistant for the negative outcome. Recall that one of the primary allegations against physical therapists, physical therapist assistants, or students is the failure to refer or seek consultation.

Infection Control

Infection control has to do with preventing the spread of infections to other patients. If the physical therapist or physical therapist assistant is working with any type of hydrotherapy devices, then the physical therapist or physical therapist assistant must ensure that the units are cleaned and perhaps sterilized between patients. There are techniques to clean the turbines, and the physical therapist, physical therapist assistant, or student must ensure that whatever supportive staff member is actually cleaning the units follows the policy and procedure for the cleaning process.

In addition, there should be plenty of clean linens available for use, and the linens should be changed after each patient. There should be clearly identified areas for clean and dirty linens so that the two are not mixed and confused. Some type of sanitizing solution should be available to wipe down all patient equipment surfaces after every use. Whenever there is any type of reported infection that could be related to a patient who received treatment in the physical therapy clinic, then whatever equipment that patient used should be cleaned before any other patient is exposed to the equipment. Remember, different bacteria have different life spans and grow or proliferate in different media. Cultures can be taken to ensure the surfaces are clean of any particular bacteria.

Recall from a study of infectious diseases that bacteria lead to infection in the human host when the number or quality of the bacteria overwhelms the host's immune system. Thus, it is possible for someone to come in contact with bacteria and not become infected. Unfortunately for litigation, if there is any way a plaintiff's attorney can make a connection between a patient becoming infected and there is some indication there was substandard infection control in the physical therapy department, then there could be allegations that the patient became infected as a result of the physical therapist's, physical therapist assistant's, or student's failure to provide infection control.

Insurance at the Appropriate Level

With regard to having adequate insurance, recall Chapter 10 and the discussion of whether the physical therapist, physical therapist assistant, or student should purchase professional malpractice insurance. As physical therapy professionals transition to entry-level health care practitioners, it seems inevitable that physical therapists and physical therapist assistants should carry professional malpractice insurance.

Based on the CNA study, it is clear that the claims against physical therapists, physical therapist assistants, and students are on the rise and it is likely the severity of the claims will increase. The risk of not carrying professional malpractice insurance is that if a claim is brought against the physical therapist, physical therapist assistant, or student, the individual therapist could find him- or herself liable to pay the damages. As an example, take the average indemnity paid for one of the nursing home physical therapy claims, $76,215.[24] Could any physical therapist or physical therapist assistant afford to pay that claim without insurance?

However, the problem that is created, as previously discussed, is that if the physical therapist or physical therapist assistant did not have professional malpractice insurance, there is a greater likelihood the physical therapist or physical therapist assistant might not be named in the lawsuit. Consequently, the physical therapist or physical therapist assistant must make a personal decision about whether to carry professional malpractice insurance. The downside of not carrying professional malpractice insurance is that with physical therapy claims on the rise, and with the severity of the claims rising, it is more likely that the physical therapist or physical therapist assistant will be individually named in a medical malpractice or negligence claim.

Informed Consent

Lastly, it is imperative that the physical therapist, physical therapist assistant, or student obtain informed consent for evaluation and treatment. For informed consent, the physical therapist or physical therapist assistant should explain in detail what the proposed treatment is and what the risks and benefits of the treatment are. This is especially true if the treatment requires the physical therapist, physical therapist assistant, or student to touch the patient. In such cases, the physical therapist, physical therapist assistant, or student must document the informed consent.

In litigation, the physical therapist, physical therapist assistant, or student can testify to what was done and how informed consent was obtained; however, the stronger evidence would be a piece of paper titled informed consent that contained a listing of the risks and benefits discussed with the patient and then the patient's signature indicating consent was granted. Otherwise, it will be the physical therapist's, physical therapist assistant's, or student's testimony against the plaintiff's testimony and the jurors will decide which witness is more credible.

SUMMARY

Risk management is a dynamic process that should be a part of the physical therapist's, physical therapist assistant's, and student's practice throughout his or her career. The simplest lapse in risk-management behavior could lead to a negative outcome that subsequently results in litigation. If the physical therapist, physical therapist assistant, or student practices in a clinic that has a history of litigation or a high-risk patient population, then he or she should understand what his or her employer's professional malpractice coverage is. Then the physical therapist, physical therapist assistant, or student should evaluate whether he or she also should carry professional malpractice insurance.

DISCUSSION QUESTIONS

1. What is risk management?
2. What is the difference between frequency of claims and severity of claims?
3. If a physical therapy student was involved in an incident that led to litigation, could the physical therapy student be sued? Would the physical therapist also be sued?
4. Why is obtaining informed consent so critical for risk management?
5. Discuss inherent risk.
6. Discuss how personnel management can reduce liability risk.
7. Discuss quality improvement.
8. Discuss some of the models for quality improvement.
9. What are some methods that can be used to reduce liability risk?
10. Discuss informed consent.
11. What can each individual clinician do to decrease liability risk?

NOTES

[1] Physical Therapy Claims Study, CNA HealthPro, 25 (December 4, 2006).
[2] *Id.*
[3] *Id.* at 9.
[4] *Id.*
[5] *Id.*
[6] *Black's Law Dictionary*, 772 (Bryan A. Gardner, ed., 7th ed., West Group 1999).
[7] Physical Therapy Claims Study, CNA HealthPro, 9 (December 4, 2006).
[8] *Id.* at 17.
[9] *Id.*
[10] *Id.*
[11] *Id.* at 18.
[12] *Id.*
[13] *Id.*
[14] *Id.*
[15] *Id.*
[16] *Id.* at 20.
[17] *Id.*
[18] *Id.* at 23.
[19] *Id.* at 24.
[20] *Id.* at 22.
[21] *Id.* at 20.
[22] *Id.*
[23] *Id.*
[24] *Id.* at 18.

CHAPTER 14

Different Types of Business Entities

There are different business entities the physical therapist, physical therapist assistant, or student can utilize to assist with the mitigation of personal liability exposure. These entities include corporations and limited liability companies. Other company structures that do not afford as much personal liability protection are professional associations, partnerships, and limited liability partnerships. Generally speaking, if the physical therapist or physical therapist assistant is trying to decide what type of business practice to operate, the physical therapist or physical therapist assistant should undertake an analysis of what he or she is trying to accomplish with any particular entity. Are they trying to limit personal liability? Perhaps they are trying to maximize tax benefits. Each different entity has risks and benefits related to personal liability and tax liability. As such, the remainder of this chapter will discuss the benefits and drawbacks of each entity.

Additionally, it should be noted that based on the CNA insurance company report discussed in detail in Chapter 13, it appears physical therapists may be migrating away from self-employment. In 1996, 64.6 percent of physical therapists reported they were self-employed, whereas in 2005 only 44.1 percent were self-employed.[1] Based on these statistics, either physical therapists are leaving the self-employment arena or the number of physical therapists carrying professional malpractice insurance practicing in nonselfemployment situations has increased at a greater rate. The latter situation seems more likely given that in 1993, only 12,371 therapists were insured, whereas in 2005, 56,971 therapists were insured.[2]

KEY CONCEPTS

Corporation
Model Business Corporation Act
Piercing the corporate veil
Limited liability company

Partnership
Shareholder
Member

GENERAL COMPANY TERMS

Before beginning a discussion about the different types of business entities, there are certain terms and concepts utilized in business that will be discussed so that a foundation about business is understood. When a business is formed, the initial money put into the business for it to begin is called capital. *Capital* is defined as "[m]oney or assets invested, or available for investment, in a business. The total assets of a business, esp[ecially] those that help generate profits. The total amount or value of a corporation's stock is also known as corporate equity."[3]

Generally speaking, a business is going to either generate profits or losses. *Profits* are defined as "[t]he excess of revenues over expenditures in a business transaction; gain,"[4] whereas loss would be the excess of debts or liabilities over revenues in a business. A *balance sheet* is "[a] statement of an entity's current financial position, disclosing the value of the entity's assets, liabilities, and owners' equity."[5] Lastly, an *income statement* is "[a] statement of all the revenues, expenses, gains, and losses that a business incurred during a given period."[6]

Generally a quick number used to gauge the health of a business is the percentage of profit or loss. The higher the percentage of profit, the more money the business is making compared to its cost. If a business has a negative percentage, loss; clearly the business is in trouble and may have to close if it continues to operate with a loss. A profit-and-loss percentage can be calculated by taking the revenues and subtracting the expenses, which is then divided by the expenses—or as an equation:

$$[\text{Revenues} - \text{Expenses}] \div \text{Expenses} \times 100\% = \text{profit or loss percentage}$$

Obviously when the expenses exceed the revenues, the percentage is a loss and when the revenues exceed the expenses, the percentage is a profit.

Each business entity's owners need to determine what profit margin the business is expected to operate within in order to determine whether the business is successful. Clearly, when a business operates with consistent losses, it will cease to run without additional capital being poured into the company.

Lastly, the physical therapist, physical therapist assistant, or student should understand the concept of a full-time equivalent employee. This also is known as 1.00 FTE (full-time equivalent). A full-time equivalent employee is calculated to work 2080 hours within a year, whereas a .75 full-time equivalent works 1560 hours per year. A

.50 full-time equivalent works 1040 hours per year, and a .25 full-time equivalent works 520 hours per year.

These become important when calculating and projecting budgets that require an estimate of the personnel (labor) a particular company will budget for the upcoming year. Additionally, the physical therapist, physical therapist assistant, or student should understand different companies have different budget years. Some budget years correlate with the calendar year; thus, these companies' fiscal years also run from January 1 through December 31. However, many companies also use a mid-year fiscal year and run from July 1 through June 30.

CORPORATION

A *corporation* is a type of business entity that is defined as "[a]n entity (usu[ally] a business) having authority under law to act as a single person distinct from the shareholders who own it and having rights to issue stock and exist indefinitely."[7] The owners of a corporation are its shareholders, and the benefit of operating a business through a corporation structure is to protect the shareholders/owners from personal liability for the acts and/or debts of the company. A *shareholder* owns or holds a share or shares in a company.

As an example, Company A is an outpatient physical therapy clinic. Company A, when it started, decided its company would have 100 shares of stock that would be issued to the owners consistent with each owner's contribution of capital to start the corporation. (A little later in this chapter will be a discussion about the value or worth of each share.) The distribution of these shares amongst the owners will determine who has a controlling interest in the company and who has a minority interest in the company. **Figure 14-1** illustrates this concept.

In this example, Shareholder 1 owns 51 shares, which means he or she is both the majority shareholder and the controlling shareholder. A *majority shareholder* "owns or

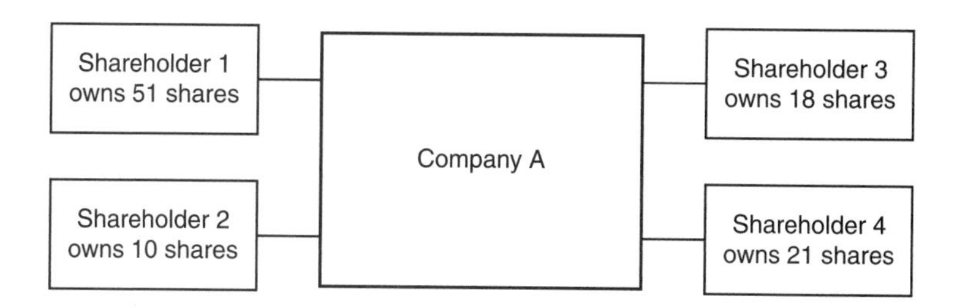

Figure 14-1 Company with Majority and Controlling Shareholder

controls more than half the corporation stock,"[8] whereas a *controlling shareholder* "is in a position to influence the corporation's activities because the shareholder either owns a majority of outstanding shares or owns a smaller percentage but a significant number of the remaining shares are widely distributed among many others."[9] Shareholders 2, 3, and 4 are minority shareholders; a *minority shareholder* "owns less than half the total shares outstanding and thus cannot control the corporation's management or single-handly elect directors."[10]

Being a majority or controlling shareholder also means the individual must act with a fiduciary duty in the performance of his or her duties as a majority or controlling shareholder. *Fiduciary duty* is defined as "[a] duty of utmost good faith, trust, confidence, and candor owed by a fiduciary (such as a lawyer or corporate officer) to the beneficiary (such as a lawyer's client or a shareholder); a duty to act with the highest degree of honesty and loyalty toward another person and in the best interests of the other person (such as the duty that one partner owes to another)."[11]

The *duty of good faith and fair dealing* is "implied in some contractual relationships, requiring the parties to deal with each other fairly, so that neither prohibits the other from realizing the agreement's benefits. This duty is most commonly implied in insurance contracts, and usu[ally] against the insurer, regarding matters such as the insurer's obligation to settle reasonable demands that are within the policy's coverage limits."[12] (Recall that acting with good faith versus bad faith was discussed in Chapter 10.)

The *duty of loyalty* is "[a] person's duty not to engage in self-dealing or otherwise use his or her position to further personal interests rather than those of the beneficiary. For example, directors have a duty not to engage in self-dealing to further his or her own personal interests rather than the interest of the corporation."[13] Lastly, the *duty of candor* is "[a] duty to disclose material facts; esp[ecially] a duty of a director seeking shareholder approval of a transaction to disclose to the shareholders all known material facts about the transaction."[14]

Now to look at this example with a little variation. **Figure 14-2** illustrates a different shareholder distribution.

In this example, Shareholder 1 owns 34 shares, Shareholder 2 owns 20 shares, Shareholder 3 owns 31 shares, and Shareholder 4 owns 15 shares. Thus, there is no controlling shareholder and no majority shareholder. Depending on how each shareholder voted during meetings, multiple outcomes could result to affect the direction of the company. This can be of critical importance when forming a corporation as well as when buying shares of companies.

The Internal Revenue Service (IRS) has classified different types of corporations for the purpose of taxation of the income derived from the corporation.[15] The most

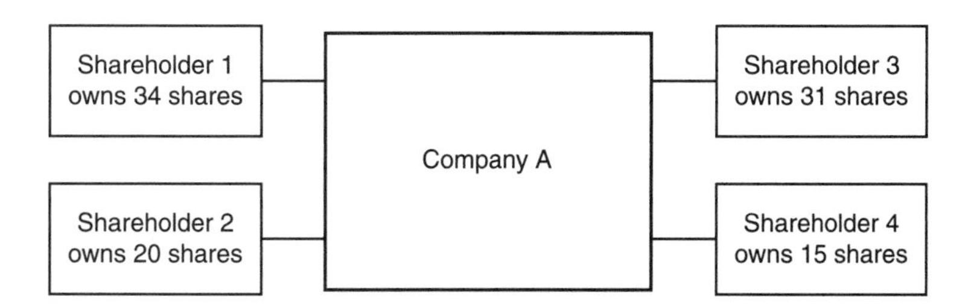

Figure 14-2 Company without Majority and Controlling Shareholder

common variations are "S" or "C" corporations. An S corporation has its income "taxed through its shareholders rather than through the corporation itself."[16] Not every corporation can elect to be an S corporation because it is restricted to those corporations with a limited number of shareholders.[17] A C corporation has its income "taxed through it [the corporation] rather than through its shareholders."[18] If the corporation does not elect S corporation status, it will automatically default to the C corporation status for purposes of the IRS.[19]

There are many formalities that must be followed when forming a business and utilizing the corporation structure. These formalities usually are set out through state-specific statutes and some states have adopted all or some of the Model Business Corporation Act[20] ("model act") as statutes for the formation and operation of corporations. Failure to follow these formalities can lead to piercing the corporate veil such that the very protection sought for the shareholders from liability for the company's acts and debts will be ignored. Piercing the corporate veil is defined as "[t]he judicial act of imposing personal liability on otherwise immune corporate officers, directors, and shareholders for the corporation's wrongful acts."[21] Thus, the shareholders could face personal liability for the acts and/or debts of the company. Accordingly, if the physical therapist, physical therapist assistant, or student is going to open a business and decides to incorporate the business, it is highly recommended he or she consult a lawyer to ensure adherence to the formalities of formation and operation.

The model act's general formalities will be discussed here. However, recall a particular state could have similar or different requirements; therefore, the physical therapist, physical therapist assistant, or student should consult an attorney or thoroughly research the state's specific requirements. Additionally, it should be pointed out that many companies form corporations in the state of Delaware and then file for foreign corporation status in other states. One of the greatest advantages to forming a corporation in Delaware is that there is significant case law in Delaware as to how a particular issue might be decided should litigation ensue.

A corporation begins with the filing and acceptance by a state of its application and supporting documents for a certificate of existence. Some states specify the form that must be used for the application. Thus, check with a particular state's secretary of state for what forms should be used. Once the certificate of existence is issued, it will specify whether the corporation is domestic or foreign. A *domestic corporation* is a corporation that was formed in that particular state, whereas a *foreign corporation* was formed in one state and has been granted corporation status to operate business in a different state.

A corporation is required to maintain articles of incorporation. Pursuant to the model act, articles of incorporation must contain[22]:

1. "[A] corporate name for the corporation that satisfies the requirement of [the model act] section 4.01;
2. [T]he number of shares the corporation is authorized to issue;
3. [T]he street address of the corporation's initial registered office and the name of its initial registered agent at that office; and
4. [T]he name and address of each incorporator"

Some of the items the articles of incorporation may contain include[23]:

1. "[T]he names and addresses of the individuals who are to serve as the initial directors;
2. [P]rovisions not inconsistent with law regarding;
   a. [T]he purpose or purposes for which the corporation is organized;
   b. [M]anaging the business and regulating the affairs of the corporation;
   c. [D]efining, limiting and regulating the powers of the corporation, its board of directors and shareholders;
   d. [A] par value for authorized shares or classes of shares; and
   e. [T]he improvisation of personal liability on shareholders for the debts of the corporation to a specified extent and upon specified conditions"

There are other things the articles of incorporation may set forth but those details are beyond the purpose of this book.

Once the corporation has been incorporated (which occurs after the secretary of the state issues the certificate of existence), the shareholders hold an organizational meeting and determine who will be named the directors of the corporation. The directors collectively form the corporation's board of directors. Once the directors are selected, they hold an organizational meeting and appoint officers, adopt bylaws, and carry on other business of the corporation. There are times when the directors will be selected prior to the completion of the incorporation process; therefore, the directors' meeting will take place without the necessity of there being a shareholders' meeting to determine the directors.

In small corporations, it is not unusual for the shareholders also to be the directors and officers of the company. When that happens, the individual or individuals must be very cautious and conscious to ensure the corporate structure formalities are maintained to defeat subsequent litigation attempts to pierce the corporate veil. Generally, the board of directors will have a chairperson and may have other or no other designated positions. The board of directors will appoint the officers of the corporation, which usually include a president or chief executive officer, vice president or chief operating officer, secretary, and treasurer or chief financial officer. The officers of the corporation select department heads and employees for the corporation. Lastly, both the directors on the board and the officers of the corporation are generally held to a duty (standard) to act with good faith and in a manner that is reasonably within the best interest of the business.

One of the last formalities of the corporate structure is to hold meetings at least annually. It is during these shareholders' meetings that business is conducted that affects the whole company. It is the duty of the officers of the corporation to perform and oversee the day-to-day operations of the company and the duty of the board of directors to oversee the performance of the officers and the oversight of the company. The shareholders vote for changes to how the officers and board of directors are taking the company.

Lastly, the physical therapist, physical therapist assistant, or student should have an understanding of piercing the corporate veil. Recall that one of the advantages of incorporating a company is protection of the shareholders from personal liability for the acts of the company and the debts of the company. However, there are occasions when a court will allow a party to sue the shareholders of a corporation because the party has successfully pled and obtained evidence to support the corporate structure was nothing more than a hoax for some type of other activity.

There are numerous cases involving piercing the corporate veil and each state's case law could be different. Thus, if a physical therapist, physical therapist assistant, or student formed a corporation, he or she should not only understand the formalities required by his or her state's corporation laws, but also have a general sense of how the courts in his or her state have decided conduct that allows parties to pierce the corporate veil.

It is the various conduct wherein the state's courts have allowed piercing of the corporate veil that the physical therapist, physical therapist assistant, or student should be knowledgeable of so as to avoid that conduct in your company. The goal of any corporate structure is to stay intact and withstand a potential attack in litigation. The physical therapist, physical therapist assistant, or student should understand what conduct enables piercing the corporate veil in the state in which he or she practices and/or forms a company. Incorporating may protect personal assets from being attacked during litigation. Thus, during a lawsuit, the physical therapist, physical therapist assistant, or student wants a party suing the company to only be able to sue the company and not sue the individual as a shareholder, director, or officer of the corporation. Further, the physical therapist, physical therapist assistant, or student does not want him- or herself as a shareholder, officer, or director of the company being held liable for debts of the company should the business not do well. **Figure 14-3** illustrates this schematic.

CORPORATE VEIL

As seen from the schematic drawing, one of the main purposes of incorporation is to shield the owners (or shareholders) of the company from liability related to lawsuits and/or debts of the company.

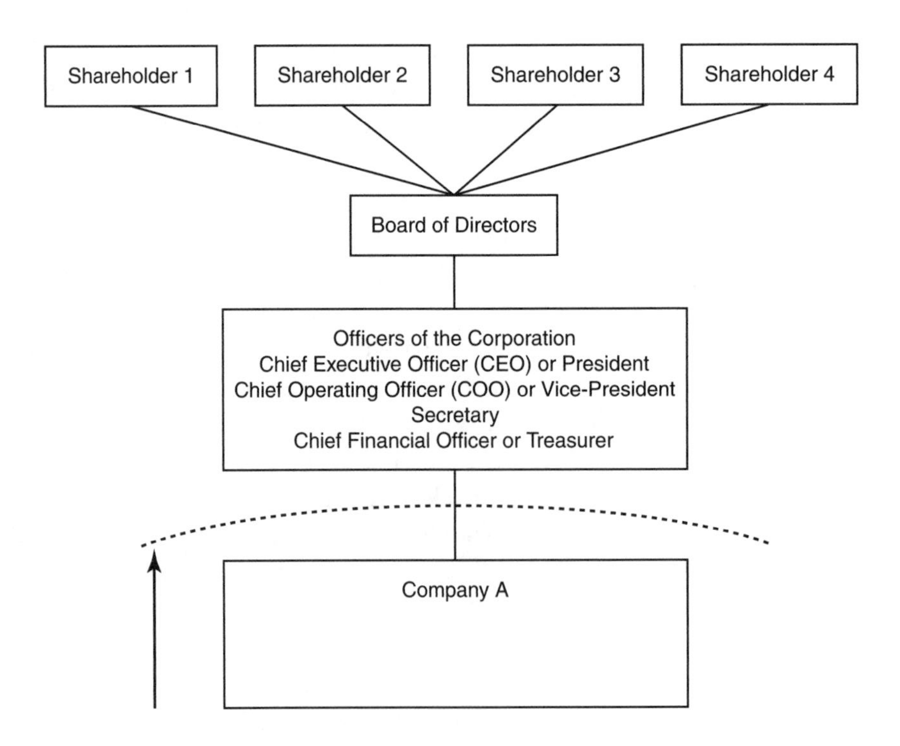

Figure 14-3 Corporate Veil

There are times when a corporation may want to trade its shares publicly versus hold them privately. When that occurs, the company must meet additional requirements and comply with the Security Exchange Act of 1934, which is administered through the Security Exchange Commission (SEC), a federally run organization. (Again the details of taking a company from private to public are beyond the scope of this book.)

Some of the classic cases dealing with piercing the corporate veil will be discussed. In *Bartle v. Home Owners Cooperation*,[24] the plaintiff attempted to hold the defendant (Home Owners Cooperation) liable for the debts of its subsidiary, Westerlea Builders, Inc. Home Owners Cooperation was formed in 1947 to provide low-cost housing to its members, who were mainly veterans.[25] When the Home Owners Cooperation was unable to find contractors to do the construction of the homes, the Home Owners Cooperation Company formed another company, Westerlea Builders, Inc., in 1948 to provide the contractor and construction needs of the Home Owners Cooperation Company.[26]

However, the company had financial difficulties such that the creditors, through an agreement, took over the construction responsibilities approximately 6 months later.[27] Four years later, Westerlea Builders, Inc. was found bankrupt despite the parent company, Home Owners Cooperation, contributing funds in addition to the original capital funds.[28] Thus, the plaintiff asserted the corporation structure of Westerlea Builders, Inc., should be pierced such that Home Owners Cooperation should be liable for the debts of its subordinate company.[29] The plaintiff's argument was an attempt to pierce the corporate veil. The court found that despite Home Owners Cooperation owning the stock of Westerlea Builders, Inc., and controlling its affairs, the outward operation of the two companies as separate companies had been maintained throughout the period of time that creditors were granting credit.[30]

Significant findings of the court that prevented the plaintiff from piercing the corporate veil included: (1) that Westerlea Builders, Inc., did not mislead creditors; (2) that Westerlea Builders, Inc., did not commit fraud; and (3) that Home Owners Cooperation did not deplete the assets of Westerlea Builders, Inc., so as to cause harm to the creditors.[31] Lastly, the court reiterated that the purpose of incorporating a company is for the exact purpose of avoiding personal liability.[32] Thus, the court examined whether the company, Westerlea Builders, Inc., committed fraud, misrepresentation, or some activity that was illegal to allow the plaintiff to pierce the corporate veil of Westerlea Builders. In this case, the court did not find Westerlea Builders had committed any of the prohibited conduct; therefore, it denied the plaintiff's request to pierce the corporate veil, which would have allowed the plaintiff to hold the parent company, Home Owners Cooperation, liable for the debts of Westerlea Builders, Inc.

Now to look at a piercing the corporate veil case that involved a physical therapy company. In *Nursing Home Group Rehabilitation Services, LLC v. Suncrest Healthcare, Inc., et. al.*,[33] a therapy company sued a nursing home and its sole owner for an outstanding bill.[34] The owner of the nursing home, Suncrest Healthcare, Inc., employed an administrator and management company to run the home's day-to-day operations.[35] The owner obtained a line of credit for which he was personally liable, but where all deposits into the account would automatically be applied to any outstanding balance of the credit line until it was paid in full.[36]

The administrator and management company of the nursing home entered into a contract with a therapy company, Nursing Home Group Rehabilitation Services, LLC, for the provision of therapy services to the nursing home residents.[37] Unfortunately, the nursing home had financial difficulties and eventually ceased operation.[38] Thereafter, the Nursing Home Group sued Suncrest Healthcare and the owner for not paying its outstanding invoices.[39] The therapy company argued it should be allowed to pierce the corporate veil of Suncrest Healthcare, Inc., and hold the sole owner liable for outstanding debts of the nursing home despite it being a corporation.[40] At trial, the sole owner of the nursing home lost and subsequently appealed the verdict against him.[41]

The appellate court reversed the trial court's decision.[42] The appellate court found that the owner of the nursing home had not committed any fraud and found no evidence the sole owner acted illegally.[43] The plaintiff's argument was that the sole owner deposited Medicare and Medicaid funds after the nursing home ceased operation that could have been used to pay the therapy company's outstanding bill.[44] Thus, by depositing the funds, the sole owner reaped the benefit of that act because it reduced his personal liability for the credit line; hence, he used corporate assets for his personal benefit and to the detriment of the nursing home's creditors.[45]

The appellate court disagreed and stated the corporate funds were not used to personally benefit the sole owner; therefore, there was no evidence of a fraudulent act and no evidence of an illegal act.[46] It should be noted, however, the case might have had a different outcome in another state. Other judges might have opined the personal benefit to the sole nursing home owner of reducing the debt for which he was going to be liable, established self-dealing for the shareholder's personal benefit at the expense of the corporation's creditors.

LIMITED LIABILITY COMPANY

A limited liability company (LLC) is "[a] company, statutorily authorized in certain states, that is characterized by limited liability, management by members or managers, and limitations on ownership transfer."[47] There are advantages and disadvantages to being incorporated versus being a limited liability company, with the decision usually being based on tax laws. The greatest advantage of the limited liability company is that it is taxed like a partnership and yet still offers its owners limited liability. One of the differences between corporations and limited liability companies is that the owners are called members and not shareholders. There is no board of directors and there are fewer management formalities.

Just like a corporation, an LLC is created by filing documents with a particular state's secretary of state. Each state may have different forms for this application, but generally when the LLC files its articles of organization with the secretary, it is deemed to have created a limited liability company. Notice it is called articles of organization and not articles of incorporation.

Pursuant to the Uniform Limited Liability Company Act, the articles of organization must include[48]:

1. The name of the company
2. The address of the company
3. The name and street address of the initial agent for service of process
4. The name and address of each organizer
5. Whether the company is to be a term company and, if so, the term specified
6. Whether the company is to be manger-managed, and, if so, the name and address of each initial manager
7. Whether one or more of the members of the company are to be liable for its debts and obligations

The articles of organization may include:

1. Provisions permitted to be set forth in an operating agreement
2. Other matters not inconsistent with law

Just like corporations, there has been a model act created to assist with the uniformity of states' laws governing the formation and operation of LLCs. For LLCs, the model act is called the Uniform Limited Liability Company Act. The Uniform Limited Liability Company Act (ULLCA) was promulgated by the National Conference of Commissioners on Uniform State Laws in 1996. The stated purposes of ULLCA are:

> To allow for the formation of limited liability companies. An LLC is a single business entity which provides limited liability protection for the partners, as well as providing all the owners of the business with federal partnership taxation. This differs from general and limited partnerships, which offer federal partnership taxation, but make at least one general partner bear personal

> liability for the debts and obligations of the business. This act incorporates the best features of existing, yet disparate, state legislation, modern law practice and the most recent developments in tax rulings.[49]

A schematic drawing of what a limited liability company looks like is found in **Figure 14-4**.

PARTNERSHIPS

Partnerships are defined as "[a] voluntary associations of two or more persons who jointly own and carry on a business for profit."[50] As with corporations and limited liability companies, there is a uniform partnership act that attempts to create uniformity in the laws governing partnerships. Partnerships are different from corporations and limited liability companies because the owners (partners) share proportionally in the profits as well as the losses and can be held personally liable for the debts of the partnership.

Every partner in a partnership acts as an agent for the partnership in conducting and carrying out the business of the partnership.[51] Of note, if a partner acts in a way that does not purport to be in the furtherance of the partnership business, that partner's acts do not bind the other partners unless the other partners authorized the particular act.[52]

The thing that makes partnerships very different from corporations and limited liability companies is that each partner is liable not just proportionally for the debts and liabilities of the partnership but also they can be held completely liable for the partnership debts and liabilities.[53] What is meant by proportionally is that if the partner

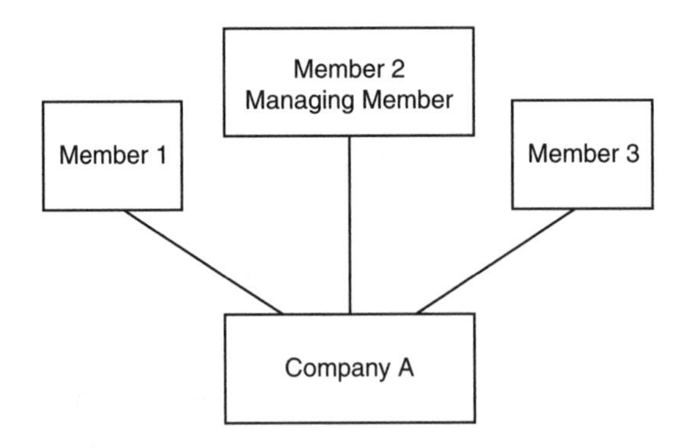

Figure 14-4 Schematic for Limited Liability Company

contributed 35 percent to the beginning capital of the partnership, then that partner has 35 percent ownership. Thus, that partner can be held liable for 35 percent of the debts and liabilities of the partnership. However, the partner will also be held jointly liable for the remaining 65 percent of the debts and liabilities of the partnership if the other partners are unable to pay. This is known as joint and several liability. *Joint and several liability* is defined as "[l]iability that may be apportioned either among two or more parties or to only one or a few select members of the group, at the adversary's discretion. Thus, each liable party is individually responsible for the entire obligation, but a paying party may have a right of contribution and indemnity from nonpaying parties."[54]

There are some variations to the partnership structure. There can be a general partnership (GP), a limited liability partnership (LLP), or a limited partnership (LP). A *general partnership* is "[a] partnership in which all partners participate fully in running the business and share equally in profits and losses (though the partners' monetary contributions may vary)."[55] A *limited liability partnership* is "[a] partnership in which a partner is not liable for a negligent act committed by another partner or by an employee not under the partner's supervision. All states have enacted statutes that allow a business (typically a law firm or accounting firm) to register as this type of partnership."[56]

A *limited partnership* is defined as "[a] partnership composed of one or more persons who control the business and are personally liable for the partnership's debts (called general partners), and one or more persons who contribute capital and share profits but who cannot manage the business and are liable only for the amount of their contribution (called limited partners). The chief purpose of a limited partnership is to enable persons to invest their money in a business without taking an active part in the managing of the business, and without risking more than the sum originally contributed, while securing the cooperation of others who have ability and integrity but insufficient money."[57]

PROFESSIONAL ASSOCIATION

A *professional association* (PA) is defined as "[a] group of professionals organized to practice their profession together, though not necessarily in corporate or partnership form."[58] Note there will not be any liability limited for any of the owners of a professional association. PAs are usually used for physician groups and law firms; the reason being these individuals cannot shield themselves from liability for the acts of themselves or their employees.

SUMMARY

There are various business entity structures that can be utilized when forming a business. Usually the two key factors that determine which business entity to form involves personal liability shelter for the owner(s) and tax liability for the owner(s). The business entity that is best for a physical therapy clinic will depend on the goals of the owner(s) forming the business.

DISCUSSION QUESTIONS

1. Why would someone want to incorporate or form a limited liability company?
2. What is the biggest advantage to being incorporated or having a limited liability company over a professional association?
3. Discuss and define a corporation.
4. Discuss and define a limited liability company.
5. Discuss and define a partnership.
6. Discuss and define a professional association.
7. How can a plaintiff pierce the corporate veil?
8. Why would a plaintiff want to pierce the corporate veil?

NOTES

[1] Physical Therapy Claims Study, CNA HealthPro, 2 (December 4, 2006).
[2] *Id.* at 3.
[3] *Black's Law Dictionary*, 200 (Bryan A. Gardner, ed., 7th ed., West Group 1999).
[4] *Id.* at 1226.
[5] *Id.* at 138.
[6] *Id.* at 768.
[7] *Id.* at 341.
[8] *Id.* at 1381.
[9] *Id.* at 1380–1381.
[10] *Id.* at 1381.
[11] *Id.* at 523.
[12] *Id.*
[13] *Id.*
[14] *Id.* at 522.
[15] *Id.* at 341.
[16] *Id.* at 344.
[17] *Id.*
[18] *Id.* at 341.

[19] *Id.*

[20] The Model Business Corporation Act was created and revised by the Committee on Corporate Laws, which is a permanent committee of the Section of Business Law of the American Bar Association.

[21] *Black's Law Dictionary,* 1168 (Bryan A. Gardner, ed., 7th ed., West Group 1999).

[22] *Statutory Supplement to Cases and Materials on Corporations Including Partnership and Limited Liability Companies,* 108 (Robert W. Hamilton, 7th ed., West Group 2001).

[23] *Id.* at 108–109.

[24] *Bartle v. Home Owners Coop.,* 127 N.E. 2d 832 (Court of Appeals NY 1955).

[25] *Id.*

[26] *Id.*

[27] *Id.*

[28] *Id.*

[29] *Id.*

[30] *Id.*

[31] *Id.*

[32] *Id.*

[33] *Nursing Home Group Rehabilitation Services, LLC v. Suncrest Healthcare, Inc., et. al.,* 2005 WL 1819378 (Ohio Ct. App., 9th Dist., August 3, 2005).

[34] Andrews Litigation Reporter, *Sole Shareholders of Ohio Home Not Liable for Therapy Firm's Bill,* page 11, September 16, 2006.

[35] *Id.*

[36] *Id.*

[37] *Id.*

[38] *Id.*

[39] *Id.*

[40] *Id.*

[41] *Id.*

[42] *Id.*

[43] *Id.*

[44] *Id.*

[45] *Id.*

[46] *Id.*

[47] *Black's Law Dictionary,* 275 (Bryan A. Gardner, ed., 7th ed., West Group 1999).

[48] *Uniform Limited Liability Company Act, § 203; and Statutory Supplement to Cases and Materials on Corporations Including Partnership and Limited Liability Companies,* 108 (Robert W. Hamilton, 7th ed., West Group 2001).

[49] *Corporations Including Partnerships and Limited Liability Companies Cases and Materials,* 189 (Robert W. Hamilton, 7th ed., West Group 2001).

[50] *Black's Law Dictionary,* 1142 (Bryan A. Gardner, ed., 7th ed., West Group 1999).

[51] *Statutory Supplement to Cases and Materials on Corporations Including Partnership and Limited Liability Companies,* 5 (Robert W. Hamilton, 7th ed., West Group 2001).

[52] *Id.*

[53] *Id.* at 7.
[54] *Black's Law Dictionary,* 926 (Bryan A. Gardner, ed., 7th ed., West Group 1999).
[55] *Id.* at 1142.
[56] *Id.*
[57] *Id.* at 1142–1143.
[58] *Id.* at 119.

CHAPTER 15

Legal Issues Particular to Practice Ownership

One of the goals for physical therapy under Vision 2020 is that more physical therapists will be clinic owners. Private clinic owners will face the challenges of reducing reimbursement with increased expenses, especially the salary demands of physical therapists who are graduating with doctoral degrees and believe they should be paid more money than baccalaureate- or master's-prepared physical therapists. The private practice owner will face the clinical, legal, financial, and operational challenges created by this.

As the private clinic owner goal is realized, physical therapists and physical therapist assistants also must acknowledge that with clinic ownership comes not just more responsibility and financial risk, but also more risk or exposure to lawsuits. These risks include not only negligence in the treatment of patients individually but also liability for the act(s) and/or omission(s) of any employee. Additionally, as a clinic owner, the physical therapist or physical therapist assistant could be liable for injuries sustained as a result of the premises or from equipment and could be held liable for various corporate compliance violations. Medical malpractice, also called negligence, was discussed in Chapter 5. Liability for an employee's act(s) and/or omission(s) is called vicarious liability or *respondeat superior*, which was discussed in Chapter 7. This chapter will examine premises liability, equipment injuries, corporate compliance, and county/city laws.

KEY CONCEPTS

Premises liability
Equipment issues
Supervision and delegation

PREMISES LIABILITY

Premises liability is defined as "[a] landowner's or landholder's tort liability for conditions or activities on the premises."[1] Thus, if a patient trips and falls on a rug in the physical therapy waiting area, the physical therapy clinic owner could be held liable for the damages flowing from any injuries related to the fall. Likewise, if some defect in the physical therapy premises caused an injury to an employee, patient, or visitor, the physical therapy clinic owner can be held liable for the damages resulting from the defect.

With premises liability, there are sometimes different duties owed to various classifications of individuals who might enter the physical therapy clinic. The various classifications can be generally identified as: (1) invitee; (2) licensee; or (3) trespasser. The *invitee* is defined as "[a] person who has an express or implied invitation to enter or use another's premises, such as a business visitor or a member of the public to whom the premises are held open. The occupier has a duty to inspect the premises and to warn the invitee of dangerous conditions."[2]

A *licensee* is defined as "[o]ne to whom a license is granted. One who has permission to enter or use another's premises, but only for one's own purposes and not for the occupier's benefit. The occupier has a duty to warn the licensee of any dangerous conditions known to the occupier but unknown to the licensee."[3]

Lastly, a *trespasser* is defined as "[o]ne who commits a trespass; one who intentionally and without consent or privilege enters another's property. In tort law, a landholder owes no duty to unforeseeable trespassers."[4] However, there could be some exceptions to this if the trespasser is a child. Physical therapy clinics that utilize pools should consult with a lawyer as to what duty is owed a potential child trespasser in relation to the pool.

Thus, the physical therapy patient is an invitee of the physical therapy clinic and therefore the clinic owner owes his or her patients a duty to inspect the premises and to warn the patients of any danger. Understand, this duty is different than the duty to treat the patient appropriately. If the patient was injured as a result of a premises defect, then the potential lawsuit would plead the duty as that of an invitee to the physical therapy clinic and not as that of what a reasonable physical therapist would do in like circumstances. However, depending on insurance coverage, a plaintiff might plead alternative theories in a lawsuit in an attempt to obtain the largest dollar for the lawsuit. Usually premises liability insurance coverage will be less than professional malpractice.

Likewise, if the physical therapy clinic owner decided to host a meeting or a marketing event at the clinic, then the physical therapy clinic owner would owe the guests of the event the duty of a licensee. If someone breaks into the physical therapy clinic, essentially the physical therapy clinic owner owes no duty to the trespasser.

The classification of the person establishes the legal duty the physical therapy clinic owner owes the person. Please note that plaintiffs' attorneys will choose to use the highest duty possible in litigation; therefore, in premises liability the plaintiffs' lawyers will want to assert the physical therapy clinic owner owed a duty to inspect the premises and warn of potential dangers. Conversely, the defense lawyer prefers to use the lowest duty, that of trespass; however, that will be the rare occurrence.

An interesting case involving a physical therapist and premises liability, but not as a physical therapy clinic owner, is *Jenner v. the Board of Education of the North Syracuse Central School District*. In this case, a physical therapist was working at an elementary school and allegedly slipped on a loose rug and fell down some stairs.[5]

While the case's ruling is not related to premises liability, it demonstrates how the owner (landlord) of property (school) can be held liable for any injury sustained on the property. In *Jenner*, the physical therapist alleged there was a loose rug on the school premises and because it was loose, the physical therapist slipped and fell down some stairs. One of the injuries asserted included the development of visual problems. If the lawsuit was ultimately successful, the school might have to pay for all of the physical therapist's medical expenses as a result of the fall, lost wages, and, if the vision problems prevented the physical therapist from working permanently, the school might have to pay future lost wages as well as compensation for the loss of an organ.

The best protection against premises liability is to routinely inspect the premises and repair damaged items immediately. If an item cannot be repaired immediately, then appropriate and conspicuous warnings should be posted to warn individuals about the defect. The warning may or may not subsequently eliminate liability, but it should mitigate damages. One of the aggravating factors in premises liability lawsuits is when the premises owner knew of a defect and simply failed to repair it. The ignoring of the premise defect could equate to conscious disregard. Recall that conscious disregard is the standard for punitive damages.

EQUIPMENT INJURIES

A physical therapy clinic owner also will be held liable for injuries sustained as a result of equipment in the clinic. Just like with premises liability, the physical therapy clinic owner is liable for injuries that are the result of equipment in the physical therapy clinic. A case that demonstrates this concept is *Pulaski v. Healthsouth Rehabilitation Center of Connecticut*. This case was examined in Chapter 5 for alleged malpractice against the physical therapist. However, in this case the plaintiff also asserted that the Cybex machine malfunctioned.[6]

Thus, in the *Pulaski* case, there were allegations of a physical therapist's negligence as well as equipment malfunction.[7] Regarding the equipment malfunction, the plaintiff asserted that his shoulder was strapped into the Cybex unit and that the machine malfunctioned.[8] Specifically, the plaintiff asserted that the machine "rapidly jerk[ed] his arm and caus[ed] him severe pain."[9] Thus, the case had a claim for negligence and/or malpractice as well as an assertion of equipment malfunction for which the clinic owner—in this case Healthsouth—could be held liable.

Some ways to manage the risk associated with equipment is to routinely clean, inspect, and calibrate the equipment in the physical therapy clinic. Cleaning the equipment is essential for infection control. This cleaning should take place in the morning, after any patient's use, after each patient's treatment, and at the end of the day. If linens are used between equipment and the patient, it does not eliminate the need to clean the equipment. However, there is some equipment, like the hydrocollator unit, that it is impractical to clean daily; still, such equipment should have an appropriate cleaning schedule. All cleaning should be documented and made part of the clinic's operational policy and procedures.

Inspection also should be done routinely and should be part of the operational policy and procedures. Among the things to consider when inspecting are whether the equipment functions as designed, whether any parts are broken or cracked, whether there are any frayed parts, whether the equipment parts fit together properly, and whether there are any odors emanating from the equipment. Electrical outlets in the physical therapy clinic also should be inspected routinely, at least annually. It is common for electrical outlet plate covers to get broken. When this occurs, the outlet should not be used until the cover is replaced.

Calibration is the process of checking a piece of equipment to ensure its sensors or output meet the manufacture's specifications. Generally speaking, the usual equipment in a physical therapy clinic includes plinths, ultrasound, electrical stimulation, hot packs, cold packs, exercise equipment, whirlpools, mats, weights, bikes, balls, and assistive devices. All of these items should be cleaned before and after each patient's use except hot and cold packs, and these should be cleaned at least monthly. The items that should be calibrated at least yearly include ultrasound machines, electrical stimulation machines, hot-pack units, cold-pack units, and any exercise equipment. However, if at any time a piece of equipment does not appear to be operating correctly, take it out of use and have it checked.

A case involving physical therapy equipment that allegedly malfunctioned is *Fernandez v. Eleman*.[10] Although the physical therapist was not sued in this case, based on the facts of the case, it appears the plaintiff simply got wrong who was the proper party to sue or the physical therapist had no insurance so the plaintiff chose to sue another party. In this case, the plaintiff allegedly received an electrical shock during an electrical stimulation treatment by the physical therapist.[11] The plaintiff then sued the physician who ordered the plaintiff to continue with his plan of treatment with physical therapy.[12]

In the complaint, the plaintiff alleged the physician failed to "maintain, inspect and repair the equipment."[13] Thereafter, the physician demonstrated "he did not own the subject equipment, and had no responsibility to inspect, maintain or repair."[14] Thus, the court dismissed the complaint against the physician because the physician had no responsibility relative to the electrical stimulation equipment.[15]

Consequently, what should be learned from this case is that had the plaintiff sued the correct party (most probably the physical therapist and/or the clinic owner), the results would have been different. Then the plaintiff would have had to establish whether the physical therapist or physical therapy clinic breached his or her duty related to the equipment or in the treatment of the patient.

CITY/COUNTY ORDINANCES

An *ordinance* is defined as "[a]n authoritative law or decree; esp[ecially] a municipal regulation. Municipal governments can pass ordinances on matters that the state government allows to be regulated at the local level."[16] Some of the city or county ordinances with which a physical therapy clinic may need to comply are business license or occupational license regulations. Contact the local city and county government agencies and ask what, if any, licenses are needed to operate a physical therapy clinic.

OTHER LAWS TO CONSIDER WHEN BILLING THIRD PARTIES

There are other laws that a private physical therapy clinic owner should be aware of and have systems in place to prevent violation of these laws. These laws are health care fraud, theft or embezzlement, false statements, false claims, obstruction of criminal investigations, frauds and swindles, and fraud by television, radio or wire. Each will be discussed in the next several paragraphs. *Health care fraud* is defined as:

> Whoever knowingly; and willfully executes, or attempts to execute, a scheme or artifice; to defraud any health care benefit program; or to obtain, by means of false or fraudulent pretenses, representations, or promises; any of the money or property owned by, or under the custody or control of, any health care benefit program; in connection with the delivery of or payment for health care benefits, items, or services.[17]

The potential sanction (penalty) for a violation of this law is mandatory in nature and could result in a fine, imprisonment up to 10 years, or both.[18] However, if the violation resulted in serious bodily harm, then the person violating the law can be subjected to a fine, imprisonment up to 20 years, or both.[19]

Theft or *embezzlement* associated with health care is defined as "[w]hoever knowingly and willfully embezzles, steals, or otherwise without authority converts to the use of any person other than the rightful owner, or intentionally misapplies any of the moneys, funds, securities, premiums, credits, property, or other assets of a health care benefit program."[20] The penalty for violation of this law is a potential fine, imprisonment up to 10 years, or both.[21] However, if the property was valued less than $100, then the potential sanction is a fine, imprisonment up to 1 year, or both.[22]

False statements associated with health care are defined as "[w]hoever, in any matter involving a health care benefit program, knowingly and willfully (1) falsifies, conceals, or covers up by any trick, scheme, or device a material fact; or (2) makes any materially false, fictitious, or fraudulent statements or representations, or makes or uses any materially false writing or document knowing the same to contain any materially false, fictitious, or fraudulent statement or entry, in connection with the delivery of or payment for health care benefits, items, or services."[23] The penalty for violation of this law is to be fined, imprisonment up to 5 years, or both.[24]

There is also a law against false claims. *False claims* are defined as any person who[25]:

1. knowingly presents, or causes to be presented, to an officer or employee of the United States Government or a member of the Armed Forces of the United Sates a false or fraudulent claim for payment or approval;
2. knowingly makes, uses, or causes to be made or used, a false record or statement to get a false or fraudulent claim paid or approved by the Government;
3. conspires to defraud the Government by getting a false or fraudulent claim allowed or paid;
4. has possession, custody, or control of property or money used, or to be used, by the Government and, intending to defraud the Government or willfully to conceal the property, delivers, or causes to be delivered, less property than the amount for which the person receives a certificate or receipt;
5. authorized to make or deliver a document certifying receipt of property used, or to be used, by the Government and, intending to defraud the Government, makes or delivers the receipt without completely knowing that the information on the receipt is true;

6. knowingly buys, or serves as a pledge of an obligation or debt, public property from an officer or employee of the Government, or a member of the Armed Forces, who lawfully may not sell or pledge the property; or
7. knowingly makes, uses, or causes to be made or used, a false records or statement to conceal, avoid, or decrease an obligation to pay or transmit money or property to the Government."

The penalty for a violation of this law is a fine (civil penalty) between $5000 and $10,000 as well as three times the damages that were sustained by the government.[26]

Obstruction of criminal investigations related to health care offenses is defined as "[w]hoever willfully prevents, obstructs, misleads, delays or attempts to prevent, obstruct, mislead, or delay the communication of information or records relating to a violation of a Federal health care offense to a criminal investigator shall be fined under this title or imprisoned not more than five years, or both."[27]

> *Frauds* and *swindles* are defined as "[w]hoever having devised or intending to devise any scheme or artifice to defraud, or for obtaining money or property by means of false or fraudulent pretenses, representations, or promises, or to sell, dispose of, loan, exchange, alter, give away, distribute, supply, or furnish or procure for unlawful use any counterfeit or spurious coin, obligation, security, or to the article, or anything represented to be or intimated or held out to be such counterfeit or spurious article, for the purpose of executing such scheme or artifice or attempting so to do, places in any post office or authorized depository for mail matter, any matter or thing whatever to be sent or delivered by the Postal Service, or deposits or causes to be deposited any matter or thing whatever to be sent or delivered by any private or commercial interstate carrier, or takes or receives therefrom, any such matter or thing, or knowingly causes to be delivered by mail or service carrier according to the direction thereon, or at the place at which it is directed to be delivered by the person to whom it is addressed, any such matter or thing."[28] The penalty for violation of this law is a fine, imprisonment up to 20 years, or both.[29] However, if the violation involves or affects a financial institution, then the penalty will be a fine up to $1,000,000, imprisonment up to 30 years, or both.[30]

Fraud by television, radio, or wire is defined as "[w]hoever, having devised or intending to devise any scheme or artifice to defraud, or for obtaining money or property by means of false or fraudulent pretenses, representations, or promises, transmits or causes to be transmitted by means of wire, radio, or television communication in interstate or foreign commerce, any writings, signs, signals, pictures, or sounds for the purpose of executing such scheme or artifice."[31] The sanction for violation of this law is a fine, imprisonment up to 20 years, or both.[32] Again, if the violation affects any type of financial institution, then the penalty is a fine, imprisonment up to 30 years, or both.[33]

There are also times when a health care provider can be excluded from participation in the Medicare or Medicaid program. When this occurs, other health care providers have to have systems in place to ensure it is not conducting business with an excluded provider. Title 42 of the U.S. Code, section 1320a-7 provides the law for "[e]xclusion of certain individuals and entities from participation in Medicare and State health care programs." There are mandatory exclusions and permissive exclusions. The Office of the Inspector General is responsible for the surveillance of excluded entities and individuals. The easiest way to check whether an individual or entity has been excluded from participation in the Medicare or Medicaid program is to go to www.oig.hhs.gov. Once there, select Fraud Prevention and Detection, then select Exclusion Program, and then an online search may be conducted.

SUPERVISION AND DELEGATION

The issues related to supervision and delegation are commonly debated. Usually a question is how much supervision is required for physical therapist assistants or supportive staff and what can be delegated to a physical therapist assistant or physical therapy aide. The APTA published Medicare's supervision requirements for the physical therapist assistant based on clinical settings. These requirements are as follows[34]:

Type of Setting	Supervision Ruling
Certified Rehabilitation Agency (CRA)	CRAs are required to have qualified personnel provide initial direction and periodic observation of the actual performance of the function and/or activity. If the person providing services does not meet the assistant-level practitioner qualifications in 485.705, then the physical therapist must be on the premises.
Comprehensive Outpatient Rehabilitation Facility (CORF)	The services must be furnished by qualified personnel. If the personnel do not meet the qualifications in 485.705, then the qualified staff must be on the

	premises and must instruct these personnel in appropriate patient care service, techniques, and retain responsibility for their activities. A qualified professional representing each service made available at the facility must be either on the premises of the facility or must be available through direct telecommunications for consultation and assistance during the facility's operating hours.
Home Health Agencies (HHA)	Physical therapy services must be performed safely and/or effectively only by or under the general supervision of a skilled therapist. General supervision has been traditionally described in HCFA manuals as requiring the initial direction and periodic inspection of the actual activity. However, the supervisor need not always be physically present or on the premises when the assistant is performing services.
Inpatient Hospital Services	Physical therapy services must be those services that can be safely and effectively performed only by or under the supervision of a qualified physical therapist. Because the regulations do not specifically delineate the type of direction required, the provider must defer to his or her physical therapy state practice act.
Outpatient Hospital Services	Physical therapy services must be those services that can be safely and effectively performed only by or under the supervision of a qualified physical therapist. Because the regulations do not specifically delineate the type of direction required, the provider must defer to his or her physical therapy state practice act.
Physical Therapist in Private Practice (PTPP)	Physical therapy services must be provided by or under the **direct** supervision of the physical therapist in private practice. CMS has generally defined direct supervision to mean that the supervising private practice therapist must be present in the office suite at the time the service is performed.

Physician's Office	Services must be provided under the direct supervision of a physical therapist who is enrolled as a provider under Medicare. A physician cannot bill for the services provided by a physical therapist assistant. The services must be billed under the provider number of the supervising physical therapist. CMS has generally defined direct supervision to mean that the physical therapist must be in the office suite when an individual procedure is performed by supportive personnel.
Skilled Nursing Facility (SNF)	Skilled rehabilitation services must be provided directly or under the general supervision of skilled rehabilitation personnel. General supervision is further defined in the manual as requiring the initial direction and periodic inspection of the actual activity. However, the supervisor need not always be physically present or on the premises when the assistant is performing services.

However, even with these published guidelines, remember the APTA is only an organization that interprets the rules and regulations promulgated by Medicare. Further, because Medicare is a federal agency, its rules and regulations regarding supervision and delegation will not trump or excuse a physical therapist's or physical therapist assistant's failure to comply with state practice act laws.

First and foremost, the physical therapist and physical therapist assistant must comply with their state physical therapy practice act regarding supervision and delegation. If the Medicare rules and regulations are stricter, then there is no conflict. However, if the Medicare guidelines are more lenient than the state physical therapy practice act, the physical therapist or physical therapist assistant must adhere to the state physical therapy practice act.

Additionally, the physical therapist or physical therapist assistant should specifically verify with his or her intermediary what its supervision requirements are. An *intermediary* is defined as "a third party that offers intermediation services between two trading parties. The intermediary acts as a conduit for goods or services offered by a supplier to a consumer. Typically the intermediary offers some added value to the transaction that may not be possible by direct trading."[35] Each intermediary has contracted with Medicare (Centers for Medicare and Medicaid Services) to pay claims. These intermediaries have the autonomy to interpret the Medicare rules and regulations within reason. Consequently, to ensure compliance, the physical therapist or physical therapist assistant should know the intermediaries' requirements.

SUMMARY

There are many things a private practice clinic owner must consider in the operation of a physical therapy clinic. Some of these considerations include methods to reduce liability exposure and ensure compliance with various federal, state, and local laws. It is imperative that any physical therapist or physical therapist assistant understand the rules with which a private clinic must comply in order to avoid criminal sanctions and civil liability exposure.

DISCUSSION QUESTIONS

1. Discuss at least three federal laws and the potential penalty for each violation.
2. Discuss premises liability.
3. Discuss equipment injuries and liability for equipment injuries.
4. Discuss methods to reduce liability risks associated with premises liability.
5. Discuss methods to reduce liability risks associated with equipment.
6. What is health care fraud?
7. What is health care theft or embezzlement?
8. What are health care false statements?
9. What is obstruction of criminal investigations?
10. What are frauds and swindles?
11. What is fraud by television, radio, or wire?

NOTES

[1] *Black's Law Dictionary*, 1199 (Bryan A. Gardner, ed., 7th ed., West Group 1999).
[2] *Id.* at 832.
[3] *Id.* at 932.
[4] *Id.* at 1510.
[5] *Id.*
[6] *Pulaski v. Healthsouth Rehabilitation Center of Connecticut, LLC*, 2005 WL 941419 (Conn. Super. 2005).
[7] *Id.*
[8] *Id.* at 1.

[9] *Id.*
[10] *Fernandez v. Eleman*, 809 N.Y.S.2d 513 (N.Y. Sup. 2006).
[11] *Id.* at 514.
[12] *Id.*
[13] *Id.*
[14] *Id.* at 515.
[15] *Id.*
[16] *Black's Law Dictionary,* 1125 (Bryan A. Gardner, ed., 7th ed., West Group 1999).
[17] 18 U.S.C. § 1347 (2006).
[18] *Id.*
[19] *Id.*
[20] 18 U.S.C. § 669.
[21] *Id.*
[22] *Id.*
[23] 18 U.S.C. § 1035.
[24] *Id.*
[25] 31 U.S.C. § 3729.
[26] *Id.*
[27] 18 U.S.C. § 1518.
[28] 18 U.S.C. § 1341.
[29] *Id.*
[30] *Id.*
[31] 18 U.S.C. § 1343.
[32] *Id.*
[33] *Id.*
[34] www.apta.org.
[35] www.dictionary.com.

CHAPTER 16

Ethical Dilemmas

No legal book would be complete without a discussion of the ethical issues physical therapists, physical therapist assistants, and students face every day in the clinic, any of which may present legal issues as well. Generally, when a physical therapist, physical therapist assistant, or student is attempting to make a decision in physical therapy, there is a hierarchy of authority he or she can follow in making any decision.

The hierarchy is to first consider whether the impending decision is a decision that should be made based on the laws, rules, and regulations that govern the practice of physical therapy. If the answer is no, then the physical therapist, physical therapist assistant, or student first should consider the ethical guidelines for practicing physical therapy, then the laws, rules, and regulations of other relevant disciplines. If the answer for the decision still has not been found, then the physical therapist, physical therapist assistant, or student should consult the *Guide to Physical Therapy Practice* and lastly the policies and position papers of the American Physical Therapy Association for guidance of how to make the right decision.

Thus, when facing a decision and trying to find guidance on making the correct decision, first look to the statutes (laws) of the physical therapist's, physical therapist assistant's, or student's state for the answer. If the statutes do not provide an answer, then the physical therapist, physical therapist assistant, or student should look to the rules and regulations governing the practice of physical therapy in that therapist's state.

If the answer cannot be found in the laws, rules, and regulations of the state, then look to the ethical guidelines governing the practice of physical therapy. If the question to be answered involves an issue or issues outside the scope of physical therapy (other disciplines or agencies), then the physical therapist, physical therapist assistant, or student should look to the other agencies' laws, rules, and regulations. If no answer is found, then look to the *Guide to Physical Therapy Practice* and lastly look to the policies and position papers of the APTA.

The laws, rules, and regulations governing physical therapy were covered in this book in Chapter 4; thus, the ethical guidelines as well as the policies and position statements of the APTA will be presented in this chapter and some specific ethical issues will be discussed.

KEY CONCEPTS

Hierarchy for decisions
APTA's ethical guidelines for physical therapists and physical therapist assistants
Core values
Standards of practice for physical therapy
Interpreting ethical principles for physical therapists
Interpreting ethical standards for physical therapist assistants

HIERARCHY FOR PHYSICAL THERAPY DECISIONS

As discussed in the opening comments of this chapter, the highest authority or foundation for making physical therapy decisions should be the laws of the state in which the physical therapist, physical therapist assistant, or student is practicing. Usually the laws governing physical therapy practice of a state are broad and, as such, may not provide answers to a specific question. When that occurs, the next authoritative material the physical therapist, physical therapist assistant, or student should look to are the rules and regulations promulgated by the board of physical therapy in his or her state.

If the answer cannot be found in the laws, rules, and regulations governing the practice of physical therapy in the state, then the physical therapist, physical therapist assistant, or student should turn to the ethical guidelines of the APTA. However, if the question or concern involves another discipline or agency, the physical therapist, physical therapist assistant, or student should look to the other discipline's laws, rules, and regulations.

Lastly, if the answer cannot be found in any of these mentioned materials, then the physical therapist, physical therapist assistant, or student should refer to the policies and position statements that have been published by the APTA. Thus, a schematic drawing of this hierarchy is found at **Figure 16-1**.

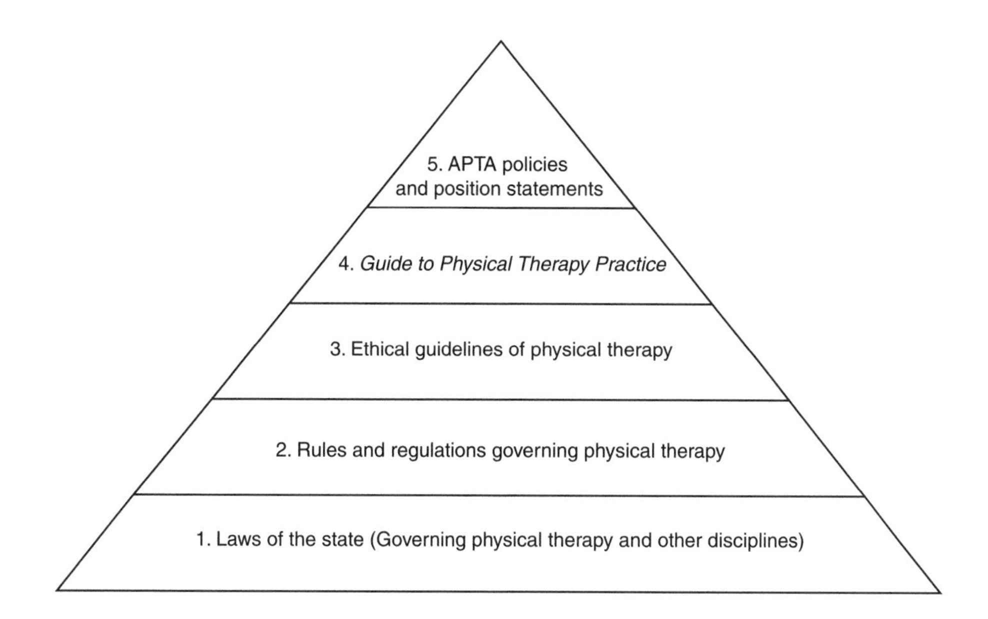

FIGURE 16-1 Hierarchy for Physical Therapy Decisions

STANDARDS OF PRACTICE FOR PHYSICAL THERAPY

Before discussing the ethical guidelines for physical therapists and physical therapist assistants, the standards of practice for physical therapy should first be reviewed. These standards have been adopted by the APTA as a way to establish what every physical therapist, physical therapist assistant, student, and physical therapy support staff should strive to deliver in the provision of physical therapy services. The standards of practice for physical therapy are[1]:

> Preamble
>
> The physical therapy profession's commitment to society is to promote optimal health and function in individuals by pursuing excellence in practice. The American Physical Therapy Association attests to this commitment by adopting and promoting the following *Standards of Practice for Physical Therapy*.* These Standards are the profession's statement of conditions and performances that are essential for provision of high quality professional service to society, and provide a foundation for assessment of physical therapist practice.

*Reprinted with permission by the American Physical Therapy Association.

I. Ethical/Legal Considerations

A. Ethical Considerations

The physical therapist practices according to the *Code of Ethics* of the American Physical Therapy Association.

The physical therapist assistant complies with the *Standards of Ethical Conduct for the Physical Therapist Assistant* of the American Physical Therapy Association.

B. Legal Considerations

The physical therapist complies with all the legal requirements of jurisdictions regulating the practice of physical therapy.

The physical therapist assistant complies with all the legal requirements of jurisdictions regulating the work of the assistant.

II. Administration of the Physical Therapy Service

A. Statement of Mission, Purposes, and Goals

The physical therapy service has a statement of mission, purposes, and goals that reflects the needs and interests of the patients/clients served, the physical therapy personnel affiliated with the service, and the community. The physical therapy service has a written organizational plan.

B. Policies and Procedures

The physical therapy service has written policies and procedures that reflect the operation, mission, purposes, and goals of the service, and are consistent with the Association's standards, policies, positions, guidelines, and *Code of Ethics*.

C. Administration

A physical therapist is responsible for the direction of the physical therapy service.

D. Fiscal Management

The director of the physical therapy service, in consultation with physical therapy staff and appropriate administrative personnel, participates in the planning for and allocation of resources. Fiscal planning and management of the service is based on sound accounting principles.

E. Improvement of Quality of Care and Performance

The physical therapy service has a written plan for continuous improvement of quality of care and performance of services.

F. Staffing

The physical therapy personnel affiliated with the physical therapy service have demonstrated competence and are sufficient to achieve the mission, purposes, and goals of the service.

G. Staff Development

The physical therapy service has a written plan that provides for appropriate and ongoing staff development.

H. Physical Setting

The physical setting is designed to provide a safe and accessible environment that facilitates fulfillment of the mission, purposes, and goals of the physical therapy service. The equipment is safe and sufficient to achieve the purposes and goals of physical therapy.

I. Collaboration

The physical therapy service collaborates with all disciplines as appropriate.

III. Patient/Client Management

A. Patient/Client Collaboration

Within the patient/client management process, the physical therapist and the patient/client establish and maintain an ongoing collaborative process of decision making that exists throughout the provision of services.

B. Initial Examination/Evaluation/Diagnosis/Prognosis

The physical therapist performs an initial examination and evaluation to establish a diagnosis and prognosis prior to intervention.

C. Plan of Care

The physical therapist establishes a plan of care and manages the needs of the patient/client based on the examination, evaluation, diagnosis, prognosis, goals, and outcomes of the planned interventions for identified impairments, functional limitations, and disabilities.

The physical therapist involves the patient/client and appropriate others in the planning, implementation, and assessment of the plan of care.

The physical therapist, in consultation with appropriate disciplines, plans for discharge of the patient/client, taking into consideration achievement of anticipated goals and expected outcomes, and provides for appropriate follow-up or referral.

D. Intervention

The physical therapist provides or directs and supervises the physical therapy intervention consistent with the results of the examination, evaluation, diagnosis, prognosis, and plan of care.

E. Reexamination

The physical therapist reexamines the patient/client as necessary during an episode of care to evaluate progress or change in patient/client status and modifies the plan of care accordingly or discontinues physical therapy services.

F. Discharge/Discontinuation of Intervention

The physical therapist discharges the patient/client from physical therapy services when the anticipated goals or expected outcomes for the patient/client have been achieved.

The physical therapist discontinues intervention when the patient/client is unable to continue to progress toward goals or when the physical therapist determines that the patient/client will no longer benefit from physical therapy.

G. Communication/Coordination/Documentation

The physical therapist communicates, coordinates, and documents all aspects of patient/client management including the results of the initial examination and evaluation, diagnosis, prognosis, plan of care, interventions, response to interventions, changes in patient/client status relative to the interventions, reexamination, and discharge/discontinuation of intervention and other patient/client management activities.

IV. Education

The physical therapist is responsible for individual professional development. The physical therapist assistant is responsible for individual career development.

The physical therapist and the physical therapist assistant, under the direction and supervision of the physical therapist, participate in the education of students.

The physical therapist educates and provides consultation to consumers and the general public regarding the purposes and benefits of physical therapy.

The physical therapist educates and provides consultation to consumers and the general public regarding the roles of the physical therapist and the physical therapist assistant.

V. Research
The physical therapist applies research findings to practice and encourages, participates in, and promotes activities that establish the outcomes of patient/client management provided by the physical therapist.

VI. Community Responsibility
The physical therapist demonstrates community responsibility by participating in community and community agency activities, educating the public, formulating public policy, or providing pro bono physical therapy services.

ETHICAL GUIDELINES OF PHYSICAL THERAPY PRACTICE

Ethics are defined as "a set of principles of right conduct; a theory or system of moral values."[2] Therefore, physical therapists, physical therapist assistants, and students have to understand that just because something is legal does not mean it is ethical. Thus, an analysis for decision making cannot stop with simply the conclusion that something is legal. The physical therapist, physical therapist assistant, or student must analyze whether the proposed decision or action is ethical. Hence, the APTA has promulgated through its policy-making mechanism, the House of Delegates, the code of ethics for physical therapists*. The code of ethics is as follows[3]:

Preamble

This Code of Ethics of the American Physical Therapy Association sets forth principles for the ethical practice of physical therapy. All physical therapists are responsible for maintaining and promoting ethical practice. To this end, the physical therapist shall act in the best interest of the patient/client. This Code of Ethics shall be binding on all physical therapists.

PRINCIPLE 1
A physical therapist shall respect the rights and dignity of all individuals and shall provide compassionate care.

PRINCIPLE 2
A physical therapist shall act in a trustworthy manner towards patients/clients, and in all other aspects of physical therapy practice.

*Reprinted with permission by the American Physical Therapy Association.

PRINCIPLE 3
A physical therapist shall comply with laws and regulations governing physical therapy and shall strive to effect changes that benefit patients/clients.

PRINCIPLE 4
A physical therapist shall exercise sound professional judgment.

PRINCIPLE 5
A physical therapist shall achieve and maintain professional competence.

PRINCIPLE 6
A physical therapist shall maintain and promote high standards for physical therapy practice, education and research.

PRINCIPLE 7
A physical therapist shall seek only such remuneration as is deserved and reasonable for physical therapy services.

PRINCIPLE 8
A physical therapist shall provide and make available accurate and relevant information to patients/clients about their care and to the public about physical therapy services.

PRINCIPLE 9
A physical therapist shall protect the public and the profession from unethical, incompetent, and illegal acts.

PRINCIPLE 10
A physical therapist shall endeavor to address the health needs of society.

PRINCIPLE 11
A physical therapist shall respect the rights, knowledge, and skills of colleagues and other health care professionals.

Notice these ethical principles are for physical therapists and not physical therapist assistants. Instead of the code of ethics being guidance for both the physical therapists and the physical therapist assistants, the APTA set out a code of ethics for physical therapists and standards of ethical conduct for physical therapist assistants. Further, the APTA expanded these ethical principles to establish specific behaviors that are expected of the physical therapist for each principle. These details are called *interpreting ethical principles*.

How to Interpret Ethical Principles

The APTA publishes how it interprets the ethical principles of physical therapists conduct*. The interpretations are based on "the opinions, decisions, and advice of the Ethics and Judicial Committee. These interpretations are intended to assist a physical therapist in applying general ethical principles to specific situations. They should not be considered inclusive of all situations that could evolve."[4] The specific principles are as follows[5]:

PRINCIPLE 1

A physical therapist shall respect the rights and dignity of all individuals and shall provide compassionate care.

1.1 Attitudes of a Physical Therapist

A. A physical therapist shall recognize, respect, and respond to individual and cultural differences with compassion and sensitivity.

B. A physical therapist shall be guided at all times by concern for the physical, psychological, and socioeconomic welfare of patients/clients.

C. A physical therapist shall not harass, abuse, or discriminate against others.

PRINCIPLE 2

A physical therapist shall act in a trustworthy manner towards patients/clients, and in all other aspects of physical therapy practice.

2.1 Patient/Physical Therapist Relationship

A. A physical therapist shall place the patient/client's interest(s) above those of the physical therapist. Working in the patient/client's best interest requires knowledge of the patient/client's needs from the patient/client's perspective. Patients/clients often come to the physical therapist in a vulnerable state and normally will rely on the physical therapist's advice, which they perceive to be based on superior knowledge, skill, and experience. The trustworthy physical therapist acts to ameliorate the patient's/client's vulnerability, not to exploit it.

B. A physical therapist shall not exploit any aspect of the physical therapist/patient relationship.

C. A physical therapist shall not engage in any sexual relationship or activity, whether consensual or nonconsensual, with any patient while a physical therapist/patient relationship exists. Termination of the physical therapist/patient relationship does not eliminate

*Reprinted with permission by the American Physical Therapy Association.

the possibility that a sexual or intimate relationship may exploit the vulnerability of the former patient/client.

D. A physical therapist shall encourage an open and collaborative dialogue with the patient/client.

E. In the event the physical therapist or patient terminates the physical therapist/patient relationship while the patient continues to need physical therapy services, the physical therapist should take steps to transfer the care of the patient to another provider.

2.2 Truthfulness

A physical therapist has an obligation to provide accurate and truthful information. A physical therapist shall not make statements that he/she knows or should know are false, deceptive, fraudulent, or misleading. See Section 8.2.C and D or Ethical Principles.

2.3 Confidential Information

A. Information relating to the physical therapist/patient relationship is confidential and may not be communicated to a third party not involved in that patient's care without the prior consent of the patient, subject to applicable law.

B. Information derived from peer review shall be held confidential by the reviewer unless the physical therapist who was reviewed consents to the release of the information.

C. A physical therapist may disclose information to appropriate authorities when it is necessary to protect the welfare of an individual or the community or when required by law. Such disclosure shall be in accordance with applicable law.

2.4 Patient Autonomy and Consent

A. A physical therapist shall respect the patient's/client's right to make decisions regarding the recommended plan of care, including consent, modification, or refusal.

B. A physical therapist shall communicate to the patient/client the findings of his/her examination, evaluation, diagnosis, and prognosis.

C. A physical therapist shall collaborate with the patient/client to establish the goals of treatment and the plan of care.

D. A physical therapist shall use sound professional judgment in informing the patient/client of any substantial risks of the recommended examination and intervention.

E. A physical therapist shall not restrict patients' freedom to select their provider of physical therapy.

PRINCIPLE 3

A physical therapist shall comply with laws and regulations governing physical therapy and shall strive to effect changes that benefit patients/clients.

3.1 Professional Practice

A physical therapist shall comply with laws governing the qualifications, functions, and duties of a physical therapist.

3.2 Just Laws and Regulations

A physical therapist shall advocate the adoption of laws, regulations, and policies by providers, employers, third party payers, legislatures, and regulatory agencies to provide and improve access to necessary health care services for all individuals.

3.3 Unjust Laws and Regulations

A physical therapist shall endeavor to change unjust laws, regulations, and policies that govern the practice of physical therapy. See Section 10.2 or Ethical Principles.

PRINCIPLE 4

A physical therapist shall exercise sound professional judgment.

4.1 Professional Responsibility

A. A physical therapist shall make professional judgments that are in the patient/client's best interests.

B. Regardless of practice setting, a physical therapist has primary responsibility for the physical therapy care of a patient and shall make independent judgments regarding that care consistent with accepted professional standards. See Sections 2.4 and 6.1 or Ethical Principles.

C. A physical therapist shall not provide physical therapy services to a patient/client while his/her ability to do so safely is impaired.

D. A physical therapist shall exercise sound professional judgment based upon his/her knowledge, skill, education, training, and experience.

E. Upon accepting a patient/client for physical therapy services, a physical therapist shall be responsible for: the examination, evaluation, and diagnosis of that individual; the prognosis and intervention; re-examination and modification of the plan of care; and the maintenance of adequate records, including progress reports. A physical therapist shall establish the plan of care and shall provide and/or supervise and direct the appropriate interventions. See Section 2.4 or Ethical Principles.

F. If the diagnostic process reveals findings that are outside the scope of the physical therapist's knowledge, experience, or expertise, the physical therapist shall so inform the patient/client and refer to an appropriate practitioner.

G. When the patient has been referred from another practitioner, the physical therapist shall communicate pertinent findings and/or information to the referring practitioner.

H. A physical therapist shall determine when a patient/client will no longer benefit from physical therapy services. See Section 7.1.D or Ethical Principles.

4.2 Direction and Supervision

A. The supervising physical therapist has primary responsibility for the physical therapy care rendered to a patient/client.

B. A physical therapist shall not delegate to a less qualified person any activity that requires the professional skill, knowledge, and judgment of the physical therapist.

4.3 Practice Arrangements

A. Participation in a business, partnership, corporation, or other entity does not exempt physical therapists, whether employers, partners, or stockholders, either individually or collectively, from the obligation to promote, maintain and comply with the ethical principles of the Association.

B. A physical therapist shall advise his/her employer(s) of any employer practice that causes a physical therapist to be in conflict with the ethical principles of the Association. A physical therapist shall seek to eliminate aspects of his/her employment that are in conflict with the ethical principles of the Association.

4.4 Gifts and Other Consideration(s)

A. A physical therapist shall not invite, accept, or offer gifts, monetary incentives, or other considerations that affect or give an appearance of affecting his/her professional judgment.

B. A physical therapist shall not offer or accept kickbacks in exchange for patient referrals. See Sections 7.1.F and G and 9.1.D or Ethical Principles.

PRINCIPLE 5

A physical therapist shall achieve and maintain professional competence.

5.1 Scope of Competence

A physical therapist shall practice within the scope of his/her competence and commensurate with his/her level of education, training and experience.

5.2 Self-assessment

A physical therapist has a lifelong professional responsibility for maintaining competence through ongoing self-assessment, education, and enhancement of knowledge and skills.

5.3 Professional Development

A physical therapist shall participate in educational activities that enhance his/her basic knowledge and skills. See Section 6.1 or Ethical Principles.

PRINCIPLE 6

A physical therapist shall maintain and promote high standards for physical therapy practice, education and research.

6.1 Professional Standards

A physical therapist's practice shall be consistent with accepted professional standards. A physical therapist shall continuously engage in assessment activities to determine compliance with these standards.

6.2 Practice

A. A physical therapist shall achieve and maintain professional competence. See Section 5 or Ethical Principles.

B. A physical therapist shall demonstrate his/her commitment to quality improvement by engaging in peer and utilization review and other self-assessment activities.

6.3 Professional Education

A. A physical therapist shall support high-quality education in academic and clinical settings.

B. A physical therapist participating in the educational process is responsible to the students, the academic institutions, and the clinical settings for promoting ethical conduct. A physical therapist shall model ethical behavior and provide the student with information about the Code of Ethics, opportunities to discuss ethical conflicts, and procedures for reporting unresolved ethical conflicts. See Section 9 or Ethical Principles.

6.4 Continuing Education

A. A physical therapist providing continuing education must be competent in the content area.

B. When a physical therapist provides continuing education, he/she shall ensure that course content, objectives, faculty credentials, and responsibilities of the instructional staff are accurately stated in the promotional and instructional course materials.

C. A physical therapist shall evaluate the efficacy and effectiveness of information and techniques presented in continuing education programs before integrating them into his or her practice.

6.5 Research

A. A physical therapist participating in research shall abide by ethical standards governing protection of human subjects and dissemination of results.

B. A physical therapist shall support research activities that contribute knowledge for improved patient care.

C. A physical therapist shall report to appropriate authorities any acts in the conduct or presentation of research that appear unethical or illegal. See Section 9 or Ethical Principles.

PRINCIPLE 7

A physical therapist shall seek only such remuneration as is deserved and reasonable for physical therapy services.

7.1 Business and Employment Practices

A. A physical therapist's business/employment practices shall be consistent with the ethical principles of the Association.

B. A physical therapist shall never place her/his own financial interest above the welfare of individuals under his/her care.

C. A physical therapist shall recognize that third-party payer contracts may limit, in one form or another, the provision of physical therapy services. Third-party limitations do not absolve the physical therapist from making sound professional judgments that are in the patient's best interest. A physical therapist shall avoid underutilization of physical therapy services.

D. When a physical therapist's judgment is that a patient will receive negligible benefit from physical therapy services, the physical therapist shall not provide or continue to provide such services if the primary reason for doing so is to further the financial self-interest of the physical therapist or his/her employer. A physical therapist shall avoid overutilization of physical therapy services. See Section 4.1.H or Ethical Principles.

E. Fees for physical therapy services should be reasonable for the service performed, considering the setting in which it is provided, practice costs in the geographic area, judgment of other organizations, and other relevant factors.

F. A physical therapist shall not directly or indirectly request, receive, or participate in the dividing, transferring, assigning, or rebating of an unearned fee. See Sections 4.4.A and B or Ethical Principles.

G. A physical therapist shall not profit by means of a credit or other valuable consideration, such as an unearned commission, discount, or gratuity, in connection with the furnishing of physical therapy services. See Sections 4.4.A and B or Ethical Principles.

H. Unless laws impose restrictions to the contrary, physical therapists who provide physical therapy services within a business entity may pool fees and monies received. Physical therapists may divide or apportion these fees and monies in accordance with the business agreement.

I. A physical therapist may enter into agreements with organizations to provide physical therapy services if such agreements do not violate the ethical principles of the Association or applicable laws.

7.2 Endorsement of Products or Services

A. A physical therapist shall not exert influence on individuals under his/her care or their families to use products or services based on the direct or indirect financial interest of the physical therapist in such products or services. Realizing that these individuals will normally rely on the physical therapist's advice, their best interest must always be maintained, as must their right of free choice relating to the use of any product or service. Although it cannot be considered unethical for physical therapists to own or have a financial interest in the production, sale, or distribution of products/services, they must act in accordance with law and make full disclosure of their interest whenever individuals under their care use such products/services.

B. A physical therapist may receive remuneration for endorsement or advertisement of products or services to the public, physical therapists, or other health professionals provided he/she discloses any financial interest in the production, sale, or distribution of said products or services.

C. When endorsing or advertising products or services, a physical therapist shall use sound professional judgment and shall not give the appearance of Association endorsement unless the Association has formally endorsed the products or services.

7.3 Disclosure

A physical therapist shall disclose to the patient if the referring practitioner derives compensation from the provision of physical therapy.

PRINCIPLE 8

A physical therapist shall provide and make available accurate and relevant information to patients/clients about their care and to the public about physical therapy services.

8.1 Accurate and Relevant Information to the Patient

A. A physical therapist shall provide the patient/client accurate and relevant information about his/her condition and plan of care. See Section 2.4 or Ethical Principles.

B. Upon the request of the patient, the physical therapist shall provide, or make available, the medical record to the patient or a patient-designated third party.

C. A physical therapist shall inform patients of any known financial limitations that may affect their care.

D. A physical therapist shall inform the patient when, in his/her judgment, the patient will receive negligible benefit from further care. See Section 7.1.C or Ethical Principles.

8.2 Accurate and Relevant Information to the Public

A. A physical therapist shall inform the public about the societal benefits of the profession and who is qualified to provide physical therapy services.

B. Information given to the public shall emphasize that individual problems cannot be treated without individualized examination and plans/programs of care.

C. A physical therapist may advertise his/her services to the public. See Section 2.2 or Ethical Principles.

D. A physical therapist shall not use, or participate in the use of, any form of communication containing a false, plagiarized, fraudulent, deceptive, unfair, or sensational statement or claim. See Section 2.2 or Ethical Principles.

E. A physical therapist who places a paid advertisement shall identify it as such unless it is apparent from the context that it is a paid advertisement.

PRINCIPLE 9

A physical therapist shall protect the public and the profession from unethical, incompetent, and illegal acts.

9.1 Consumer Protection

A. A physical therapist shall provide care that is within the scope of practice as defined by the state practice act.

B. A physical therapist shall not engage in any conduct that is unethical, incompetent or illegal.

C. A physical therapist shall report any conduct that appears to be unethical, incompetent, or illegal.

D. A physical therapist may not participate in any arrangements in which patients are exploited due to the referring sources' enhancing their personal incomes as a result of referring for, prescribing, or recommending physical therapy. See Sections 2.1.B, 4, and 7 or Ethical Principles.

PRINCIPLE 10

A physical therapist shall endeavor to address the health needs of society.

10.1 Pro Bono Service

A physical therapist shall render pro bono public (reduced or no fee) services to patients lacking the ability to pay for services, as each physical therapist's practice permits.

10.2 Individual and Community Health

A. A physical therapist shall be aware of the patient's health-related needs and act in a manner that facilitates meeting those needs.

B. A physical therapist shall endeavor to support activities that benefit the health status of the community. See Section 3 or Ethical Principles.

PRINCIPLE 11

A physical therapist shall respect the rights, knowledge, and skills of colleagues and other healthcare professionals.

11.1 Consultation

A physical therapist shall seek consultation whenever the welfare of the patient will be safeguarded or advanced by consulting those who have special skills, knowledge, and experience.

11.2 Patient/Provider Relationships
A physical therapist shall not undermine the relationship(s) between his/her patient and other healthcare professionals.

11.3 Disparagement
Physical therapists shall not disparage colleagues and other health care professionals. See Section 9 and Section 2.4.A.

THE STANDARDS OF ETHICAL CONDUCT FOR THE PHYSICAL THERAPIST ASSISTANT*

As previously discussed, the ethical conduct for a physical therapist assistant is promulgated by the APTA as standards of ethical conduct. These standards are as follows[6]:

PREAMBLE
This document of the American Physical Therapy Association sets forth standards for the ethical conduct of the physical therapist assistant. All physical therapist assistants are responsible for maintaining high standards of conduct while assisting physical therapists. The physical therapist assistant shall act in the best interest of the patient/client. These standards of conduct shall be binding on all physical therapist assistants.

STANDARD 1
A physical therapist assistant shall respect the rights and dignity of all individuals and shall provide compassionate care.

STANDARD 2
A physical therapist assistant shall act in a trustworthy manner towards patients/clients.

STANDARD 3
A physical therapist assistant shall provide selected physical therapy interventions only under the supervision and direction of a physical therapist.

STANDARD 4
A physical therapist assistant shall comply with laws and regulations governing physical therapy.

*Reprinted with permission by the American Physical Therapy Association.

STANDARD 5
A physical therapist assistant shall achieve and maintain competence in the provision of selected physical therapy interventions.

STANDARD 6
A physical therapist assistant shall make judgments that are commensurate with their educational and legal qualifications as a physical therapist assistant.

STANDARD 7
A physical therapist assistant shall protect the public and the profession from unethical, incompetent, and illegal acts.

The student physical therapist or physical therapist assistant should follow the ethical principles or standards for whichever profession the student is studying.

INTERPRETING ETHICAL STANDARDS FOR PHYSICAL THERAPIST ASSISTANTS

Just like with physical therapists, the APTA publishes how it interprets the ethical standards of physical therapist assistants' conduct*. The interpretations are based on "the opinions, decisions, and advice of the Ethics and Judicial Committee. These interpretations are intended to assist a physical therapist assistant in applying general ethical principles to specific situations. They should not be considered inclusive of all situations that could evolve."[7] The specific standards are as follows[8]:

STANDARD 1
A physical therapist assistant shall respect the rights and dignity of all individuals and shall provide compassionate care.

1.1 Attitude of a physical therapist assistant

A. A physical therapist assistant shall recognize, respect and respond to individual and cultural difference with compassion and sensitivity.

B. A physical therapist assistant shall be guided at all times by concern for the physical and psychological welfare of patients/clients.

C. A physical therapist assistant shall not harass, abuse, or discriminate against others.

*Reprinted with permission by the American Physical Therapy Association.

STANDARD 2

A physical therapist assistant shall act in a trustworthy manner towards patients/clients.

2.1 Trustworthiness

A. The physical therapist assistant shall always place the patient's/client's interest(s) above those of the physical therapist assistant. Working in the patient's/client's best interest requires sensitivity to the patient's/client's vulnerability and an effective working relationship between the physical therapist and the physical therapist assistant.

B. A physical therapist assistant shall not exploit any aspect of the physical therapist assistant–patient/client relationship.

C. A physical therapist assistant shall clearly identify him/herself as a physical therapist assistant to patients/clients.

D. A physical therapist assistant shall conduct him/herself in a manner that supports the physical therapist–patient/client relationship.

E. A physical therapist assistant shall not engage in any sexual relationship or activity, whether consensual or nonconsensual, with any patient/client entrusted to his/her care.

F. A physical therapist assistant shall not invite, accept, or offer gifts or other considerations that affect or give an appearance of affecting his/her provision of physical therapy interventions. See Section 6.3, Interpreting Ethical Standards for Physical Therapist Assistants.

2.2 Exploitation of Patients

A physical therapist assistant shall not participate in any arrangements in which patients/clients are exploited. Such arrangements include situations where referring sources enhance their personal incomes by referring to or recommending physical therapy services.

2.3 Truthfulness

A. A physical therapist assistant shall not make statements that he/she knows or should know are false, deceptive, fraudulent, or misleading.

B. Although it cannot be considered unethical for a physical therapist assistant to own or have a financial interest in the production, sale, or distribution of products/services, he/she must act in accordance with law and make full disclosure of his/her interest to patients/clients.

2.4 Confidential Information

A. Information relating to the patient/client is confidential and shall not be communicated to a third party not involved in that patient's/client's care without the prior consent of the patient/client, subject to applicable law.

B. A physical therapist assistant shall refer all requests for release of confidential information to the supervising physical therapist.

STANDARD 3

A physical therapist assistant shall provide selected physical therapy interventions only under the supervision and direction of a physical therapist.

3.1 Supervisory Relationship

A. A physical therapist assistant shall provide interventions only under the supervision and direction of a physical therapist.

B. A physical therapist assistant shall provide only those interventions that have been selected by the physical therapist.

C. A physical therapist assistant shall not provide any interventions that are outside his/her education, training, experience, or skill, and shall notify the responsible physical therapist of his/her inability to carry out the intervention. See Sections 5.1 and 6.1B, Interpreting Ethical Standards for Physical Therapist Assistants.

D. A physical therapist assistant may modify specific interventions within the plan of care established by the physical therapist in response to changes in the patient's/client's status.

E. A physical therapist assistant shall not perform examinations and evaluations, determine diagnoses and prognoses, or establish or change a plan of care.

F. Consistent with the physical therapist assistant's education, training, knowledge, and experience, he/she may respond to the patient's/client's inquiries regarding interventions that are within the established plan of care.

G. A physical therapist assistant shall have regular and ongoing communication with the physical therapist regarding the patient's/client's status.

STANDARD 4

A physical therapist assistant shall comply with laws and regulations governing physical therapy.

4.1 Supervision

A physical therapist assistant shall know and comply with applicable law. Regardless of the content of any law, a physical therapist assistant shall provide services only under the supervision and direction of a physical therapist.

4.2 Representation

A physical therapist assistant shall not hold him/herself out as a physical therapist.

STANDARD 5

A physical therapist assistant shall achieve and maintain competence in the provision of selected physical therapy interventions.

5.1 Competence

A physical therapist assistant shall provide interventions consistent with his/her level of education, training, experience, and skill. See Sections 3.1C and 6.1B, Interpreting Ethical Standards for Physical Therapist Assistants.

5.2 Self-assessment

A physical therapist assistant shall engage in self-assessment in order to maintain competence.

5.3 Development

A physical therapist assistant shall participate in educational activities that enhance his/her basic knowledge and skills.

STANDARD 6

A physical therapist assistant shall make judgments that are commensurate with their educational and legal qualifications as a physical therapist assistant.

6.1 Patient Safety

A. A physical therapist assistant shall discontinue immediately any interventions(s) that, in his/her judgment, may be harmful to the patient/client and shall discuss his/her concerns with the physical therapist.

B. A physical therapist assistant shall not provide any interventions that are outside his/her education, training, experience, or skill and shall notify the responsible physical therapist of his/her inability to carry out the intervention. See Sections 3.1C and 5.1, Interpreting Ethical Standards for Physical Therapist Assistants.

C. A physical therapist assistant shall not perform interventions while his/her ability to do so safely is impaired.

6.2 Judgments of Patient/Client Status

If in the judgment of the physical therapist assistant, there is a change in the patient/client status he/she shall report this to the responsible physical therapist. See Section 3.1, Interpreting Ethical Standards for Physical Therapist Assistants.

6.3 Gifts and Other Considerations

A physical therapist assistant shall not invite, accept, or offer gifts, monetary incentives or other consideration that affect or give an appearance of affecting his/her provision of physical therapy interventions. See Section 2.1F, Interpreting Ethical Standards for Physical Therapist Assistants.

STANDARD 7

A physical therapist assistant shall protect the public and the profession from unethical, incompetent, and illegal acts.

7.1 Consumer Protection

A physical therapist assistant shall report any conduct that appears to be unethical or illegal.

7.2 Organizational Employment

A. A physical therapist assistant shall inform his/her employer(s) and/or appropriate physical therapist of any employer practice that causes him or her to be in conflict with the Standards of Ethical Conduct for the Physical Therapist Assistant.

B. A physical therapist assistant shall not engage in any activity that puts him or her in conflict with the Standards of Ethical Conduct for the Physical Therapist Assistant, regardless of directives from a physical therapist or employer.

POSITION STATEMENTS OF THE APTA

There are many situations when there will be no law, rule, or regulation that provides an answer to a physical therapist's, physical therapist assistant's, or student's question and after a review of the ethical guidelines, there still will be no answer. The next place to look is within the policies, positions, and guidelines of the American Physical Therapy Association. These may be found online at www.apta.org under the publications sections, resource catalog, and then go to policies, positions, and guidelines. Some examples of policies, positions, and guidelines available are: Criteria for Standards of Practice for Physical Therapy; Disciplinary Action Procedural Document;

Guidelines for Recognizing and Providing Care for Victims of Child Abuse; Guidelines for Recognizing and Providing Care for Victims of Domestic Violence; Guidelines for Recognizing and Providing Care for Victims of Elder Abuse; and Guidelines: Physical Therapy Documentation of Patient/Client Management.

CORE VALUES*

As discussed in Chapter 1, professionalism is defined as "professional character, spirit, or methods. [T]he standing practice or methods of a professional as distinguished from an amateur."[9] The APTA identified seven core values of professionalism in physical therapy as:

1. Accountability
2. Altruism
3. Compassion/Caring
4. Excellence
5. Integrity
6. Professional duty
7. Social responsibility[10]

Some of the sample indicators of each of these values as published by the APTA are as follows:

Accountability

Accountability as defined by the association is "active acceptance of the responsibility for the diverse roles, obligations, and actions of the physical therapist including self-regulation and other behaviors that positively influence patient/client outcomes, the profession and the health needs of society."[11] Some of the sample indicators of accountability are[12]:

1. Responding to patient's/client's goals and needs;
2. Seeking and responding to feedback from multiple sources;
3. Acknowledging and accepting consequences of his/her actions;
4. Assuming responsibility for learning and change;
5. Adhering to code of ethics, standards of practice, and policies/procedures that govern the conduct of professional activities;

---

*Reprinted with permission by the American Physical Therapy Association.

6. Communicating accurately to others (payers, patients/clients, other health care providers) about professional actions;
7. Participating in the achievement of health goals of patients/clients and society;
8. Seeking continuous improvement in quality of care;
9. Maintaining membership in APTA and other organizations; and
10. Educating students in a manner that facilitates the pursuit of learning.

Altruism

Altruism is defined by the APTA as "the primary regard for or devotion to the interest of patients/clients, thus assuming the fiduciary responsibility of placing the needs of the patient/client ahead of the physical therapist's self interest."[13] Some of the sample indicators for altruistic behavior are[14]:

1. Placing patient's/client's needs above the physical therapist's;
2. Providing pro bono services;
3. Providing physical therapy services to underserved and underrepresented populations;
4. Providing patient/client services that go beyond expected standards of practice; and
5. Completing patient/client care and professional responsibility prior to personal needs.

Compassion/Caring

Compassion has been defined by the APTA as "the desire to identify with or sense something of another's experience; a precursor of caring."[15] *Caring* is defined by the association as "the concern, empathy, and consideration for the needs and values of others."[16] The sample indicators for compassion and care are[17]:

1. Understanding the socio-cultural, psychological and economic influences on the individual's life in their environment;
2. Understanding an individual's perspective;
3. Being an advocate for patient's/client's needs;
4. Communicating effectively, both verbally and non-verbally, with others taking into consideration individual differences in learning styles, language, and cognitive abilities, etc.;
5. Designing patient/client programs/interventions that are congruent with patient/client needs;
6. Empowering patients/clients to achieve the highest level of function possible and to exercise self-determination in their care;

7. Focusing on achieving the greatest well-being and the highest potential for a patient/client;
8. Recognizing and refraining from acting on one's social, cultural, gender, and sexual biases;
9. Embracing the patient's/client's emotional and psychological aspects of care;
10. Attending to the patient's/client's personal needs and comforts; and
11. Demonstrating respect for others and considers others as unique and value.

Excellence

The APTA defines *excellence* as "physical therapy practice that consistently uses current knowledge and theory while understanding personal limits, integrates judgment and the patient/client perspective, embraces advancement, challenges mediocrity, and works toward development of new knowledge."[18] Some of the sample indicators of excellence are[19]:

1. Demonstrating investment in the profession of physical therapy;
2. Internalizing the importance of using multiple sources of evidence to support professional practice and decisions;
3. Participating in integrative and collaborative practice to promote high quality health and educational outcomes;
4. Conveying intellectual humility in professional and interpersonal situations;
5. Demonstrating high levels of knowledge and skill in all aspects of the profession;
6. Using evidence consistently to support professional decisions;
7. Demonstrating a tolerance for ambiguity;
8. Pursuing new evidence to expand knowledge;
9. Engaging in acquisition of new knowledge throughout one's professional career;
10. Sharing one's knowledge with others; and
11. Contributing to the development and shaping of excellence in all professional roles.

Integrity

Integrity, as defined by the APTA, is "the possession of and steadfast adherence to high ethical principles or professional standards."[20] Some of the sample indicators of integrity are[21]:

1. Abiding by the rules, regulations, and laws applicable to the profession;
2. Adhering to the highest standards of the profession (practice, ethics, reimbursement, Institutional Review Board (IRB), honor code, etc);
3. Articulating and internalizing stated ideals and professional values;

4. Using power (including avoidance of use of unearned privilege) judiciously;
5. Resolving dilemmas with respect to a consistent set of core values;
6. Being trustworthy;
7. Taking responsibility to be an integral art in the continuing management of patients/clients;
8. Knowing one's limitations and acting accordingly;
9. Confronting harassment and bias among ourselves and others;
10. Recognizing the limits of one's expertise and making referrals appropriately;
11. Choosing employment situations that are congruent with practice values and professional ethical standards; and
12. Acting on the basis of professional values even when the results of the behavior may place oneself at risk.

Professional Duty

The APTA defines *professional duty* as "the commitment to meeting one's obligations to provide effective physical therapy services to individual patients/clients, to serve the profession, and to positively influence the health of society."[22] Some of the sample indicators for meeting one's professional duty include[23]:

1. Demonstrating beneficence by providing "optimal care";
2. Facilitating each individual's achievement of goals for function, health, and wellness;
3. Preserving the safety, security and confidentiality of individuals in all professional contexts;
4. Involved in professional activities beyond the practice setting;
5. Promoting the profession of physical therapy;
6. Mentoring others to realize their potential; and
7. Taking pride in one's profession.

Social Responsibility

Social responsibility is defined by the APTA as "the promotion of a mutual trust between the profession and the larger public that necessitates responding to societal needs for health and wellness."[24] The sample indicators for social responsibility are[25]:

1. Advocating for the health and wellness needs of society including access to health care and physical therapy services;
2. Promoting cultural competence within the profession and the larger public;

3. Promoting social policy that affects function, health, and wellness needs of patient/client;
4. Ensuring that existing social policy is in the best interest of the patient/client;
5. Advocating for changes in laws, regulations, standards, and guidelines that affect physical therapist service provision;
6. Promoting community volunteerism;
7. Participating in political activism;
8. Participating in achievement of societal health goals;
9. Understanding of current community wide, nationwide and worldwide issues and how they impact society's health and well-being and the delivery of physical therapy.
10. Providing leadership in the community;
11. Participating in collaborative relationships with other health practitioners and the public at larger; and
12. Ensuring the blending of social justice and economic efficiency of services.

TREATING WHEN NOTHING TO TREAT

As an example of an ethical dilemma that can encompass all of the ethical principles, interpretation, and professional core values is treating when the treatment is nothing more than a placebo. Placebos are sometimes used in medicine because nothing else seems to work for a patient. With regard to physical therapy, a placebo would be an inactive treatment that has no value. Although not standard, sometimes a placebo treatment is what will really work for a patient. Nonetheless, physical therapists and physical therapist assistants should not utilize placebo treatments and, if they do, they should not bill for the services.

As an example, the physical therapist, physical therapist assistant, or student may have a patient who has met all the goals of the plan of treatment but really would like to receive ongoing massages because it makes the patient "feel better." The astute physical therapist, physical therapist assistant, or student informs the patient he or she no longer requires the skills of the therapist to perform the services; therefore, it would be inappropriate for the physical therapy services to continue. However, if the patient agreed to pay for the massage services privately, there really should be no unethical or illegal situation. This patient will just become a private-pay patient for the massage services and the physical therapist, physical therapist assistant, or student will need to comply with his or her particular state's requirement for physician orders.

SUMMARY

Ethical conduct in physical therapy should be the goal of every physical therapist, physical therapist assistant, and student. Situations will arise wherein consultation may be needed with the laws, rules, regulations, or other materials to determine the correct decision or course of action. The tenet to remember is that just because something is legal does not always make it ethical.

DISCUSSION QUESTIONS

1. What are ethics?
2. If a physical therapist or physical therapist assistant does not belong to the American Physical Therapy Association, does the physical therapist or physical therapist assistant have to abide by the code of ethics or standards of conduct?
3. What are core values?
4. List and discuss the core values.

NOTES

[1] www.apta.org; Core Documents; Criteria for Standards of Practice for Physical Therapy.
[2] www.thefreedictionary.com.
[3] www.apta.org; Core Documents; Code of Ethics.
[4] *Id.*
[5] *Id.*
[6] *Id.*
[7] *Id.*
[8] *Id.*
[9] www.dictionary.com.
[10] The American Physical Therapy Association web page at www.apta.org, Professionalism in Physical Therapy: Core Values.
[11] *Id.*
[12] *Id.*
[13] *Id.*
[14] *Id.*
[15] *Id.*
[16] *Id.*
[17] *Id.*
[18] *Id.*
[19] *Id.*
[20] *Id.*
[21] *Id.*

[22] *Id.*
[23] *Id.*
[24] *Id.*
[25] *Id.*

CHAPTER 17

Legal Opportunities for the Physical Therapist

Physical therapists have unique skills, knowledge, and experience that allow for the development of expertise. Most, if not all, medical malpractice lawsuits require an expert to establish the standard of care that should have been followed and how a particular practitioner breached or did not breach the prevailing standard. As such, physical therapists have the opportunity to become experts who can be utilized not only in cases involving physical therapists, physical therapist assistants, or students, but also in cases involving other health care providers.

KEY CONCEPTS

How to become an expert witness
Fee consideration
Working with a lawyer
Credibility

MEDICAL MALPRACTICE CASES

Generally speaking, the first thing an attorney does when a potential plaintiff walks in the door with an alleged medical malpractice issue is to request a copy of the plaintiff's medical records. To obtain these records, the lawyer will have the potential plaintiff execute an authorization allowing the records to be obtained and sent directly to the lawyer. Once received, the lawyer usually retains an expert to review the records to provide opinions about whether the duty or standard of care was breached in any way.

One thing that should be noted is that the lawyer is not looking for serious or egregious breaches in the standard of care, although these types of breaches would be welcomed; instead, the lawyer is looking for an identification of all the breaches of the standard of care, regardless of the severity. Then the lawyer will attempt to match breaches in the standard of care to bad outcomes (damages) or harm. Thus, the expert is reviewing the records and identifying all breaches in the prevailing standard of care and how each breach in the standard of care may have led to harm of the patient.

Once the review of records is complete, an expert usually will have a telephone conference or an in-person meeting with the attorney who retained the expert. The expert will enumerate his or her opinion(s) and what documentation, or lack thereof, is being used to support his or her opinion.

As an example, return to the hot-pack burn example that has been used throughout this book. The patient arrives at the lawyer's office complaining he was burned during a physical therapy treatment with a hot pack. The patient's records are requested and forwarded to a physical therapist expert for review and rendering of opinion(s). After reviewing the records, the expert might opine the physical therapist breached the standard of care to evaluate sensation before placing a hot pack on the patient. The support for this opinion is based on the lack of documentation in the evaluation or prior to placement of the hot pack demonstrating sensation was tested, cleared, and then documented.

Thus, the physical therapist expert opines the patient would not have received a hot-pack burn had the therapist tested sensation. Additionally, the physical therapist expert notes a physical therapist assistant documented the treatment on the date of the burn. Therefore, the physical therapist expert also opines the physical therapist failed to appropriately supervise the physical therapist assistant.

The plaintiff's lawyer's argument is that, because the physical therapist did not test sensation as evidenced by a lack of documentation, the hot pack burned the patient because insufficient padding was placed between the hot pack and the patient. Thus, had the physical therapist tested sensation, as would be evidenced by documentation in the chart, then the physical therapist would have known to either not use the hot-pack modality or the physical therapist would have put additional padding between the hot pack and the patient. This breach in duty resulted in the patient being burned when treated with the hot pack.

The damages are for medical expenses to treat the burn and the subjective pain and suffering of the patient (plaintiff). Hence, the physical therapy expert provides identification of the breach in duty that could have resulted in the problem of which the plaintiff was complaining. The lawyer uses the information to piece together the evidence necessary to support the elements of the cause of action for negligence (medical): duty, breach of duty, causation, and damages.

OTHER PROFESSIONS AS EXPERTS

Physicians are often hired and used in medical negligence cases to establish what the applicable standard of care is for the case. Both plaintiffs and defendants will hire experts. Many times the case revolves around what is termed the battle of the experts. Thus, the physician experts testify as to the duty owed by the health care practitioner to the patient, how the health care practitioner breached the prevailing standard of care, and how that breach led to or caused the patient's damages. Hence, the question will obviously present itself: Can a physician testify as to the prevailing standard of care that a physical therapist owes a patient?

Historically physicians have been hired to testify as to standard of care owed from other health care practitioners, including nurses. However, in January 2006, the American Association of Legal Nurse Consultants published a position statement as to whom it felt could or should provide expert testimony regarding nursing care.[1] The position statement came after a review of literature and case law identified that physician experts were being utilized to provide expert testimony on the nursing standard of care.[2] The conclusion of the statement was "that when applicable nursing standards need to be established through expert testimony, that the expert shall be a licensed, registered nurse. Further, the only expert competent to testify on clinical and administrative nursing issues is a licensed, registered nurse."[3]

Thus, it seems appropriate that a licensed physical therapist should be the only expert competent to render an opinion as to what applicable duty is owed a patient in the delivery of physical therapy services. Likewise, it would seem a physical therapist would be the only expert competent to render an opinion as to what duty is owed a patient in the delivery of any physical therapy service regardless of the setting. Thus, if the physical therapy services are delivered in a physician's office, under the supervision of the physician, a physical therapist would be the only expert competent to render an opinion as to the applicable standard of care owed in the delivery of those services, especially if the physician's office was billing for the services under physical therapy codes. Hence, physical therapists could evolve their practice to include rendering expert opinions.

EXPERTISE NECESSARY TO PROVIDE EXPERT TESTIMONY

In order for a physical therapist to become an expert witness, the physical therapist will need to know what duty a physical therapist owes a patient in a given practice area. In other words, a physical therapist practicing in pediatrics would likely be unable to provide expert testimony as to the duty a physical therapist owes a knee ligament reconstruction patient. Likewise, an orthopedic physical therapist would probably be unable to provide expert testimony as to the duty a physical therapist owes a student in a school setting practice.

Additionally, the physical therapist will need to be well versed in a particular state's physical therapy practice act, a particular state's administrative codes regulating the practice of physical therapy, and any practice statements generated through the associations within the physical therapy arena such as the American Physical Therapy Association and/or any specialty subgroup.

HOW TO GET STARTED

The first step toward becoming an expert witness is to fully understand and comprehend the different statutes, regulations, and positions regarding the practice of physical therapy. First, the physical therapist should update a resume or curriculum vitae and send it with an introduction letter to law firms practicing in the area of medical malpractice. Along with this introduction letter should go a fee schedule for the services the physical therapist is willing and able to provide as an expert.

Usually this would include a fee per hour for the reviewing of medical records, a fee for consultation time, a fee for providing deposition testimony including any applicable travel expense, and a fee for providing trial testimony and any applicable travel expenses. It is common for the fee for medical record review and consultation to be at the same rate per hour, whereas the fee for deposition testimony and trial testimony is usually a little higher. Some experts also have a separate fee for preparation time. Thus, the therapist also needs to establish whether the fee for a particular item includes time for preparation or is exclusive of preparation time and that the lawyer clearly knows such time will be billed separately. It is up to the individual whether these introduction letters would only be sent to plaintiff lawyers or only to defense lawyers or both.

Some defense lawyers, when looking for an expert, like to find someone who has rendered opinions for both plaintiffs and defendants. This balance can add credibility to the expert versus looking like an expert who is for hire for one side or the other. Inevitably, it is fairly easy to find expert witnesses for the plaintiff, but it can be a real challenge on the defense side.

Usually, a law firm, after receipt of the introduction letter, may put the information into its pool of potential experts and, when the right case comes along, contact the expert via a phone call to see if the expert is willing to review some medical records and render an opinion. If the assignment is accepted, the law firm usually will give a time frame within which the review must be completed and schedule a telephone or in-person conference. At the telephone or in-person conference, the physical therapist will need to be prepared to render his or her preliminary opinions along with providing the evidence used to establish the opinions.

Returning to the hot-pack burn example, one opinion might be that the physical therapist breached the prevailing standard of care because the physical therapist did not evaluate the patient's sensation. The basis for that opinion would be the particular's state's physical therapy practice act wherein it likely provides something to the effect that the physical therapist will implement an appropriate plan of treatment after evaluation, as well as the applicable administrative code that likely will state something similar, and the *Guide to Physical Therapy Practice* that identifies one of the tests and measurements utilized by the physical therapist is sensory integrity, which includes sensory testing to incorporate into the development and implementation of interventions.[4] Thus, all of these (state's practice act, administrative code, and the *Guide to Physical Therapy Practice*) would establish the duty the physical therapist owed the patient.

The expert then would need to identify where the records demonstrate that the physical therapist breached this standard of care. One example would be the physical therapy evaluation where sensation was not documented. Thus, again referring to the tenet most frequently used in medical malpractice cases: not documented, not done. Therefore, the conclusion would be because there was no documentation regarding the patient's sensation, the physical therapist did not evaluate the patient's sensation before planning and implementing the use of hot packs as an intervention in that patient's care.

The next opinion would be because there was no sensation documented and the hot packs were put into the plan of care, the physical therapist breached the prevailing standard of care and that led to the hot packs being used and burning the patient. This is obviously the case that the physical therapist expert would be building for the plaintiff's side of the case. This opinion would be strengthened with the billing records, if the physical therapist billed for an evaluation, and if the evaluation form had a place for the recording of sensation. The opinion would be strengthened even further if there was something in the patient's medical history that would heighten the concern for abnormal sensation such as the patient was diabetic. Thus, the physical therapist expert would go through all the records provided and identify these types of things in the documentation to support each of the opinions being provided.

It will be up to the hiring law firm whether the physical therapist expert is to provide any kind of a written report regarding the opinions rendered. Once the telephone conference or in-person meeting is over, it is recommend a bill for those services be submitted for payment. Along with the invoice for services, the physical therapist expert will need to provide a W-9 income form, tax identification number, or social security number so that the law firm at the end of the year can report to the physical therapist expert on a 1099 form income paid to the expert for services rendered.

It is debatable whether after the physical therapist receives payment for the services rendered should the physical therapist maintain any records as to the amount of time billed and the amount of money paid for the rendering of the expert services. The physical therapist will need to check with the particular law firm as to its particular practice. However, in some views, an expert loses some credibility when asked if these records have been maintained and the expert testifies they have not. The next usual question will be "why were the records not kept?" The implied reason is going to be because the physical therapist expert is trying to hide something, whether it is the amount of money that has been paid or the small amount of time actually billed and put into the records review to develop his or her opinions.

Further, after the physical therapist has done several of these cases, the physical therapist may get familiar with lawyers and may be asked why he would not keep the records when he knew it will be a question that will be asked every time. The downside to keeping records is that the information will be attached to depositions and possibly shown to a jury. However, in some opinions, it is better to show the jury and be upfront than to try and explain it is not the expert's general practice to keep these records once payment is received. However, the expert should check with the law firm that retained the expert for the work and get an idea from the law firm whether it is recommended to keep these records.

Once the physical therapist expert has met with the hiring attorney and rendered opinions, the physical therapist expert may not hear from the law firm ever again or months or even years later, because these cases generally take some time to be litigated. Additionally, if the case settles early, the physical therapist expert may not get advised about the settlement until the physical therapist expert asks about the case at a later date. It is not uncommon for an expert to have to rereview the file materials prior to a second meeting with the hiring attorney or before deposition testimony because of the amount of time between the first review and a second utilization of the information.

If the hiring attorney decides to disclose the physical therapist expert as an expert in the matter, it is likely the opposite side will want to schedule the physical therapist expert's deposition. Usually, the professional and courteous thing that will happen is the physical therapist expert will receive a phone call from the hiring attorney's office advising that the opposing counsel wants to schedule a deposition. From that, the physical therapist expert will be asked when is a good day and time to be deposed. This may also include a request for the scheduling of a predeposition conference with the hiring attorney. At the deposition, depending on what the opposite side requests, the physical therapist expert may be asked to bring the entire litigation file. At the deposition, the opposite side's attorney may choose to attach as an exhibit the physical therapist expert's entire file.

Once the court reporter takes the file materials and has them attached, the original records likely will be returned to the physical therapist expert. An expert deposition can last anywhere from 15 minutes to several days, depending on how much information the physical therapist expert has and how critical the expert's testimony is to the case. The hiring attorney should be able to give some idea of how long the deposition will take. Thereafter, if the case proceeds to trial, the physical therapist expert will be advised what date he or she can expect to be called at the trial so that he or she does not have to be at the courthouse every day waiting to testify.

If the physical therapist expert is hired by an out-of-town or out-of-state law firm, the physical therapist expert should be paid for travel time as well as all expenses related to the travel. Once the trial is over and a verdict is rendered, the physical therapist expert should be advised whether to return the records to the hiring attorney or execute a document confirming the documents have been destroyed.

CREDIBILITY

What is credibility? According to Black's Law Dictionary, *credibility* is "[t]he quality that makes something (as a witness or some evidence) worthy of belief."[5] For an expert, it is everything. Once an expert has been discredited in the giving of expert testimony, it is rare that the expert will be utilized again. Most lawyers keep databases of deposition and trial testimony of experts. When an expert then is disclosed, the lawyers will go back and review prior testimony and look for inconsistencies that can be highlighted during testimony.

This makes it difficult when an expert works for both sides, plaintiff and defense, because if the expert as an expert ever offers an absolute opinion and then tries to retract that absolute, the likelihood of success in the retraction is slim to none. Thus, although most experts do not keep copies of their own testimony, the physical therapist as an expert should expect the opposing lawyer to do his or her homework and review as many of the expert's prior transcripts of testimony as can be found. It is recommended any expert testifying maintain credibility. Once an expert has lost credibility, it is unlikely he or she will be hired again because they have been discredited and if done during testimony, it is possible an opposing counsel will be able to get the expert stricken so that he or she will be unable to offer any testimony.

What does it mean it be consistent with testimony? An example may help explain this concept of consistency so that credibility is maintained. Return to the hot-pack example. The plaintiff retained a physical therapist to review the medical records and offer opinions about whether the standard of care was breached. The physical therapist reviewed the records and opined the standard of care was breached because the physical therapist did not document assessment of sensation on the evaluation. The expert physical therapist's opinion is that had the physical therapist evaluated the patient's sensation, then the physical therapist would have known the patient had impaired sensation and not utilized hot packs in the plan of care or modified the standard number of layers between the patient and the hot pack. Thus, because the physical therapist did not evaluate sensation, it led to a burn on the patient; thus, damages.

Now, in another hot-pack burn case, the same physical therapist expert is hired for the defense. The expert physical therapist reviews the medical records and opines the physical therapist did not breach the standard of care; however, again there was no documentation that the physical therapist evaluated sensation on the patient. Thus, the expert now has provided in essence opposite opinions based on the same set of facts. The plaintiff's counsel in this latter example, if he or she is able to get a copy of the prior opinion or testimony from the expert physical therapist, will attempt to discredit the expert because it appears the expert is giving an opinion based on who has retained him or her versus the standards of care for the practice and the facts from the records.

In this latter example, if the expert physical therapist was discredited, it is unlikely the expert would ever be retained again to offer opinions as an expert for the standard of care owed from a physical therapist. Thus, if the physical therapist plans to offer expert opinions regarding the practice of physical therapy, the physical therapist must maintain credibility.

DEVELOPING A FEE SCHEDULE

Before a physical therapist decides to undertake the review of a case, he or she should develop a fee schedule. The fee schedule should include his or her price per hour for review of records, conference time with an attorney, deposition and trial testimony, travel time, and confirmation that expenses of travel will be covered. If the physical therapist is uncertain what to charge for his or her time, it is recommended to discuss with other experts in the geographical area what he or she charges. Usually the hourly rate for records review is less than the fee per hour for depositions testimony. Trial testimony time is usually the most expensive and it is not uncommon for this to be a one-half-day or full-day fee. This is because much time is lost when waiting to testify at trial and this allows for the physical therapist not to lose revenue because he or she is waiting to provide testimony at trial.

MEETINGS WITH LAWYERS

When the expert has completed a review of the records, it is time to schedule either an in-person or a telephone conference with the lawyer. Usually a lawyer will want to meet personally with the expert the first time so that an assessment can be made of how the expert might present in court before a jury. After that, lawyers usually conduct telephone conferences for the convenience of time and to reduce costs.

At the meeting with the lawyer, the physical therapist expert needs to be ready to present opinions and explain on what those opinions are based. As an example, if the physical therapist expert opined that the physical therapist breached the prevailing standard of care when allowing an aide to put a hot pack on the patient without testing sensation, the expert might use the *Guide to Physical Therapy Practice* as the basis of the duty to test sensation before application of the hot pack.

The physical therapist expert should be ready to discuss with the attorney any and all violations in the standard of care or offer opinions to refute those of the plaintiff. The conversations between the attorney who retained the physical therapist expert and the expert are confidential and should not be discussed with anyone other than the lawyer who retained the expert. However, the exception is when giving deposition or trial testimony. The conversations between the attorney who retained the expert and the expert are not protected pursuant to the attorney work product privilege; however, the analysis used in working through various theories of the case are protected. Thus, the expert should be very careful not to put anything in writing unless asked to do so by the attorney who retained the expert.

The physical therapist expert should retain the records provided by the retaining attorney until such time as requested to return those records or receipt of confirmation the case is over and the records should be destroyed. In working with the records, the physical therapist expert must maintain the patient's confidentiality of health care information pursuant to HIPAA rules and regulations.

SUMMARY

Becoming an expert witness provides professional growth and opportunities for a physical therapist. In order to become an expert witness, physical therapists must obtain expertise in their field. One of the key factors in being an expert witness, regardless of the side that retained the physical therapist as an expert, is to always maintain credibility.

DISCUSSION QUESTIONS

1. Why is credibility in an expert witness critical?
2. Can a newly graduated physical therapist provide expert testimony? Why?
3. With what documents should an expert physical therapist be familiar in order to provide expert physical therapy testimony?
4. Discuss what an expert does when evaluating a medial malpractice case.
5. In order to become an expert witness, what should the physical therapist do?
6. What are some of the consideration in giving expert opinion testimony?

NOTES

[1] Position Statement Providing Expert Nursing Testimony published by the American Association of Legal Nurse Consultants in January 2006.

[2] *Id.*

[3] *Id.*

[4] *Guide to Physical Therapy Practice*, 90–91 (American Physical Therapy Association, 2nd ed., 2003).

[5] Black's Law Dictionary, 374 (Bryan A. Gardner, ed., 7th ed., West Group 1999).

Index of Cases

Glossary of Terms

Administrative law addresses the executive branch of government and related agencies as well as the interactions and relationship between the executive branch and the legislative and judicial branches, and between the executive branch and the public.

Affirmative defenses provide facts that mitigate a defendant's culpability or liability, even if the facts the plaintiff alleges are true or proven. Self-defense is a clear illustration of an affirmative defense.

Affirmative duty is a duty to take a positive step to do something, for example, a duty imposed on therapists to warn a potential victim of intended harm by the client.

Age discrimination occurs when discrimination, particularly with regard to employment, is based on age. Federal regulations prohibit discriminating against people who are age 40 or older in employment.

Aggravated battery occurs when circumstances such as the use of a deadly weapon or severe bodily harm increase the severity of an act of criminal battery.

Appeal occurs when a party seeks review from a higher court of a lower court's decision, for example, with a claim that the trial of the lower court was conducted improperly.

Arbitration is a method for resolving disputes. The two disputing parties agree to allow a neutral third party (the arbitrator) to resolve the dispute and, in binding arbitration, agree to be bound by the arbitrator's decision.

Assault occurs when a threat or use of force on another person causes that person to have a reasonable belief or fear that he or she may suffer harm, offensive bodily contact, or battery.

Attorney work product is "[t]angible material or its intangible equivalent—in unwritten or oral form—that was either prepared by or for a lawyer or prepared for litigation, either planned or in progress. Work product is generally exempt from discovery or other compelled disclosure. The term is also used to describe the products of a party's investigation or communications concerning the subject matter of a lawsuit if made (1) to assist in the prosecution or defense of a pending suit, or (2) in reasonable anticipation of litigation."[1]

Balance sheet provides a statement of the current financial position of some entity—for example, a business—including the value of the entity's assets, liabilities, and owners' equity.

Battery occurs when a person applies force to another person, resulting in harmful or offensive contact. Typically, battery is a misdemeanor and is less severe than assault or, especially, aggravated assault.

But-for test is the cause necessary for an event to occur.

Capital is the money or assets in a business, typically those that can help generate profits.

Causation is the thing that produced an effect or result.

Cause of action is the part of a claim (e.g., for damages) that the plaintiff or prosecutor must prove in order for the claim to succeed.

Civil law is not a criminal litigation, but, instead, is an action meant to enforce or protect or redress a private right or a civil right.

Clear and convincing standard requires that the thing to be proved is highly probable or reasonably certain. In criminal trials, the standard is "beyond a reasonable doubt," and in most civil trials, the standard is "preponderance of the evidence." The clear and convincing standard is more stringent than the former, and less stringent than the latter.

Closing argument is a lawyer's final statement to the judge or jury before the judge or jury begins deliberations. Both the defendant's lawyer and the plaintiff's lawyer or the prosecutor ask the judge or jury to consider the evidence presented during the trial and to apply the law in a particular way. In a jury trial, the judge may instruct the jury on the law relevant to the case.

Contingency fee arrangement occurs when an attorney only charges for his or her services if the lawsuit is successful or is favorably settled out of court. Most commonly, contingency fees are a percentage of the amount of money the client recovers (e.g., 25% of the recovery if the case is settled, and 33% if the case is won at trial).

A **contract** is an agreement between two or more parties. A contract creates obligations that are enforceable or otherwise recognizable at law.

Contractual duty is a duty that arises as a result of a particular contract.

Corporation is a type of business entity that has the authority under the law to act as a single person. The corporation is distinct from the shareholders who own it.

Credibility is the quality that makes something worthy of belief. For example, a witness or a body of evidence may be credible (have credibility).

Declaratory judgment is "[a] binding adjudication that establishes the rights and other legal relations of the parties without providing for or ordering enforcement."[2]

Discovery is fact-finding, i.e., the event, act, or process of learning something that was unknown.

Discrimination occurs when a law or established practice fails to treat all persons equally or confers on or denies privileges to a certain class of persons, typically because of race, age, sex, nationality, religion, or handicap. Federal law, including Title VII of the Civil Rights Act, court decisions, and many state and local laws, prohibit employment discrimination based on those characteristics and also prohibit discrimination in voting rights, housing, credit extension, public education, and access to public facilities.

Duty is an obligation, particularly a legal obligation that one party owes to another party; the latter has a right that corresponds to the former's duty.

Duty of loyalty requires that a person not use his or her position to further personal interests rather than the interests of the entity who (for example) is employing that person.

Duty to act requires a person to take some action to prevent harm to another person or persons. Depending on the relationship and arrangement between the parties and on the circumstances, failure to act may be a cause for liability.

Duty of candor requires a person to disclose material facts relevant to the matter at hand.

Duty to speak requires a person to say something to correct another party's false impression.

Element is one of the major parts of a claim that must be proved for the claim to succeed.

Employee works for another person (the employer). A contract, either expressed or implied, sets the terms of the work, and the employer has the right to control the details of the work performance.

Employer hires and/or controls and directs the work of an employee. A contract, either expressed or implied, sets the terms of the work, and the employer has the right to control the details of work performance and pays the worker's salary or wages.

Employment contract is between an employer and employee. Such a contract details the terms and conditions of employment, including the compensation and, as relevant, the details of work performance.

Employment at will is employment without a contract. Either party, employer or employee, may terminate such employment at any time, without cause.

Equal Employment Opportunity Commission (EEOC) is "[a] federal agency created under the Civil Rights Act of 1964 to end discriminatory employment practices and to promote nondiscriminatory employment programs. The EEOC investigates alleged discriminatory employment practices and encourages mediation and other nonlitigious means of resolving employment disputes. A claimant is required to file a charge of discrimination with the EEOC before pursuing a claim under Title VII of the Civil Rights Act and certain other employment related statutes."[3]

Equal Pay Act of 1963 requires that women and men receive the same compensation while working in substantially the same job and for the same workplace.

Excessive insurance is defined as an agreement to indemnify against any loss that exceeds the amount of coverage under another policy.

Fair Labor Standards Act was passed in 1938 (29 USCA §§ 201–219); it regulates employment conditions, including the minimum wage, overtime pay, and the employment of minors.

False advertising is advertising that is misleading, deceptive, or untrue.

Federalism addresses the relationship and distribution of power between the national and (in the United States) state governments.

Felony is a serious crime (as opposed to a misdemeanor, for example). A felony is punishable by imprisonment for more than one year or, in some cases and in some jurisdictions, by death.

Fiduciary duty is "[a] duty of utmost good faith, trust, confidence, and candor owed by a fiduciary (such as a lawyer or corporate officer) to the beneficiary (such as a lawyer's client or a shareholder); a duty to act with the highest degree of honesty and loyalty toward another person and in the best interests of the other person."[4]

Foreseeability is the quality of being able to be anticipated. Both foreseeability and causation are elements of proximate cause in tort law.

Fraud includes the knowing misrepresentation of the truth. Fraud also includes concealing a fact in order to induce another person to act in a way that is detrimental to that person.

General partnership is where all partners are active participants in running the business and share in monetary contributions, profits, and losses.

Gender discrimination is synonymous with sex discrimination and is defined as discrimination based on gender. Typically, gender discrimination refers to discrimination against women.

Good faith and fair dealing is "[a] duty that is implied in some contractual relationships, requiring the parties to deal with each other fairly, so that neither prohibits the other from realizing the agreement's benefits. This duty is most commonly implied in insurance contracts, and usu[ally] against the insurer, regarding matters such as the insurer's obligation to settle reasonable demands that are within the policy's coverage limits."[5]

Income statement is a statement of all of a business's revenues, expenses, gains, and losses; an income statement typically covers a specific given period.

Indemnity is a sum paid by one party to a second party in order to compensate the second party for a particular loss. It is not necessary that the indemnifying party be responsible for the loss suffered by the indemnified party.

Insurance is an agreement by which the insurer commits to do something of value for the insured upon the occurrence of some specified contingency; particularly an agreement by which the insurer assumes a risk faced by the insured in return for a premium payment.

Judgment notwithstanding the verdict (JNOV) occurs when a judge reverses a jury's verdict, because there were insufficient facts on which the jury could base a verdict or because the verdict did not correctly apply the law in some way.

Jury deliberations are the process by which a jury weighs and discusses evidence and considers issues and options in order to reach a verdict.

Jury instructions are the instructions, directions, or guidelines the judge provides to a jury concerning the law that is relevant to the matter in front of the jury.

Legal duty occurs through a contract or by operation of the law; breaching a legal duty is legally wrong.

Lien is "[a] legal right or interest that a creditor has in another's property, lasting usu[ually] until a debt or duty that it secures is satisfied."[6]

Limited liability company (LLC) is statutorily authorized in certain states. An LLC is characterized by limited liability, management by members or managers, and limitations on ownership transfer.

Limited liability partnership is a partnership in which a partner is not liable for a negligent act committed by another partner or by an employee not under the partner's supervision.

Limited partnership is a "partnership composed of one or more persons who control the business and are personally liable for the partnership's debts (called general partners), and one or more persons who contribute capital and share profits but who cannot manage the business and are liable only for the amount of their contribution (called limited partners). The chief purpose of a limited partnership is to enable persons to invest their money in a business without taking an active part in the managing the business, and without risking more than the sum originally contributed, while securing the cooperation of others who have ability and integrity but insufficient money."[7]

Majority shareholder owns or controls more than half the stock in a corporation.

Malicious conduct is an act or conduct accompanied by ill will or spite, or for the purpose of injuring another person.

Malpractice insurance indemnifies a person such as a doctor or lawyer against claims of negligence.

Mediation is a method of resolving disputes. The disputing parties utilize a neutral third party to attempt to reach a mutually agreeable solution. A mediator's recommendations are nonbinding.

Minority shareholder owns less than half the total shares in a business entity. Such shareholders cannot control the corporation's management or elect directors single-handedly.

Motion for summary judgment is "[a] request that the court enter judgment without a trial because there is no genuine issue of material fact to be decided by a fact-finder—that is, because the evidence is legally insufficient to support a verdict in the nonmovant's favor."[8]

Murder is generally defined as taking a human life with malice aforethought.

Non-compete clauses are contracts under which one party (employee) agrees to not pursue a similar profession or trade in competition against another party (employer).

Opening statement is given by an attorney at the outset of a trial and provides a preview of the case and of the evidence; an opening statement does not contain an argument about the case or evidence.

Ordinance is "[a]n authoritative law or decree; esp[ecially] a municipal regulation. Municipal governments can pass ordinances on matters that the state government allows to be regulated at the local level."[9]

Partnership is a voluntary association of two or more persons. In business, the partners own the business jointly and operate it for profit.

Personal jurisdiction is "[a] court's power to bring a person into its adjudicative process; jurisdiction over a defendant's personal rights, rather than merely over property interests."[10]

Piercing the corporate veil is "[t]he judicial act of imposing personal liability on otherwise immune corporate officers, directors, and shareholders for the corporation's wrongful acts."[11]

Premises liability is "[a] landowner's or landholder's tort liability for conditions or activities on the premises."[12]

Preponderance of the evidence means the greater weight of the evidence. It is not required that the weight of the evidence be beyond reasonable doubt, only that a fair and impartial person would regard the evidence as stronger one way than the other. In a civil trial, as opposed to a criminal trial, "preponderance of the evidence" is the burden of proof.

Principal authorizes another person or entity to act on his or her behalf.

Products liability is "[a] manufacturer's or seller's tort liability for any damages or injuries suffered by a buyer, user, or bystander as a result of a defective product. Products liability can be based on a theory of negligence, strict liability, or breach of warranty."[13]

Professional association is a group of persons who practice a profession and who form an organization around that practice, although the organization is not necessarily a corporation or partnership.

Profits are revenues that exceed expenditures in a business enterprise or transaction.

***Pro se* litigant** is a person who represents himself or herself in a court proceeding. A *pro se* litigant does not utilize an attorney's services or assistance.

Proximate cause, also known as the legal cause, is the cause that directly produces an event. Without the proximate cause, the event would not have occurred.

Quality assurance privilege, also known as peer-review privilege, is "[a] privilege that protects from disclosure the proceedings and reports of a medical facility's peer-review committee, which reviews and oversees the patient care and medical services provided by the staff."[14]

Racial discrimination is discrimination based on race. In a similar vein, invidious discrimination, including invidious racial discrimination, is discrimination that is offensive or objectionable, typically because of prejudice or stereotyping.

Reasonable doubt is "[t]he doubt that prevents one from being firmly convinced of a defendant's guilt, or the belief that there is a real possibility that a defendant is not guilty."[15]

Reckless behavior creates the substantial and unjustifiable risk of harm to others. Reckless behavior is more serious than negligence; it is characterized by a conscious disregard for or indifference to the risk of harm to others. The disregard may be deliberate and deviates significantly from what a reasonable person would do.

Reprimand is a disciplinary action. It is imposed after formal charges have been brought, and evidence has been investigated and weighed. In the case of physical therapy, a reprimand identifies the therapist's behavior as improper but does not prevent the physical therapist from practicing.

Reservation of rights means "[a] contract (supplementing a liability-insurance policy) in which the insured acknowledges that the insurer's investigation or defense of a claim against the insured does not waive the insurer's right to contest coverage later."[16]

Res ipsa loquitor ("the thing speaks for itself") is the doctrine asserting that, in some circumstances, the fact that an accident occurred implies a prima facie case that negligence was involved.

Retaliatory discharge is made by an employer in retaliation for an employee's conduct, e.g. when an employee reports unlawful activity by the employer. Retaliatory discharges violate public policy, and, in some jurisdictions, employees who are so dismissed can recover damages.

Reverse discrimination is defined as preferential treatment of a minority person or group in a way that adversely affects members of a majority group.

Settlement is an agreement ending a dispute or lawsuit.

Sexual battery is "[t]he forced penetration of or contact with another's sexual organs or the sexual organs of the perpetrator."[17]

A **shareholder** owns or holds a share or shares in a business enterprise or company.

Simple battery is criminal battery that is not accompanied by aggravating circumstances such as a weapon and does not result in serious bodily harm.

Spoliation of evidence is "[t]he intentional destruction, mutilation, alteration, or concealment of evidence, usu[ally] a document. If proved, spoliation may be used to establish that the evidence was unfavorable to the party responsible."[18]

Statute of limitations establishes a time limit for suing in a civil case, based on the date when an injury occurred or was discovered.

Strict liability for products is "[p]roducts liability arising when the buyer proves that the goods were unreasonably dangerous and that (1) the seller was in the business of selling goods, (2) the goods were defective when they were in the seller's hands, (3) the defect caused the plaintiff's injury; and (4) the product was expected to and did reach the consumer without substantial change in condition."[19]

Subject matter jurisdiction is jurisdiction over the nature of the case and the type of relief or damages sought. Subject matter jurisdiction restricts a court's ability to make decisions or hear cases on the conduct of persons or the status of things.

Subrogation is "[t]he substitution of one party for another whose debt the party pays, entitling the paying party to rights, remedies, or securities that would otherwise belong to the debtor. The principle under which an insurer that has paid a loss under an insurance policy is entitled to all the rights and remedies belonging to the insured against a third party with respect to any loss covered by the policy."[20]

Title VII of the Civil Rights Act of 1964 prohibits employment decisions that are discriminatory based on race, color, religion, sex or national origin.

Respondeat superior is the principle holding an employer liable for an employee's wrongful acts committed within the scope of the employment. The same principle holds with regard to a principal and an agent.

Venue is the appropriate place for the trial of a lawsuit. The venue may have some connection (e.g., geographical, subject matter) with the events under consideration.

Vicarious liability is the liability that a supervisory party bears with regard to a subordinate or associate because of the relationship between the two parties; for example, an employer may bear vicarious liability for an employee's actions.

Voir dire is the preliminary examination of a prospective juror by a judge or lawyer. During this examination, the attorneys and judge determine whether the prospective is qualified and suitable for jury service.

Workers' compensation provides benefits to an employee for injuries occurring on the job.

Wrongful termination is discharge from employment for reasons that are illegal or that violate public policy.

NOTES*

[1] Black's Law Dictionary, 1600–1601 (Bryan A. Gardner, ed., 7th ed., West 1999).
[2] *Id.* at 846.
[3] *Id.* at 557.
[4] *Id.* at 523.
[5] *Id.* at 701.
[6] *Id.* at 933.
[7] *Id.* at 1142–1143.
[8] *Id.* at 1033.
[9] *Id.* at 1125.
[10] *Id.* at 857.
[11] *Id.* at 1168.
[11] *Id.* at 1199.
[13] *Id.* at 1225.
[14] *Id.* at 1216.
[15] *Id.* at 1272.
[19] *Id.* at 1082.
[19] *Id.* at 1377.
[19] *Id.* at 1409.
[19] *Id.* at 1226.
[20] *Id.* at 1440.

*Reprinted from Black's Law Dictionary, pages listed, with permission of Thomas West.

Index

Page numbers followed by "t" or "f" in italics denote tables or figures respectively.

A

D

E

F

G

H

I

J

K

L

M

O

P

Q

R

S

T

U